Endometriosis For Dummies®

Asking Your Doctor the Right Questions

Your doctor may already ask you the appropriate questions before she can give the correct diagnosis of endometriosis. However, to be on the safe side, use the following questions (and follow the advice that follows each of them) if she does diagnose your problems as endometriosis:

- **How can I reduce the pain?** Be sure to keep a diary of treatments you have already tried and how they made you feel.

- **Is my irregular cycle a serious problem?** Keep a menstrual calendar; doing so can help your doctor decide on treatment.

- **How can I make sex better?** Let your doctor know about discomfort and other trouble with sex. Be sure to let her know where you feel discomfort and when it happens in your cycle.

- **What treatments may be best for me and why?** Tell your doctor what symptoms bother you and people close to you the most. That way she can concentrate on these problems first.

- **Do these treatments have options?** If you don't want to use certain medications or have surgery, ask about alternatives.

- **Is surgery right for me?** Be sure to tell your doctor about previous surgical experience and any problems you may have had. Also, be sure to let her know of any other medical problems you have.

- **Will my endometriosis prevent me from getting pregnant?** Be prepared; have a plan for your future family growth. Tell your doctor if and when you want to start a family or if you don't want to get pregnant. These choices affect the approach to treatment.

- **What can I do to get pregnant?** Keep a record of how often and at what time in your cycle you have intercourse. Let your doctor know about previous pregnancies or attempts at getting pregnant, of yours or your partner's, and their outcomes.

- **Can my boss (or anyone else I deal with) tell that I have endometriosis?** If you worry about other people knowing about your problem, ask your doctor about this. Rest assured that endometriosis isn't visible to others, although your pain may be.

- **Will my endometriosis get worse over time?** Let your doctor know of your fears so she can address them and you can get some answers.

- **Does having endometriosis mean I'm more likely to get cancer?** Be sure to ask this question if this worries you; let your doctor know of any family history of cancer.

- **Is endometriosis curable?** Ask your doctor what to expect over time so you can adjust your life style if necessary.

- **What can my partner or family do to help?** Let your doctor know how your endometriosis is affecting other people and what solutions you may have already tried.

Identifying the Most Common Places to Have Endometriosis

- Ovaries
- Fallopian tubes
- Uterus
- Cul de sac
- Pelvic peritoneum
- Bladder
- Bowel
- Appendix

For Dummies: Bestselling Book Series for Beginners

Endometriosis For Dummies®

Keeping in Contact

Use the following chart to keep track of important names and numbers.

Contact/Name	Address	Number
Partner		
Children's school		
General doctor		
Gynecologist		
Pharmacy		
Hospital		
ER		
Endometriosis Association	www.endometriosisassn.org	414-355-2200
Endometriosis Research Center	www.endocenter.org	561-274-7442

Helping Yourself When You Have Endometriosis

When the pain gets unbearable or when you anticipate an episode of endometriosis coming on, keep the following pointers in mind to help you function better:

- **Take nonsteroidal anti-inflammatory drugs (NSAIDs), like ibuprofen.** They can help decrease pain and inflammation.

- **Anticipate pain and take medication before it starts.** Getting a jump on pain usually lessens its severity.

- **Reduce stress.** Take a deep breath. We know it's easy to say, hard to do, but try.

- **Accept your limitations.** Accept that you sometimes have to say *no* to events and activities.

- **Explain to your family, friends, and loved ones what's happening with your disease.** They're more likely to be supportive if they know what's going on.

- **Don't blame yourself.** Nobody gives herself endometriosis!

- **Join a support group.** Listening to the support of other people can be comforting.

- **Get enough sleep.** Your body can heal and your immune system can function better when you're not sleep-deprived.

- **Eat right.** Occasional indulgences are still okay, but they shouldn't be a diet staple!

- **Take vitamins and minerals.** A good multivitamin contains everything you need.

- **Avoid toxins.** They're everywhere. Become aware so you can cut down on your exposure to them.

- **Don't ignore allergies.** They're common in people with autoimmune disorders, such as endometriosis.

- **Keep a diary.** Remembering the details of your symptoms is difficult without an accurate record.

- **See your doctor.** She can be your greatest ally in fighting endometriosis — and winning!

For Dummies: Bestselling Book Series for Beginners

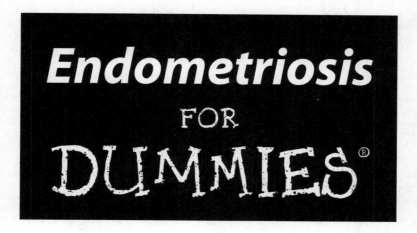

Endometriosis FOR DUMMIES®

by **Joseph W. Krotec, MD**

Former Director of Endoscopic Surgery at Cooper Institute
for Reproductive Hormonal Disorders

and **Sharon Perkins, RN**

Coauthor of *Osteoporosis For Dummies*

BICENTENNIAL
1807
WILEY
2007
BICENTENNIAL

Wiley Publishing, Inc.

Endometriosis For Dummies®

Published by
Wiley Publishing, Inc.
111 River St.
Hoboken, NJ 07030-5774
www.wiley.com

Copyright © 2007 by Wiley Publishing, Inc., Indianapolis, Indiana

Published by Wiley Publishing, Inc., Indianapolis, Indiana

Published simultaneously in Canada

For general information on our other products and services, please contact our Customer Care Department within the U.S. at 800-762-2974, outside the U.S. at 317-572-3993, or fax 317-572-4002.

For technical support, please visit www.wiley.com/techsupport.

Wiley also publishes its books in a variety of electronic formats. Some content that appears in print may not be available in electronic books.

Library of Congress Control Number: 2006392696

ISBN-13: 978-0-470-05047-7

ISBN-10: 0-470-05047-0

Manufactured in the United States of America

10 9 8 7 6 5 4 3 2 1

1B/RR/RQ/QW/IN

WILEY

About the Authors

Dr. Joseph W. Krotec from Philadelphia, Pennsylvania, has practiced general gynecology, reproductive endocrinology, and gynecologic surgery specializing in endoscopic surgery. He has instructed peers, residents, and students for more than 25 years and has been Chair of Obstetrics and Gynecology, Chief of Gynecology, and Director of Endoscopic Surgery at various institutions. Dr. Krotec recently won the Milton Goldrath, M.D. Award for excellence in teaching.

Sharon Perkins is an RN with 20 years of experience in maternal child health. She currently works for retinal specialists. Sharon has five children, two daughters-in-law, one son-in-law, and two perfect grandchildren. Oh, and a retired husband. This is her fourth *For Dummies* book.

Dedication

To all the women with endometriosis we've known and treated and to all the women who've suffered without knowing why.

Authors' Acknowledgments

I thank my wife, Susan and my children, Joshua, Alexis, and Nicholas, for their love, support, and patience — and Sharon Perkins for her ideas, writing, persistence, and nagging to get it done.

—Joseph Krotec

Many people helped me write this book, and most of them don't even know it. On days when I was discouraged, tired, and grouchy, a phone call from a family member, a smile from a patient, kind words from a co-worker, or an encouraging word from someone at church gave me the energy to get back to writing. For all the people who have crossed my path and lifted me up when I needed it badly, I thank you — even if you don't know who you are, I do.

My family just assumes I can do this without a lot of effort, and even though it isn't true, I appreciated their confidence. I was fortunate to grow up with parents who supported everything I did, and I'm blessed to have a mom who still does. Thanks, Mom! (And Dad, I'm sure you're watching and applauding still.) To all the rest of my family, thanks for being there when I need you. And to Matthew and Emma, my wonderful grandchildren — you'll never know what a joy to my life you are.

Thanks, Josh, for being willing to take on this task at a tough time; we've been through some interesting times together. You're a good doc.

—Sharon Perkins

Both of us want to say thanks to our acquisitions editor, Stacy Kennedy; our indomitable project editor, Chad Sievers; copy editor Pam Ruble; technical editor Dr. William Hurd; and our medical illustrator Kathryn Born. Another great Wiley team!

Publisher's Acknowledgments

We're proud of this book; please send us your comments through our Dummies online registration form located at www.dummies.com/register/.

Some of the people who helped bring this book to market include the following:

Acquisitions, Editorial, and Media Development

Project Editor: Chad R. Sievers

Acquisitions Editor: Stacy Kennedy

Copy Editor: Pam Ruble

Editorial Program Coordinator: Erin Calligan

Technical Editor: William Hurd, MD, Professor of Obstetrics and Gynecology, Wright State University School of Medicine

Editorial Manager: Michelle Hacker

Cartoons: Rich Tennant (www.the5thwave.com)

Illustrations: Kathryn Born, M.A.

Composition

Project Coordinator: Heather Kolter

Layout and Graphics: Stephanie D. Jumper, Barbara Moore, Barry Offringa, Lynsey Osborn, Laura Pence, Alicia South

Proofreader: Techbooks

Indexer: Techbooks

Publishing and Editorial for Consumer Dummies

Diane Graves Steele, Vice President and Publisher, Consumer Dummies

Joyce Pepple, Acquisitions Director, Consumer Dummies

Kristin A. Cocks, Product Development Director, Consumer Dummies

Michael Spring, Vice President and Publisher, Travel

Kelly Regan, Editorial Director, Travel

Publishing for Technology Dummies

Andy Cummings, Vice President and Publisher, Dummies Technology/General User

Composition Services

Gerry Fahey, Vice President of Production Services

Debbie Stailey, Director of Composition Services

Contents at a Glance

Table of Contents

Part II: Digging Deeper into Endometriosis 81

Chapter 5: Understanding Your Menstrual Cycle (And Its Relationship to Endometriosis) 83

Chapter 6: Looking Closer at How Endometriosis Also Affects Other Body Parts 97

Introduction

*E*ndometriosis is a chronic disease that, until recently, didn't get the attention it deserves. In fact, not too long ago, medical personnel and laymen often dismissed the symptoms of endometriosis as being more psychological than physical in origin. Fortunately, times are changing, and interest in endometriosis research has never been higher.

But the more researchers uncover about endometriosis, the more complicated this disease seems to be. For example, some researchers believe that endometriosis isn't one, but several different diseases. And many researchers believe that endometriosis is closely related to autoimmune disease.

If you're one of the millions of women suffering from endometriosis or if you suspect your symptoms are from endometriosis, you may not care much about research; you just want your symptoms to go away! We want you to feel better too, but we also look forward to the day when researchers discover what causes endometriosis — so they can figure out how to cure it.

Endometriosis is far more than just cramps. Millions of dollars are lost in the workplace each year because of absences and surgeries related to endometriosis. Endometriosis symptoms can cause everything from headaches to chest pain — in addition to the more common symptoms of cramps, painful sex, and abnormal bleeding. Many women with endometriosis have suffered for years without realizing they had a serious disease (and may have been called *malingerers,* fakers who use illness to avoid work) because their disease wasn't visible! Too often these women have given up on getting help.

We hope you read *Endometriosis For Dummies* saying, "That's me! I never knew endometriosis caused that!" In addition, we hope to help you find ways to live a more pain-free life. If you want kids, we want to show you that pregnancy and endometriosis aren't mutually exclusive. To sum up, we want to show you that endometriosis doesn't have to rule — or ruin — your life.

About This Book

We wrote this book realizing that many women never know that their pain and suffering (often dismissed as *all in the head* by family, friends, and doctors alike) stem from a real disease with symptoms so diverse that it sometimes defies diagnosis. Our goal is to inform you about endometriosis and to help you understand what it is and how it affects many body systems, not just your reproductive organs. We also want to show you how to live with endometriosis as painlessly as possible and how to modify the effect endometriosis has on your life.

We cover all the bases in this book, starting with the basic information on what endometriosis is, what the symptoms are, and who gets it. If you don't know much about endometriosis or about the reproductive system in general, start at the beginning of the book and read straight through. After the basics, we delve a little deeper into how endometriosis affects specific areas of your life and discuss the treatments for endometriosis. We also help you decide whether medication, surgery, or alternative medicine options are best for you.

Conventions Used in This Book

In this book, we use the following conventions to help make the information consistent and easier to understand. The last thing we want to do is confuse you!

- ✔ All Web addresses appear in `monofont`.
- ✔ **Bold** text indicates key words in bulleted lists and highlights the action parts of numbered steps.
- ✔ *Italics* identify new terms that are beside easy-to-understand definitions.

What You're Not to Read

Although we hope you, our dear reader, cherish every word in this book, we know better. Sometimes you're just looking for quick answers, but other times you want to discover everything possible about endometriosis, even the technical stuff. We've designated some information as *interesting-but-not-essential-to-read*. Feel free to read it, but if you skip it, you're not missing anything vital. Optional sections are

✔ **Text in sidebars:** This text is in shaded boxes that appear throughout the book. The information in sidebars may be anything from personal stories to technical information. The common denominator is that the information isn't essential to understanding or dealing with endometriosis.

✔ **Anything with a *Technical Stuff* icon attached:** This information is interesting, but not essential — unless you're planning on doing your doctorate thesis on endometriosis. (For more information on icons, check out "Icons Used in This Book" later in this Introduction.)

✔ **The stuff on the copyright page:** The attorneys require that we have this information. Unless you're an aspiring lawyer, feel free to skip it.

Foolish Assumptions

We assume that you're reading this book because you want to know more about endometriosis. We also assume that you want to

✔ Understand the basic biology of what endometriosis is and why it develops

✔ Understand how endometriosis affects different body systems

✔ Discover what medical options are available for treating endometriosis

✔ Be up-to-date on the latest surgical treatments for endometriosis

✔ Find out how you can get pregnant if you have endometriosis

✔ Figure out how to manage the pain of endometriosis

Endometriosis doesn't have to mean the end of a good life for you; you can figure out how to manage pain, minimize symptoms, and keep endometriosis from taking over your life. Our greatest hope is that this book takes the clout out of endometriosis and gives you the tools to live your life as symptom-free as possible.

How This Book Is Organized

Endometriosis For Dummies is divided into six parts. As with every *For Dummies* book, this one is designed to help you find the information you need quickly and easily, without having to read the book cover-to-cover. The following explanations can help you find the information you need with a minimum of effort.

Part I: Endometriosis: What It Is and Isn't

What exactly is endometriosis and what causes it? Who gets endometriosis and why? In these chapters, we explore the mysteries behind endometriosis, its typical symptoms, the biology behind it, and the most common risk factors for developing it.

Part II: Digging Deeper into Endometriosis

In these chapters, we look at how endometriosis affects various body systems, such as the menstrual cycle, digestive system, and the urinary tract. We also delve into the complicated relationship between endometriosis and infertility and describe the tests that determine whether you really have endometriosis or another disease. Finally, we help you find a doctor who's willing to treat you as an equal partner and make a diagnosis based on your symptoms.

Part III: Treating Endometriosis

You may already know you have endometriosis. Now the big question is, "How do you treat it?" These chapters describe numerous treatments, from traditional to alternative, from medications and surgeries to massages and acupuncture. We also talk about the way endometriosis affects teens and pre-teens and how their treatment differs from that of adults.

Part IV: Living with Endometriosis

Life goes on, even when you have a chronic disease such as endometriosis. In these chapters, we talk about how to cope with work, family, and friends when you're in pain. We also give you suggestions for changing your lifestyle to minimize the impact of endometriosis, including how to eat better, exercise more, and avoid toxins. Finally we provide a chapter specifically for your friends and family that helps them better understand you and your disease.

Part V: The Part of Tens

We have nothing long-winded in the Part of Tens chapters — they're short and sweet, giving you a lot of information in little bites. These chapters dispel some of the most common myths about endometriosis, give some insight into the future of endometriosis diagnosis and treatment, and list some quick ways to decrease pain when you're down and out with endo.

Part VI: Appendixes

This section contains two appendixes. The first is a glossary that defines all the undecipherable (and unpronounceable!) Latin medical terms as well as other terms in this book that may be unfamiliar to you. The second appendix is a list of resources to help you find out more about endometriosis, support groups, and online information sources.

Icons Used in This Book

Icons are the strange-looking symbols that appear occasionally in the margins next to the text. We include them to let you know that a topic or information is special in some way. *Endometriosis For Dummies* includes the following icons:

This icon identifies information that's helpful and can save you time or trouble.

This icon highlights key points in the section you're reading.

This icon stresses information that describes potentially serious issues, such as side effects to medication or other dangerous problems. Pay attention to warnings — they can keep you out of trouble!

This icon signals information that's interesting but not essential to understanding endometriosis, unless you're a scientist or medical student.

This icon shows up when a situation requires you to — you guessed it! — notify your doctor. The situation can include symptoms or side effects.

This icon appears next to information straight from the doctor's mouth — in this case, from Dr. Krotec. You can find personal stories and suggestions here from his years of treating patients with endometriosis.

Where to Go from Here

Enough talk about the book — time to read it already! If this were a novel, you'd start at Chapter 1 and read straight through. But it's not a novel, and it's not a textbook, where each chapter builds on the one before. You can open this book at any point and be able to understand the information there.

For example, you may suspect you have endometriosis, but you're not sure. Turn to Chapter 2 to read about the most common symptoms of endometriosis. Feeling a little technical today? Turn to Chapter 3 for an in-depth look at the biology behind endometriosis.

The point is, you don't have to read everything (although you certainly can, and you may discover something you never knew before)! Just flip to the Table of Contents or Index, find a subject that interests you, and turn to that chapter. It's not essential to read everything — just what interests you and helps you.

Endometriosis For Dummies is a resource, a guide that presents the practical information in a fun, easy-to-read-and-understand format. Read a chapter a day or a chapter a year, or keep it in the bathroom for frequent browsing. But however you choose to use this book, we hope it's helpful.

Part I
Endometriosis: What It Is and Isn't

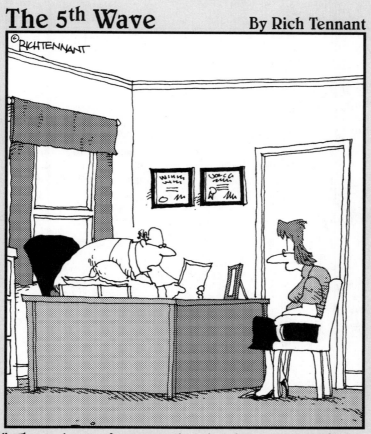

The 5th Wave — By Rich Tennant

"The pain you're experiencing is normal. It's as normal as walking down the street with say, an inflated truck tire in your pelvis."

In this part . . .

*E*ndometriosis is a long word derived from Greek, as many medical words are, but what is it? In this part, we look at the complicated disease of endometriosis: what it is, what the typical symptoms are, and how common it is. We cover some biology to give you a good understanding of how all your inner parts interrelate. And we look at the reasons some women get the disease and others don't.

Chapter 1

The Lowdown on Endometriosis: A Quick Run-Through

In This Chapter

▶ Understanding endometriosis basics

▶ Educating the public about endometriosis

▶ Knowing who's who in endometriosis

▶ Counting the real costs of endometriosis

▶ Answering the big question: A self-test

*P*eople generally don't understand endometriosis very well. Until recently, you didn't even hear about it — unless you were at a gynecology convention! But new research and better publicity have brought endometriosis to the public's attention, making many women wonder whether this is the nameless disease they've had since puberty.

In this chapter, we talk about the little-known disease of endometriosis: what it is, who it affects, and why it's received so little attention (despite the fact that it costs millions of dollars a year in lost wages and productivity). We also include a self-test to see whether you may have this disease.

Defining Endometriosis

If you tell someone you have endometriosis, you probably get a blank look in return. Unfortunately most people are pretty clueless when it comes to this disease. (Check out the nearby sidebar, "The roots of endometriosis," for some background on the word itself.)

The roots of endometriosis

Endometriosis (en-doe-meet-ree-*oh*-sis) has six syllables, but don't let its size intimidate you. Just put the accent on the *oh* and you'll impress your gynecologist. (Maybe he'll even warm the speculum for you next time.) The roots of the syllables break it down — in Greek, *Endo* means *inside,* and *metros* means *uterus.* So *endometrium* essentially means *inside the uterus.* The *-is* suffix means *an abnormal state,* like gastrit*is,* cystit*is,* and sinusit*is.*

So what *does* having endometriosis mean? The following basics can give you a better grasp of it:

- ✔ Every woman has a uterus with an *endometrium* (the uterine lining).
- ✔ When this lining implants outside the uterus, the abnormal condition is called *endometriosis.*
- ✔ Endometriosis consists of *endometrial tissue* (pieces of endometrium) containing glands (just like sweat glands and saliva glands) and *stroma* (supporting tissue) growing where it doesn't belong — anywhere *outside* the endometrial cavity.

Sounds fairly clear so far, right? However, endometriosis isn't quite so simple. This section looks a bit closer at the complexities of endometriosis, including how endometriosis moves to different parts of the body and why it hurts.

Figuring out why endometriosis moves

You think you're starting to understand endometriosis, but you may be wondering how pieces of a uterus get into places they don't belong. After all, parts of your nose or ears don't wander to other places in your body, so why do parts of your uterus travel around to lodge in your lungs, intestines, bladder, ovaries, or even your brain?

Unfortunately, the simple answer is this: Doctors and researchers still don't know. In Chapter 4, we delve into the mysteries of endometriosis and some theories of why it travels to strange places.

Understanding why endometriosis hurts

Endometriosis is painful because the endometrial tissue in other locations behaves just like the endometrium inside your uterus. The endometrium normally becomes thicker during your menstrual cycle and then sheds off the wall, flowing out through the cervix and vagina as menstrual bleeding. (See Chapter 5 for a more detailed description of the menstrual cycle.)

The endometrial tissue in your ovaries or fallopian tubes also bleeds during your cycle, but the blood has no place to go. The trapped blood irritates nearby tissue by stretching the lining (like a pimple stretches the skin), making it tender. In addition, localized inflammatory factors, such as prostaglandins, interleukin, and tumor necrosis factor (we talk about these in detail in Chapter 4) also irritate tissue. These inflammatory factors can cause severe, painful reactions even when very small areas are involved.

But wait, we're not done. Irritation and inflammation month after month can lead to *nodules* (or cysts) that form on ovaries or other organs. Over time, these nodules can turn into *adhesions* (scar tissue) that cause organs and tissue to stick together, also causing pain. And when the misplaced endometrial tissue releases chemical irritants over long periods of time, a chronic irritation develops, forming extensive scar tissue and — you guessed it — chronic pain. In other words, every month *is* a vicious cycle of pain or other symptoms.

Endometriosis lesions, or *implants,* range in size from too small to see with the naked eye to as large as a grapefruit. Most implants are fairly small, the size of a pencil eraser or smaller. The implants can grow throughout the pelvis and may be singular (rare) or number in the hundreds (also rare). In Chapter 3, we cover the most and least common areas for endometriosis to occur, along with the consequences for each location.

Another factor that makes endometriosis difficult to understand is the amount of endometrial tissue versus the amount of pain a woman feels. For example, you may have a neighbor who has just a few spots of endometriosis but experiences a lot of pain each month, but your sister, who was diagnosed with many endometrial implants during an appendectomy, may have no pain at all.

It's never too late for endometriosis

A 40-year-old patient came to my office because her family practitioner had tested her and diagnosed a cyst in her left ovary. (Her symptoms had been pain with bowel movements.) Because she was in her 40s, my initial concern was cancer. This woman had never had any symptoms related to endometriosis; she had no painful periods and no pain with sex,

and she had delivered three children without any problems. What did we find? Stage III (we define staging in Chapter 9) endometriosis with a large chocolate cyst (see Chapter 3 for more on these not-so-yummy cysts!). No doctor would ever consider endometriosis from her history. And that's the problem — endometriosis isn't always the obvious diagnosis.

Going Public: Why Don't People Know About Endometriosis?

With endometriosis being one of the most common gynecologic problems that women face, you would expect everyone to know about it. So why don't you see ads about endometriosis on television and national telethons to raise money for research?

This section covers some of the reasons for the relative anonymity of endometriosis. Sadly, some of these reasons are all too familiar to many women.

Endometriosis is a women's disease

Even though women have come a long way, baby, they haven't come all the way. Gynecologic diseases, especially non-life-threatening ones, don't get the respect, research dollars, or media play that other diseases do. Is this somewhat puritan? Yes. Unfair? Absolutely. Remediable? Of course, but change takes public awareness.

Simply put, government agencies, insurance companies, and even pharmaceutical companies shortchange female problems. Consider the dozens and dozens of blood pressure medications, diabetes treatments, cold remedies, and, yes, erectile dysfunction treatments (men must be men!), but modern science provides few therapeutic options for most female problems. One reason? The United States is still male-dominated. As a result, according to documented studies, medical research and treatment for women receive far fewer dollars than they do for men.

Endometriosis symptoms are "all in your head"

Guess what — the naysayers are partly right. Endometriosis really *may* be in your head — and in your lungs, appendix, and ovaries, too! But for years, health professionals have ignored or minimized the symptoms of endometriosis due to a variety of misunderstandings. For example:

✔ They thought the symptoms were mere exaggerations of the monthly menstrual cycle.

✔ They thought the woman was a hypochondriac, depressed, or simply seeking attention.

✔ They thought that women were meant to suffer in silence, especially with traditionally taboo topics, such as menstrual pain.

✔ Too many women believed (because their moms said so) that all women suffer during their periods, so they didn't bother their doctors with their symptoms.

In fact, many women who seek help for infertility often have a long history of painful periods, irregular periods, painful sex, and so on (all signs of endometriosis). But, too often that history includes a doctor who ignored the patient's symptoms or made her feel that the symptoms were normal. (Check out Chapter 7, which discusses the relationship between endometriosis and fertility.)

Endometriosis is invisible until you have surgery

When a disease has obvious signs (markings on the skin, abnormal EKG, and so on), the patient usually has confidence in the diagnosis. Unfortunately, endometriosis has no outward signs and no accurate diagnostic test. As Chapter 9 discusses, an accurate diagnosis occurs only when a doctor can visually observe the endometriosis during surgery or through a biopsy.

However, some doctors are hesitant to put patients under the knife for diagnostic purposes. Because surgery has risks even under ideal conditions, a doctor may decide some symptoms don't justify the risk (see Chapter 11 for more on surgery and endometriosis). This decision is especially true with young patients, who often have other problems that can mimic endometriosis. (Chapter 14 has more on teens and their symptoms.)

Endometriosis isn't glamorous

The symptoms of endometriosis aren't dire enough or intriguing enough to draw the media attention — or big funding dollars — that support the more socially acceptable diseases. Women's diseases certainly don't make the cover of national magazines, and no movie star has broadcast that she has endometriosis — it's just not glamorous or popular.

Add to the mix that men don't *usually* get endometriosis (yup, you heard me right) and that it's not contagious, and you have a formula for widespread disinterest. So endometriosis remains in the background — a disease that today's society just doesn't bother to promote or treat.

Speaking of sex . . .

I can't count the number of patients over the years that have refused to discuss sex in medical terms. I try to inquire about their sex lives, orgasms, pain, lubrication, and basic enjoyment, but most women are too embarrassed to talk even with a gynecologist about these issues. Most times I hear, "It's okay," or "If my husband/boyfriend wants it. . . ." In addition, most women have very little understanding of their sexual and reproductive organs. Because of this taboo against discussing sex and genitals, too many women have a hard time bringing up the symptoms of endometriosis, even when a doctor encourages them to. No wonder this disease and its symptoms often go undiagnosed.

Who Gets Endometriosis?

Does endometriosis find its way to all countries in equal numbers, or is it more of an industrial society's problem? Obviously, in developing countries, where women need to worry more about their family's next meal than mid-cycle bleeding, endometriosis isn't a high priority to diagnose or treat. In addition, endometriosis is less common in women who have many children and at a young age (which is also more typical in third-world societies).

This section takes a look at the number of people endometriosis affects worldwide, and it discusses age and pregnancy — two of the important factors in determining the total number.

Counting the women with endometriosis

How many women have endometriosis? The numbers may surprise you. Because determining the number of women with endometriosis can be difficult, estimates worldwide range from as little as 2 to as much as 40 percent. Based on a relatively conservative estimate then, endometriosis affects one out of every ten women of childbearing age.

So what women have endometriosis? The following facts provide some insight:

✔ More than 5.5 million women in North America alone suffer from endometriosis.

✔ Race and socioeconomic status don't seem to influence the incidence of endometriosis in any meaningful way.

✔ Women with lower socioeconomic status (regardless of race) are less likely to be diagnosed.

✔ Women with more education and a higher socioeconomic status generally seek medical care sooner, read more, ask their doctors more questions, and, therefore, are more likely to be diagnosed with endometriosis. And, because they're more likely to delay childbearing until later in life, these women have more time to develop severe symptoms, including infertility.

✔ Around 50 percent of women with new onset of severe menstrual cramps have endometriosis.

✔ At least one-third of infertile women have endometriosis.

Many women don't know they have endometriosis until they have surgery for another condition, such as a Cesarean section or tubal ligation. And this incidental diagnosis complicates the numbers issue by raising the following questions:

✔ How many other women who never have surgery have undiagnosed endometriosis?

✔ If these undiagnosed women have none of the typical endometriosis complaints, should they be part of the total number of women suffering from endometriosis?

✔ If a woman doesn't have pain, does she still have endometriosis?

✔ Is endometriosis without pain the same disease that causes so much pain in other women?

The total number of women with endometriosis is difficult to estimate because of these great variabilities in symptoms and diagnoses. An accurate diagnosis of endometriosis is possible only through a visual confirmation during surgery or by biopsy.

Looking at age and endometriosis

Women between the ages of 23 and 35 are most likely to be diagnosed with endometriosis. The average age at diagnosis in North America is 27. Table 1-1 shows data by the Endometriosis Association of more than 3,000 women with endometriosis. The percentage for each group represents the amount of women who had endometriosis symptoms begin at that age.

Is endometriosis becoming more common throughout the world?

According to a recent World Congress on endometriosis, the disease hasn't increased over the last 30 years. However, doctors are diagnosing it earlier and more effectively, probably because more medical personnel are looking for the disease. Also, because of smaller instruments, better optics, and vast improvements in anesthesia (even local anesthesia), more gynecologists feel comfortable using surgery to diagnose the disease (we talk more about surgery in Chapter 11).

Even in third-world countries, where basic surgery tools aren't available and surgery is a major risk, many doctors are treating women for endometriosis and could treat more of them if the resources were available.

Endometriosis is clearly a worldwide disease, and the estimated number of women suffering from it is at least 15 million. Nevertheless, endometriosis is still more likely to be diagnosed in industrialized countries for reasons that reflect varying social systems. For example:

- Cultural norms in some countries discourage women from complaining about pain, especially pain related to the reproductive system.

- Women in industrialized countries put off childbirth longer and have fewer children.

- Women in poorer countries and third-world countries tend to have children earlier and more often.

- Women in poorer countries don't live as long — they may even die before puberty.

- Techniques for diagnosing endometriosis aren't easily available or may be dangerous.

- The attitude may exist that, if treatment isn't available, why bother to diagnose it?

- Medical knowledge of the disease may be lacking in some areas.

- Women in industrialized countries are more likely to be exposed to toxins and hormones.

Even with the greater likelihood for it to be diagnosed in industrialized countries, endometriosis is everywhere. Medical journals of Europe, Japan, and Australia all have numerous articles on the topic. So the disease is present, but the real challenges are looking for it and diagnosing it.

Table 1-1	Age When Endometriosis Symptoms Begin
Age When Symptoms Began	*Percentage*
<15 years old	14.9
15–19 years old	25.9
20–24 years old	19.6
25–29 years old	23.3
30–34 years old	12.5
35–39 years old	4.0

Endometriosis through the ages

Endometriosis isn't a new disease, although it hasn't always had the same name. Daniel Shroen first described the symptoms in 1690 as sores throughout the stomach, bladder, and intestines as well as broad ligaments that had a tendency to form adhesions. In 1769, Arthur Duff described the intense pain of endometriosis, and it was first seen microscopically in the late 1800s. In 1921, Dr. John Sampson was the first person to hypothesize that retrograde menstruation contributed to endometriosis. (See Chapter 4 for more about the retrograde menstruation theory.)

The ages of 23 to 35 coincide with the period when many women consider pregnancy and regularly visit the gynecologist. A woman may have a problem conceiving, or she may share her symptoms with her doctor, or her physician may find a problem during the pelvic exam. Any of these scenarios may lead the doctor to suspect endometriosis (although a myriad of other problems may also cause these problems). As we note in Chapter 7, there's no law against having other diseases *and* endometriosis!

This age range also coincides with the time women work outside the home on a regular basis. At this age, the symptoms of endometriosis can alter a woman's lifestyle for the worse. For example, women who work full time may have symptoms that cause them to miss work, or they may have bad days that detract from their performance. They may now have a boss who doesn't understand why they're bent over in their chair, leave early, come in late, and miss a couple of days a month due to their recurring symptoms.

The incidence of endometriosis decreases in the 35 to 39 age range, and problems are rare for women in their 40s, unless they had severe endometriosis at a younger age. In contrast, one study found that 50 percent of younger women (teenagers especially) who had pelvic pain, bloating, painful periods, irregular periods, and other symptoms were diagnosed with endometriosis. This high percentage may be due to the aggressive nature of the disease in teens. (Check out Chapter 14 for more on treating teens and preteens with endometriosis.)

Linking pregnancy and endometriosis

Parity refers to the number of pregnancies a woman has had, so women who have never been pregnant are *nulliparous,* and women who've had at least one pregnancy are *multiparous.*

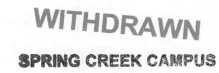

WITHDRAWN

SPRING CREEK CAMPUS

Can men ever have endometriosis?

Even though a uterus seems like a basic requirement for endometriosis, a few men have developed lesions that appear to be endometriosis after exposure to high-dose estrogen treatments for prostate cancer. The lesions developed in the prostate.

Endometriosis is

- ✔ Most common in women with no children.
- ✔ More common in women with fewer children.
- ✔ Least common in women with more children.

Linking pregnancy to endometriosis may be a chicken-egg relationship. In other words, do women who have endometriosis have fewer children because endometriosis can contribute to infertility, or do they develop endometriosis because they've had fewer pregnancies? Pregnancy does seem to have a protective and therapeutic effect on the disease (we discuss the effects of pregnancy in Chapter 4). In fact, pregnancy was one of the oldest treatments for endometriosis — but, then again, not being able to get pregnant may be part of the problem!

Furthermore, endometriosis is less common in women

- ✔ Whose first pregnancy occurred at a younger age
- ✔ Who have had multiple pregnancies

When women have their first pregnancy early and then have several children, their uterus and ovaries have longer *quiet* times — without the steady supply of irritants from the menstrual cycle, the endometriosis simply burns out.

Calculating the Cost of Endometriosis

Endometriosis literally costs millions of dollars. How ironic is it that a disease that can't be seen and doesn't kill you can still cause so many problems? Consider this: The main symptom of endometriosis is pain during your menstrual period, which shows up every month. So endometriosis is a disease that recurs, almost like clockwork, once every three to four weeks.

This pattern means that every three to four weeks endometriosis is affecting your life, maybe preventing you from going to work, probably adding to your medical bills for pain relief, and definitely challenging your relationships. This section totals some of those high costs of endometriosis.

Eying the economic costs

Being in pain once every three to four weeks may not seem bad, but that week that you're lying on the couch and taking pain relievers by the handful means you're not at work and you're not contributing to the economy. One large British study determined the following rather startling statistics on endometriosis:

- Sixty-five percent of women in the study indicated that they had initially been misdiagnosed with another condition.
- Seventy-eight percent missed an average of five days per month from work due to endometriosis.
- Thirty-six percent said that endometriosis had affected their job performance, and of this group
  - Forty-one percent had lost or given up their jobs entirely.
  - Thirty-seven percent had reduced their hours.
  - Twenty-three percent had changed jobs.
  - Six percent went on disability.

All this sick time and the resulting decreased performance cost the economy dearly. When you miss work for several days, you aren't productive. Either your company pays someone else to take your place or no one does the work. If you reduce your hours or quit, then your personal economy takes a big hit — and the government may end up paying unemployment or disability.

Furthermore, if the pain is severe, you may have major surgery. Women are typically out of work at least six weeks after such surgery, and this time off places an even greater burden on the economy. Often a woman who has major surgery (such as a hysterectomy) doesn't return to full productivity for several weeks or even months. (Some women never get back to full-time work.)

Common complications (wound infection, urinary tract infection, excessive blood loss, adhesions, bowel complications, and so on) can extend the recovery time even further. When major complications occur (and they do in a small percentage of cases, no matter how good the surgeon), the result is prolonged periods of reduced work, absence, or permanent loss of productivity.

Considering the diagnostic and treatment costs

In addition to its effect on the economy, endometriosis (its diagnosis and treatment) is hard on the wallet too. Considering the vast numbers of women with the disease, the total cost for even conservative treatments, pain medication, hormonal therapies, and the like, is enormous. One common prescription for endometriosis is more than $400 per month per woman! This amount of money is staggering to treat a disease we can't see and know so little about.

The total cost of diagnosis, surgical interventions, and extensive treatment is billions of dollars annually. For example, of the nearly 600,000 *hysterectomies* (removal of the uterus and one or both ovaries) in the United States each year, around 20 percent (100,000) are for reduction of endometriosis–associated symptoms. The hospitalization, medications, and other fees for these surgeries cost the healthcare system tens of millions of dollars — each year.

Looking at the cost on relationships

The cost of endometriosis extends far beyond money. Endometriosis is hard on relationships. Chronic illnesses, especially ones that affect sexual relations, can be a huge strain. The British study mentioned earlier in this section reported the following statistics:

- ✔ Seventy-two percent of the women studied reported they had problems with relationships due to endometriosis.

- ✔ Ten percent said that endometriosis had caused a split in a relationship.

- ✔ Thirty-four percent said it caused significant problems with their partner.

- ✔ Eleven percent said they had trouble taking care of their children.

How can you even put a price on these problems? No one can estimate a monetary number to compensate for loss of life's pleasures and love. These emotional and social problems can cause other problems. When a disease puts a strain on a relationship, any number of psychological troubles can surface. For example, depression is common for people with a chronic disease. Women can be anxious or paranoid, and they can lose self-esteem. A woman may shut herself off from other people and become reclusive. These side effects and other relational problems are all difficult to address.

Furthermore, surgeries such as hysterectomies and *oophorectomies* (removal of the ovaries) can be psychologically damaging, leading to depression and perceived loss of sexuality. Although placing a value on life's pleasures is next to impossible, the emotional and psychological costs of these losses (along with the many short- and long-term complications of major surgery) are substantial and may be more devastating to a woman and her family than the symptoms directly related to the disease.

DOCTOR'S NOTES

One woman's story: The high cost of endometriosis

One patient, Jane, had had 10 or 11 laparoscopies over the years for recurrent endometriosis. She'd have relief after each one for a year or two, but then the pain returned. When she couldn't function at work or socially, she'd have another laparoscopy. Jane had also tried all the conservative medical therapies (GnRH agonist, NSAIDs, and hormones — we cover all these in detail in Chapter 10) with either no relief or too many side effects. Finally, she demanded a hysterectomy and removal of the ovary that kept hurting, and she did feel better afterwards. Unfortunately, when the other ovary became a problem a couple of years later, she had several conservative surgeries to try and save it. Eventually it had to come out, and she is now symptom-free!

This story isn't typical, but it illustrates the great difficulty in assessing the cost of endometriosis and its effect on a woman's life. What was the total cost to treat Jane, and what was the cost of all the lost work days and life's pleasures while she was suffering? I don't even want to hazard a guess — it's staggering!

Of course, for every story like Jane's, another story exists of a woman who continues to suffer in silence or who has major surgery and then always wonders whether it was the right choice.

We're not saying that major surgery is always bad. Many women opt for this course when the more conservative approaches have failed, and the majority of women do well (see Chapter 11 for more info on the different types of surgeries). In fact, most patients who eventually have major surgery are ready for it *and* happy with the results.

Do You Have Endometriosis: A Self-Test

Statistics are interesting, but you're probably more concerned about whether you have endometriosis than about the statistics. Although only your doctor can diagnose endometriosis, the following questions help answer the question: Do I have endometriosis? You don't have to answer all the questions with a "yes" to have endometriosis, but more than one or two "yes" answers is a good reason to make an appointment with your doctor sooner rather than later.

Questions

1. **Do you have a family history of endometriosis?**

2. **Do you have painful periods?**

3. **Do you have pain during sex?**

4. Are you having trouble getting pregnant?

5. Did you start having periods at a younger age than the norm?

6. Do your periods last longer than four to five days?

7. Do your periods come more often than every four weeks?

8. Do you have heavier than normal menstrual periods?

9. Do you have allergies or autoimmune diseases such as asthma?

10. Do you have painful urination during your period?

11. Do you have tummy troubles, such as diarrhea, constipation, or pain, during your period?

12. Are you taller and thinner than average?

Answers

The following information provides some explanations for each question:

1. Endometriosis is more common in women whose close female relatives have endometriosis.

2. Painful cramping during menstrual periods is the most common symptom of endometriosis, although many women with cramps *don't* have endometriosis.

3. Endometriosis in the pelvis can make sex painful.

4. Thirty to forty percent of infertile women have endometriosis (see Chapter 7 for more info).

5–8. Any factor that causes more menstrual bleeding over the course of your lifetime is a risk factor for endometriosis. Women whose periods start at a younger age and who have longer than normal periods, heavier than normal periods, or periods closer than every four weeks are all more likely to develop endometriosis.

9. Women with endometriosis are also more likely to have allergies or other autoimmune diseases.

10. Endometriosis in the urinary tract can cause pain and bleeding.

11. Endometriosis in the intestines can cause pain, cramping, diarrhea, constipation, or rectal bleeding during your period.

12. Women who are taller and thinner than average are more likely to have endometriosis.

This test is just a starting point. If you're concerned that you may have endometriosis, don't hesitate. Make an appointment with your gynecologist.

Chapter 2

Suspecting Endometriosis: Defining the Symptoms

*I*s something wrong with you, something you — and your doctors — can't put your collective fingers on? You may wonder whether endometriosis is causing the symptoms that have been plaguing you. However, your symptoms seem so varied and elusive at times that you aren't quite sure what's wrong.

In this chapter, we help you answer the question, "Could I have endometriosis?" by discussing the most common symptoms of the disease. We also identify the less familiar problems of endometriosis so you can get a more complete picture of this complex disease. Finally, we help you get a handle on your specific situation by showing you how to keep a written record of symptoms (when they occur and under what circumstances) and other relevant information. With these facts, you can give your doctor clear and accurate descriptions that will help her help you.

Considering the Most Common Symptoms of Endometriosis

To say that endometriosis is a disease of many symptoms is an understatement. Sometimes the symptoms you're experiencing seem so odd and so unconnected that you can't believe they all relate to endometriosis.

In the next sections, we cover the most common symptoms of endometriosis (listing the most common symptoms first), tell you what other diseases may cause the same symptoms, and explain how endometriosis symptoms may differ from those of other diseases. Don't be disheartened by the length of this list; few, if any, women with endometriosis have *all* these symptoms. You're more likely to have just a few.

Dealing with painful periods

If you have painful periods, you may or may not have endometriosis. Endometriosis doesn't necessarily cause painful periods *(dysmenorrhea),* so this symptom doesn't mean you definitely have endometriosis. In fact, up to 80 percent of all women experience painful periods at some time in their lives. Around 10 percent experience pain severe enough to interfere with normal activities, such as school or work. (See more about painful periods in Chapter 5.)

If you do have painful periods, you may notice the following symptoms:

- Lower abdominal cramping
- Generalized pelvic pain
- Pain in the uterus due to contractions
- Back pain or leg pain
- Headaches
- Nausea, vomiting
- Diarrhea or constipation
- General body weakness

So how can you tell whether endometriosis is causing your painful periods? You can't. Cramping from endometriosis can occur before, during, or after your period, and you can't diagnose endometriosis by the type of cramping you have; only your doctor can make a diagnosis between the two. Painful cramps are just one symptom of endometriosis, and they're only one piece of a puzzle that makes up endometriosis. If you have painful pelvic cramping, you need to see your gynecologist.

If you have painful periods, you don't have to endure the agonizing pain any longer. Check with your doctor for a diagnosis (check out Chapter 9 for more on what your doctor will do to make a diagnosis). Even if your doctor rules out endometriosis, she may be able to identify another cause for your painful periods. Some other diseases that can cause painful periods include

- Premenstrual syndrome (PMS)
- Pelvic inflammatory disease (PID)
- Fibroids
- Ovarian cysts and polycystic ovary syndrome (PCOS)
- Stenotic (narrow) cervix
- Uterine abnormalities

Hurtin' for certain during sex

Pain during or after sex *(dyspareunia)* can cause more than physical problems. It can cause problems with your relationships, emotions, and self-esteem (not to mention infertility from lack of sex). Up to 50 percent of women experience dyspareunia at some time in their lives.

Dyspareunia is almost always a woman's problem; men don't usually experience it. Pain during sex from endometriosis is likely to cause the following symptoms:

- Pain with deep penetration; pain may last several days after intercourse
- Pain more intense during menstrual period or ovulation

Because endometriosis isn't the only condition that causes painful sex (check out the nearby sidebar "More than endometriosis can cause painful sex" for other conditions that may be causing your painful sex), how can you be certain that endometriosis is in fact causing your painful sex? Only your doctor can determine the truth. Try to give your doctor clues to the exact problems with your pain. He may ask questions such as:

- Have you always had pain with intercourse?
- Do you feel pain every time you have sex? If not, at what time in the month do you feel pain during sex?
- Do you have vaginal dryness? Do you use any lubricants?
- Do you use spermicides or condoms?
- Where do you feel the pain? Is it on entry or more during deep thrusting; on the outside, in the vagina, or in the pelvic area? Which side is the pain on, or is it on both? Is it in the front, the back, or both? Is it in the bladder or rectum?
- When do you feel the pain? Is it immediate, during, or after sex? And if after, how long after?

REMEMBER

More than endometriosis can cause painful sex

Endometriosis doesn't cause all painful sex problems, so having painful sex doesn't necessarily mean you have endometriosis. A host of other problems may be responsible, including

- **Infections**
  - Pelvic organ infections (PID)
  - Cervical infections
  - Vaginal infections
- **Vaginal irritation**
  - Dryness from decreased arousal or low estrogen
  - Allergic reaction to lubricants, condoms, spermicides, deodorants, laundry detergent, soaps, or douches
  - Medications
- **Pelvic muscle pain**
  - *Vaginismus* (muscles around the pelvis)
  - Pelvic floor muscles
  - Fibromyalgia

- **Tenderness on the vulva (the outside of the vagina)**
  - *Vulvodynia* (vulvar pain of unknown cause)
  - Vulvar infections
- **Pelvic masses**
  - Uterine fibroids
  - Ovarian cysts
- **Pelvic scar tissue (including adhesions from infection or surgery**
- **Bladder problems**
  - Urinary tract infection
  - *Interstitial cystitis* (an inflammatory bladder problem)
- **Intestine and rectum problems**
  - Large intestine disorders, such as irritable bowel syndrome (IBS) or colitis
  - Hemorrhoids
- **Emotional issues**

- How long have you been sexually active?
- Have you had an abnormal pap smear?
- Have you had a venereal disease?
- Do you have bladder or intestinal problems?
- Do you have any history of sexual abuse?
- What medications are you taking?

These questions may be embarrassing for you, but we guarantee your doctor has asked them a million times before, has heard a million different answers, and won't be surprised by anything you say. If he is surprised or shocked by anything you say, he'll have the good sense not to show it!

Dr. K. has had patients with many of these symptoms. Recently a patient had problems getting pregnant. The main complaint was that sex was so painful that she only rarely had sex. She also had bleeding with and after sex. These symptoms were so disturbing to her and her partner (he was frightened and thought he was damaging her) that they almost never had sex (and it's hard to get pregnant without it!). But the diagnosis was endometriosis that caused the pain and bleeding and *cervicitis* (a cervical infection) that killed his sperm. Dr. K. treated the cervicitis, explained different positions for sex (to decrease the discomfort endometriosis caused her), and told the couple about the proper timing of ovulation. Success! They soon achieved a pregnancy.

Feeling mid-cycle pain

Mid-cycle pain occurs about two weeks before your next period begins. This isn't always halfway between periods, so the name is a bit of a misnomer. For example, if your period occurs every 22 days, mid-cycle pain actually occurs around Day 8. If your period comes every 36 days, mid-cycle pain occurs around Day 24.

About 20 percent of women experience mid-cycle pain at some time in their lives; the pain usually lasts only a few minutes to a few hours. Women may confuse it with appendicitis when it occurs on the right side. A better name for mid-cycle pain is *ovulatory* pain because it usually occurs around the time of ovulation.

Mid-cycle pain related to endometriosis may cause all the same symptoms, but they usually get more intense and last longer over time. Most of the other reasons for mid-cycle pain don't show consistent progression of intensity and duration (check out the nearby sidebar "Identifying other causes of mid-cycle pain").

Experiencing abnormal bleeding

Abnormal uterine bleeding (AUB), sometimes called *dysfunctional uterine bleeding* (DUB), is any vaginal bleeding that is irregular or heavier than normal. (See Chapter 5 for more about AUB.) Endometriosis-induced AUB is often caused by a hormone imbalance. This imbalance may be the result of endometriosis on the ovaries, and it can cause the following conditions (Chapter 7 covers these further):

- ✔ Problems with follicular development
- ✔ Luteal phase defect
- ✔ Ovulatory dysfunction
- ✔ Association with thyroid disease
- ✔ Destruction of ovarian tissue

Identifying other causes of mid-cycle pain

Although mid-cycle pain is sometimes associated with endometriosis, many women without endometriosis experience it as well. Other causes of mid-cycle pain are

✔ **Ovulation:** The release of the follicular fluid or blood from the ruptured follicle can cause this pain (sometimes called *mittelschmertz,* which is German for *middle pain*)

✔ **Ovarian cysts:** From rupture, leakage, or stretching

✔ **Ovarian torsion** (twisting of the ovary): Can be caused by large ovarian cysts

✔ **Hormonal fluctuations:** May cause spasms in the uterus, intestines, or bladder muscles

Because the cause of AUB is often a hormone imbalance, doctors generally treat AUB first with hormones (after other causes have been eliminated). The hormones can be birth control pills (which are simple to use, familiar to most women, and relatively cheap) or other hormones, like progestins. The hormone or combination depends on many factors, including your doctor's preference and his assessment of what will work best for your particular problem.

Conceiving problems

Endometriosis is a common cause of infertility. In fact, 30 to 40 percent of infertile women have endometriosis. But that figure also means that 60 percent of patients with fertility issues *don't* have endometriosis, so infertility isn't a sure sign of endometriosis.

If you're having trouble getting pregnant, have your doctor first consider endometriosis as a possible cause in any fertility workup. Endometriosis can interfere with pregnancy in a large number of ways, such as

✔ Blocked fallopian tubes

✔ Hormone imbalances

✔ Implantation issues

✔ Production of ovarian cysts

See Chapter 7 for all the info you'll ever need on getting pregnant when you have endometriosis.

Considering other causes of abnormal uterine bleeding

Although endometriosis can cause abnormal uterine bleeding (AUB), a large number of unrelated problems can also cause AUB. Some of these causes are

- ✔ **Adenomyosis,** a condition where the lining of the uterus (the endometrium) gets into the muscle wall of the uterus.

- ✔ **Hormone imbalances**
  - ✔ Polycystic ovarian syndrome
  - ✔ Taking hormones
  - ✔ Hypothyroidism
  - ✔ Medications
  - ✔ Food supplements

- ✔ **Uterus problems**
  - ✔ Fibroids
  - ✔ Infection inside the uterus (*endometritis*)
  - ✔ Uterine cancer

- ✔ **Cervical problems**
  - ✔ Polyps (a fleshy, noncancerous growth)
  - ✔ Cervical infection (*cervicitis*)
  - ✔ Cervical precancer or cancer

- ✔ **Intrauterine device (an IUD)**
- ✔ **Injury to the vagina or cervix**

In order to make sure you have endometriosis and not one of these other problems, consult with your doctor.

Experiencing chronic pain

Pain that occurs frequently and regularly is, unfortunately, a hallmark of many diseases. Unlike *acute* pain, which occurs after a specific insult or injury, follows an expected timetable, and then disappears, *chronic* pain hangs around. *Note:* Although chronic pain may follow an injury (such as back pain), chronic pain may also indicate a chronic illness, such as endometriosis. As many as one in three Americans experience some type of chronic pain; some of the most common are headaches, back pain, muscle pain, and nerve pain.

The most common type of chronic pain from endometriosis is, not surprisingly, pelvic pain. Pelvic pain accounts for about 20 percent of all gynecologist appointments, and it's the reason for nearly half of all laparoscopies. Nearly two-thirds of patients with chronic pelvic pain are found to have endometriosis during laparoscopy; this percentage may increase as better visualization techniques during laparoscopy are developed.

Chronic pain is underdiagnosed and undertreated. Many women just live with the pain because they

- ✔ Think their doctor won't believe them
- ✔ Think chronic pain is a sign of weakness
- ✔ Have been treated like drug addicts when they asked for help
- ✔ Don't want to take opioids
- ✔ Are afraid to take too many over-the-counter medications
- ✔ Feel that chronic pain is untreatable

If you're suffering from chronic pelvic pain, check with your gynecologist. She can run the necessary tests (see Chapter 9 for diagnostic tests used in endometriosis) to determine whether endometriosis is causing your chronic pain. Other conditions besides endometriosis, such as the following, can also cause pelvic pain:

- ✔ Adhesions
- ✔ Pelvic inflammatory disease
- ✔ Fibroids
- ✔ Hernias
- ✔ Interstitial cystitis
- ✔ Irritable bowel syndrome

Your doctor can determine whether endometriosis or another condition is the reason for your chronic pain.

Facing autoimmune issues

Many studies support the idea that women with endometriosis are more likely than most to suffer from autoimmune diseases. With autoimmune diseases, the body makes antibodies that attack healthy organs or tissues, thereby causing disease. About 75 percent of the people with an autoimmune disease are women, and the disease often starts during the childbearing years.

Many autoimmune diseases exist, but researchers believe women with the following autoimmune diseases are also more likely to have endometriosis:

✔ Allergies

✔ Asthma

✔ Chronic fatigue syndrome

✔ Fibromyalgia

✔ Lupus

✔ Multiple sclerosis

✔ Rheumatoid arthritis

✔ Thyroid disease

Is endometriosis itself an autoimmune disease? Many scientists think so. (See Chapter 4 for more on autoimmune disease and endometriosis.) One study showed that as many as 28 percent of women with endometriosis had a positive response to an anti-nuclear antibody (ANA) blood test. This test indicates the presence of antibodies that cause inflammatory responses against a person's own cells (in other words, an autoimmune reaction).

Being tired all the time

Are you tired all the time? Ten percent of people say they are. No wonder the coffee houses are doing so well! Feeling tired can have physical or mental causes, and often it can be a combination of the two. Endometriosis can certainly cause exhaustion. In fact, in one large study of women with endometriosis, exhaustion was the second most common symptom.

The reasons for the extreme tiredness that sometimes comes with endometriosis aren't clear. Some theories explain exhaustion as

✔ Part of the autoimmune process

✔ A reaction to constant inflammation

✔ The result of stress from dealing with frequent pain

Endometriosis obviously isn't the only condition that causes extreme fatigue. Check out the nearby sidebar "Looking at other conditions that cause fatigue" for more info.

Looking at other conditions that cause fatigue

Although endometriosis and fatigue often go hand in hand, many other conditions can cause extreme tiredness, such as

✔ **Lack of sleep:** About half of all Americans claim sleep deprivation at any given time.

✔ **Anemia:** A decrease in red blood cells can cause fatigue and weakness.

✔ **Chronic fatigue syndrome:** Chronic fatigue can make even the smallest day-to-day functions difficult.

✔ **Depression:** People who are depressed are four times more likely to be fatigued.

✔ **Fibromyalgia:** Characteristics of this chronic illness are widespread muscle aches and fatigue.

✔ **Poor nutrition:** Lack of essential nutrients can cause weakness and fatigue.

✔ **Many medications:** Fatigue is a side effect of many medications.

✔ **Other diseases, such as hypothyroidism:** Fatigue is a common side effect of illness.

If you're fatigued, make sure you check with your doctor for a complete exam.

Noting the Not-Quite-As-Common Symptoms of Endometriosis

Although most people think of pelvic problems first when they think of endometriosis, endometrial tissue can travel quite a distance from the pelvis to wreak havoc in other areas of your body. In the next sections, we take a look at some not-quite-as-common symptoms related to endometriosis.

Living with your bowels in an uproar

There's nothing like bowel problems to keep you hopping. If your primary planning tool for vacations is the proximity of a bathroom at all times, you're not alone! Whether your problem is diarrhea, nausea, or constipation, rest assured that many women share your problems.

Endometriosis is one cause of bowel problems, but it's certainly not the only one. Around 10 percent of women with endometriosis have bowel problems caused by endometriosis.

One way to determine whether bowel problems are related to endometriosis is to keep track of their timing. Bowel symptoms from endometriosis are more likely to occur around the time of your periods and can include

- ✔ Diarrhea
- ✔ Constipation
- ✔ Nausea
- ✔ Rectal bleeding
- ✔ Bloating
- ✔ Stabbing rectal pain
- ✔ Increased gas
- ✔ Abdominal pain

See Chapter 6 for more on the way endometriosis affects your bowels.

Recognizing urinary symptoms

You may not think much about your urinary tract — until you have a problem with it. Endometriosis can be the cause of many bladder irritations, from blood in the urine to urgency. Ten to 20 percent of women with endometriosis have bladder issues.

Some symptoms of endometriosis in the bladder are

- ✔ Flank pain
- ✔ Pain with sex
- ✔ Urinary frequency
- ✔ Urinary urgency
- ✔ Burning or pain with urination
- ✔ Urinary retention
- ✔ Blood in the urine
- ✔ Fever

Check out Chapter 6 for more on how endometriosis can affect your urinary tract.

Coping with respiratory symptoms

When you think of endometriosis, you probably don't even consider breathing issues, right? However, for a small number of women with endometriosis, respiratory problems may be a big part of their symptoms each month.

Suspecting endometriosis when you're coughing up blood or having chest pains each month may seem a little ridiculous, but endometriosis can cause these symptoms if it lodges in your lungs. Endometriosis can occur in the lining of the lung (the *pleura*) or in the lung itself. Endometriosis in the pleura is about five times more common than in the lung, and the majority of occurrences are on the right side.

Pleural endometriosis causes the following:

- ✔ Shortness of breath
- ✔ Pain
- ✔ Collapsed lung (*pneumothorax*)
- ✔ Fluid on the lung (*pleural effusion*)

Endometriosis in the lung (*parenchymal* endometriosis) causes you to cough up blood. (Flip to Chapter 6 for more on how endometriosis can affect the lungs.)

Endometriosis is obviously not the first problem you should suspect if you have breathing difficulties. Many diseases can cause respiratory issues, including

- ✔ Asthma
- ✔ Respiratory infection, such as bronchitis or pneumonia
- ✔ Pleurisy or pneumothorax unrelated to endometriosis

Differentiating endometriosis of the respiratory system from other causes can be difficult and may require an MRI or surgery (see Chapter 9 for more on diagnosing endometriosis in the lungs). Interestingly, women with endometriosis also seem more likely to have asthma.

Minding endometriosis and the brain

Endometriosis of the brain, like endometriosis of the lungs, is uncommon. If you have symptoms such as headaches and seizures, other causes are far more likely than endometriosis. However, rare cases of endometriosis affecting the brain do exist.

Women with endometriosis are, according to some studies, more prone to migraine headaches than women without endometriosis. This connection may be due to *prostaglandins* (chemicals released from the uterus during your period) rather than endometrial lesions in the brain. (Check out Chapter 6 for more on how endometriosis can affect the brain.)

Writing It Down: How a Diary Can Help

Most patients are notoriously bad at describing their problems to medical personnel; "out of sight" and "out of mind" seem to describe many people's attitudes toward their symptoms. The average exchange between doctor or nurse and patient often goes like this:

> Doctor/Nurse: "When was your last menstrual period?"
>
> Patient: "Oh, I think it was two weeks ago Thursday, because I remember I was at the mall, and, no, wait, it wasn't Thursday. It was Tuesday, because I had that meeting — no, that was the month before, because I forgot to bring tampons with me, and. . . ."
>
> Doctor/Nurse: "When does the pain usually begin?"
>
> Patient: "Well, I guess it starts right before my period, well, not right before but maybe a few days before — sometimes a week before. . .and sometimes it lasts after my period stops, but not always, and then. . . ."

Do you see why doctors can get frustrated when trying to take a history? Patients don't remember important details about their experiences. Some patients are exceptions to this rule. For example, a patient may come in with a medical tome the size of New York's phone book that describes in detail every twinge she's had in the last month. There's such a thing as *too* much detail!

We hope you can come in with medical information that's neither too much nor too little, but just right. The right amount of information helps your doctor diagnose and treat you without getting bogged down in insignificant details.

How can you remember what's important? The best way is to keep a diary that can help you keep track of everything: your symptoms and your menstrual cycle, the pain and your feelings. Why a diary you ask? Because most people are too busy to remember every single pain they have each month. You can make your doctor a very happy woman and give her the accurate information she needs to treat you. You may not have kept a diary since grade school, but this section helps you get started so your next trip to the doctor's office isn't a guessing game.

Recording symptoms (and everything else important) from month to month

Keeping records in a diary is important to help your doctor make a diagnosis and develop a treatment plan for you. Diaries are practical for recording symptoms as well as all other important pieces of information because they provide dates and can cover a 12-month time period. The only way to see a trend in your symptoms (and feelings) is to record them for several months in a row. Pain can have many causes, and a pain that occurs once and never shows up again isn't likely to be endometriosis.

You don't have to be elaborate in your diary; a simple laundry list of symptoms is adequate. But you can really have fun buying a diary or journal — check out bookstores for some great ones. In fact, buying a diary to record your symptoms is probably the only fun aspect of having endometriosis, so get the most out of it!

After a few months, you may start to see trends that you haven't noticed before. Maybe you never recognized a cycle to the diarrhea that shows up three days before your period every month, or you never realized that you always have a headache right before your period starts. The cough that always shows up with your period may seem more significant when you realize that it's a monthly occurrence.

Now when you go to see your doctor, you can give him a concise list of your symptoms and their timing. Make sure you keep track of the items that are listed in the following sections.

Keeping track of your menstrual cycle

Now that you have a diary, you have no excuse for not knowing when your last period was, how long it lasted, how heavy it was, and what other symptoms occurred at the same time. Probably the last time you paid attention to menstrual flow so faithfully was in high school!

Knowing how long your period lasts, how heavy it is (yes, a tampon or pad count is acceptable and very helpful), and how many days are between the start of one cycle and the start of the next can be helpful for your doctor, especially if you're dealing with infertility issues.

Rating your pain

When you record pain, try to rate it. (*Awful* isn't a rating!) Rating pain on a scale from one to ten — with one being the least and ten the most pain possible — is effective, and doctors are familiar with that sort of pain scale. Children learn to rate pain by pointing to a face that best expresses how they're feeling; you may want to amuse your doctor by taking a pain chart like this. If you're artistic, you can even draw your own faces to express what you're feeling!

In addition to rating the pain, you need to describe it. You don't have to get too graphic — if your description sounds like it came out of a cheap novel, you've probably gotten too dramatic. Keep it simple by using the following words or similar terms: "The pain is. . ."

- ✔ Aching
- ✔ Building over time
- ✔ Burning
- ✔ Coming in waves
- ✔ Constant
- ✔ Dull
- ✔ Intense
- ✔ Intermittent
- ✔ Stabbing

Locating your pain

Knowing the location of your pain is just as important as knowing the kind of pain you're having. This description isn't as easy as it sounds. Pain is easy to locate when you feel it, but when it's gone, pain is hard to pinpoint. One way to mark the spot is with a magic marker (but marking it every day after your shower isn't really practical).

You don't have to be a great artist to make a sketch of your abdomen, back, or wherever you feel pain. Mark the painful spot on your drawing — or, better yet, just make a photocopy of a woman's body out of an anatomy book and mark the painful spots with an X.

Keeping track of the exact location of your pain will help over a few months. The pain that you *thought* was in the same spot every month may actually move from side to side!

Homing in on your feelings

In addition to recording your symptoms, pain, and how often they occur, you also need to record your feelings. Keeping track of your mood swings and your feelings may be more helpful to you than to your doctor, who doesn't live with you. You can devise a simple system to evaluate your daily moods, or you can go into great detail, especially if you're an aspiring novelist. Wording doesn't matter — the pattern does.

You can be as detailed as you care to be, although minute-by-minute mood descriptions will probably make for boring reading! A better way may be to capture your overall mood day-by-day. For example, were you unusually tired, out of sorts, achy, angry, or sleepy? Over time, you may see a pattern emerge so you can predict your mood changes ahead of time — and take measures to keep them under control.

Being aware of mood swings and feelings can help you plan big events in your life, such as weddings and vacations. No one wants to go to Hawaii at a time of the month when she knows she's going to feel somewhat depressed. On the other hand, perhaps Hawaii is just what you need to cheer yourself up!

Plotting your energy levels

Knowing your energy levels over time can also be helpful in planning your life. Although you may have some month-to-month variations, recording your energy levels can guide you on what activities you can reasonably expect to do and when you can do them. For example, a marathon in the middle of your *exhaustion* time probably won't work well.

Listing your pain treatments — both the good and the bad

Keep a record of what treatment decreases your pain. If you don't track your successes and failures, you may walk out of your doctor's office with a list of basic medications and exercises to try. This list is fine, unless you've been trying these methods without any decrease in pain for the last three months. Obviously, rehashing the same ineffective treatment isn't a good plan!

Many women are hesitant to speak up and tell a doctor that his suggestions haven't worked. Don't hesitate to simply say, "I tried that already and it doesn't work." Better yet, give him a list upfront of the treatments you've tried already so he won't suggest the same ones. When your doctor can see what you have (and haven't) done, he can provide different medications and exercises to help decrease the pain.

Chapter 3

Endometriosis: A Quick Review of Biology

The human body is amazing, and the female reproductive system is one of the most amazing parts of all. You may not have a good understanding of what exactly goes on in there — you may have spent sex education class hiding your head under your school desk and giggling with your friends.

This chapter fills in the gaps with knowledge about the female anatomy and physiology. In this chapter, we also explain what endometriosis consists of and how the condition affects different reproductive and surrounding organs.

Getting Back to Basics: Bio 101 of Female Anatomy

Whoever said "It's what's inside that counts" was right. How your body functions has very little to do with what you see on the outside — it's all about what goes on in the places you can't see. In the case of the female body, you may be familiar with many parts and their names, but maybe you're a little hazy on their exact locations and functions. So, to understand endometriosis, you first need to understand your reproductive system and the organs that surround it. Figure 3-1 is a picture that's worth a thousand words.

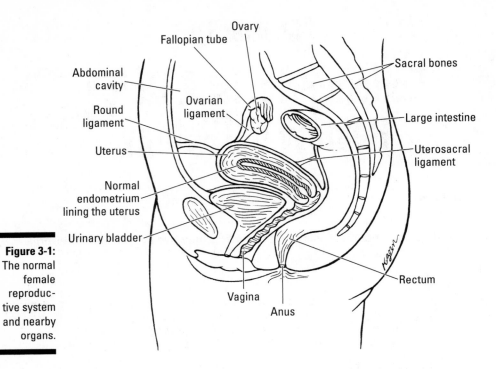

Ovary

Fallopian tube

Abdominal cavity

Round ligament

Ovarian ligament

Uterus

Normal endometrium lining the uterus

Urinary bladder

Sacral bones

Large intestine

Uterosacral ligament

Rectum

Vagina

Anus

Figure 3-1: The normal female reproductive system and nearby organs.

This section contains a part-by-part description of your reproductive system and nearby organs that endometriosis can affect.

The uterus: Your womb

The *uterus,* commonly called the *womb,* is where babies are nourished and grow for about nine months in a pregnant woman.

In women who have never been pregnant, the uterus is almost flat, but after a woman has been pregnant, her uterus becomes more pear-shaped. A uterus has three layers of tissue:

- ✔ The thin outer lining of the uterus is the *serosa,* (sometimes called the *visceral peritoneum*). This layer is part of the lining of the pelvic walls, abdominal cavity, and the intestines, forming a large area of covering tissue called the *peritoneum.*
- ✔ The middle part, or bulk, of the uterus is a muscle called the *myometrium.* This muscle causes the cramps (little contractions) women feel with their period or other bleeding, and it's responsible for the contractions of labor.

The inside of the uterus is hollow and is a *potential* space, which means that normally there's no space between the walls of the uterus; they actually touch each other.

✔ The innermost part of the uterus, the *endometrium,* grows along the inside walls of the uterus. But, when pieces of the endometrium go outside the uterus, you have endometriosis.

The endometrium consists of *glands* (tiny tubes that secrete fluid and proteins, similar to saliva glands) and two layers of *stroma* (supporting tissue). The stroma is very *vascular,* which means it has many blood vessels. The two layers of stroma are

- The *stratum basalis,* the thin inner layer that remains after each menstrual period and grows for the next cycle.

- The *stratum functionalis,* which grows from the basalis. This layer (containing glands, blood vessels, and surface epithelial cells) thickens and then is sloughed off (shed) during a menstrual period.

The inside walls of the uterus normally touch each other, except when something's inside the uterus — like a baby! Then the area inside the uterus expands as the baby does.

The uterine ligaments: The stabilizers

When discussing your uterus, we can't forget to mention the *ligaments,* or bands of cordlike tissue, which help keep the uterus in place, sort of like stabilizers. Refer to Figure 3-1 to see the relationship of the uterus to the other female reproductive parts and nearby organs. The *fundus,* or body of the uterus, sits somewhat upright (with a bend to the front or back) in the middle of the pelvic cavity, and the *cervix,* which is the opening of the uterus, protrudes into the top of the *vagina.*

Your uterus has three sets of ligaments that help keep the uterus from sliding around, including

✔ **Two round ligaments** at the top of the uterus on either side.

✔ **Two uterosacral ligaments** at the top of the cervix, where it meets the lower fundus (the bottom of the body of the uterus). These ligaments attach from the cervix to the *sacrum* (the bony end of the spine).

✔ **Two lateral (broad) ligaments** between the other two, stronger sets of ligaments. The broad ligaments are folded, flat pieces of tissue.

These three sets of ligaments consist of firm, fibrous tissue. Although the ligaments have a small amount of *give* so the uterus can move slightly, nerves running through these ligaments are often sensitive to too much stretch or movement. The cervical end of the ligaments has a collection of nerve endings called the *paracervical ganglion* (a *ganglion* is a group of neurons).

The ovaries: Your egg producers

The *ovaries,* which produce the eggs, are very near the *fallopian tubes* (see the next section and refer to Figure 3-1 for their location). This close proximity between the ovaries and fallopian tubes makes sense because eggs need to travel down the fallopian tubes to get to the uterus — where they can implant and grow into 7-pound bundles of joy.

The fallopian tubes: Your conveyor belts

The fallopian tubes are attached to the uterus — one on each side. These passages are like personal conveyor belts, transporting an egg from the ovary to the uterus. If sperm are present, the egg is fertilized at the end of the tube near the ovary. But, if there's any disruption along the path, a fertilized egg can't make its way to the uterus to implant.

Although fallopian tubes don't touch the ovaries directly, they have *fimbriae* (very fine, fingerlike projections on the end nearest the ovary) that coax the newly released egg into the fallopian tube. Their function is essential in this conveyor-belt process of getting pregnant because, if a fertilized egg floats away and doesn't get into the tube, it can result in an *ectopic pregnancy,* a pregnancy that implants a fertilized egg outside the uterus, usually in the fallopian tubes. (Check out Chapter 7 where we discuss this situation in depth.)

The vagina and cervix: The openings

The *vagina* is the muscular opening that leads from the external female genitals to the *cervix,* which is the mouth, or neck, of the uterus. Functioning as a passage between the *endometrial cavity* (the layer lining the inside of the uterus) and the vagina, the cervix is usually open just enough to let menstrual flow out and sperm in. During pregnancy, the cervix closes to keep your baby from falling out.

Other important parts

The female body has other important parts that can play a role in endometriosis. *Note:* Although males have some of the parts listed in this section, endometriosis generally only affects females (see Chapter 1 for the very rare exception of a male with endometriosis). The following body parts can be involved:

- ✔ **The pelvic cavity** is the space between the pelvic bones (which wrap around from the pubic bone in front to the *sacrum,* or tailbone, in back). The cavity holds the reproductive organs, bladder, and rectum. In addition, large amounts of small and large intestines move in and out of the pelvic cavity during digestion.

  As we mention earlier in this section, the lining of this cavity is called the *peritoneum,* which is a thin layer of cells that prevents all these organs from sticking to each other.

- ✔ **Other important areas in your pelvic cavity:**

  - **The posterior cul-de-sac** sounds like a nice place to live (no traffic!), but it's a dead end, literally, behind the uterus. The cervix, top of the vagina, rectum, and uterosacral ligaments (see the earlier section "The uterine ligaments: The stabilizers") all come together at the bottom of the posterior cul-de-sac.

  - **The anterior cul-de-sac** is between the pubic bone and the uterus. Also, the bladder is at the bottom of the anterior cul-de-sac.

- ✔ **The bladder** is the storage unit for urine. Urine comes down from the kidneys via the *ureters* (tubes) and collects in your bladder until you have a convenient and socially acceptable time to empty it.

- ✔ **The rectum** makes up the last few inches of the large intestine. Lying behind the uterus and in front of the sacrum, the rectum connects the large intestine to the *anus* (the final destination of the digestive tract and the body's exit point).

- ✔ **The large and small intestines** *(bowels)* aren't restricted to females; males obviously have them, too. But, because of their proximity to the pelvis, the intestines are common sites for endometriosis. (The names *small* and *large* may seem somewhat backwards because the uncoiled small intestine is about 20 feet long, or three to four times longer than the large intestine, which is only 5 feet long.)

  Both the small and large intestines can move in and out of both cul-de-sacs and float around in the pelvic cavity.

Finding endometriosis in unexpected places

I have seen some strange cases where pelvic endometriosis causes seemingly unrelated symptoms. A patient had right-side pain at the level of her *umbilicus* (belly button) and multiple intestinal symptoms, such as nausea, constipation, and pain after eating. She had a previous diagnosis of irritable bowel syndrome (IBS) or some other inflammatory bowel disease, but when she didn't receive any relief from other treatments, she turned to me. After much discussion, she decided on laparoscopy to try and determine the cause for her problems. Very unexpectedly, I found severe endometriosis; her intestines were stuck to her uterus and right ovary, and her appendix was literally stuck to the top of her uterus! After I cut down the adhesions and removed the appendix, her intestinal symptoms resolved.

The small intestine fills the area from the bottom of your ribs to the top of the uterus and connects the stomach to the large intestine. Meanwhile, the large intestine makes a lot of turns before reaching the anus. Starting just below the right side of the *umbilicus* (belly button), the intestine winds up toward the rib cage, makes a left turn to cross under the ribs, and takes another left to continue along the left side of the abdominal cavity and downward toward the pelvis.

✔ The **appendix** is a small, fingerlike projection near the junction of the large and small intestines.

Measuring How Endometriosis Affects Your Reproductive and Other Organs

Endometriosis lesions can act and look differently in different areas, but all are detrimental. In addition, the amount of endometriosis isn't always an indicator of the damage or pain it causes; a little endometriosis in one location can be much more damaging and painful than a lot of endometriosis somewhere else. In fact, doctors have known for a long time that the amount of visible endometriosis has very little bearing on the symptoms. In this section, we discuss the ways endometriosis can damage different organs. (See Chapter 7 to find out how these changes can affect your fertility.)

Endometriosis and your fallopian tubes

Endometriosis can implant on the outside surface of the fallopian tubes and cause scarring. Just like burn scars can lead to *contractures* that distort limbs and other body parts, the endometriosis scarring can distort the fallopian tubes so they can't function properly.

How endometriosis blocks your tubes

Endometriosis inside the fallopian tube can partially or totally block that tube. This blockage may cause infertility or ectopic pregnancy. Unfortunately, even good imaging techniques, such as X-rays or ultrasounds, can't see inside the tubes. Likewise, during surgery, doctors have a difficult time seeing directly in the narrow tubes because the instruments used to view the pelvic cavity are too big to enter the tubes.

Endometrial implants can also disrupt the function of the *fimbriae* (which means *fringe* in Latin), the ends of the tubes that pick up the egg. Endometriosis can cause these fine, delicate fimbriae to stick to each other or other structures. In the worst-case scenario, these tiny fingers are destroyed and lose all function. In that case, the chance for pregnancy in general is greatly reduced, but the risk of an ectopic pregnancy is high.

Even if the fimbriae aren't destroyed, any decrease in their functionality can lead to problems. For example, endometriosis may cause them to stick to the ovary, tube, uterus, intestines, or pelvic wall, so they can't move around to pick up an egg. Inflamed fimbriae can also be painful and can cause additional pain by adhering to another structure. This pain may be the result of the stuck tube *pulling* as a woman goes about normal activity. (Remember, tubes are usually free and can move around a bit.)

What blocks your tubes

Endometrial implants can totally block the fallopian tube by forming scar tissue that destroys the fimbriae and sticks these tiny fingers together. As these delicate fingers become distorted and stuck, the end of the tube can close off, literally, keeping sperm and egg separated.

The following three substances can damage a fallopian tube:

- **Blood:** A blocked tube filled with blood (from endometriosis in the tube or some other reason) is called a *hematosalpinx* (*hemato* means *blood* and *salpinx* means *tubes*). Visually, a hematosalpinx can look similar to an ectopic pregnancy.

- **Inflammatory fluid:** Endometriosis that totally blocks the tube near the fimbriae can lead to a swollen, chronically inflamed fallopian tube called a *hydrosalpinx*. (*Hydro* means *fluid.*)

Imagine a water balloon with fluid coming in and filling the balloon (tube). Because the end is closed, the balloon swells up. The inflammatory fluid in a blocked fallopian tube contains many chemicals, cells, and tissue that cause inflammation, which can lead to pain, fever, infertility, and even miscarriage.

✔ **Pus:** Infection is another common cause of tubal blockage, although it's not a result of endometriosis. When an infection results in tubal blockage and it fills with pus, it's called a *pyosalpinx*.

All three of the *salpinxes* (substances) can cause pain because a tube is swollen and stretched — and all of these conditions are obvious causes of infertility. (Just like having your tubes tied, the sperm and egg can't meet.) Check out Figure 3-2 for examples of how endometriosis can affect the fallopian tubes.

Endometriosis and your ovaries

Endometriosis is common on the surface of the ovaries, but it can also invade the *meat*, or interior, of the ovary. This section looks at the three ways endometriosis can affect the ovaries.

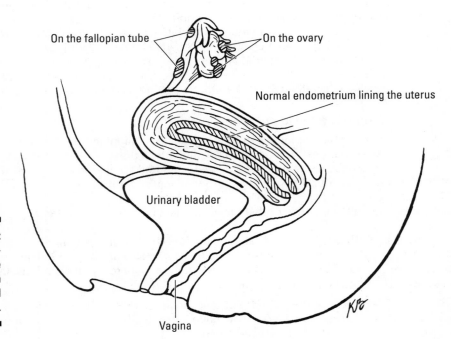

On the fallopian tube

On the ovary

Normal endometrium lining the uterus

Urinary bladder

Figure 3-2: Endometriosis on the fallopian tubes and ovaries.

Vagina

On the ovary's surface

The fact that the surface of the ovary is a very common site for endometriosis makes sense, because *retrograde menstrual flow* coming out of the tube spills right onto the ovaries. (Check out Chapter 4 for more on retrograde menstruation.) This endometrial tissue can implant onto the surface of the ovary and do all sorts of damage.

Endometriosis can also start directly from the surface cells of the ovary by a process called *metaplasia*. The resulting implants can be on any part of the ovary and cause the same problems that retrograde spills produce. (Check out Chapter 4 for more on metaplasia.)

When endometriosis develops on the surface of the ovary by retrograde menstruation or metaplasia, the inflammatory process begins and leads to *adhesions* (scar tissue). As a result, the ovary can become stuck to the tube, uterus, intestines, or pelvic wall. These adhesions (check out Figure 3-3) can cause pain and problems with the intestines and they can cause infertility.

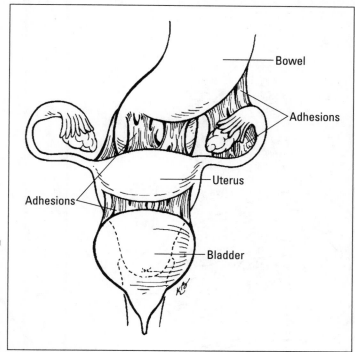

Figure 3-3:
Adhesions in the female reproductive system.

Bowel

Adhesions

Adhesions

Uterus

Bladder

In the most severe cases, all contents of the pelvis — such as the uterus, fallopian tubes, and intestines — can be stuck together in a *frozen pelvis*. In addition to causing pain and problems with the intestines, these adhesions can cause infertility.

Forming painful cysts

Another severe problem is *endometrioma* (cysts) inside the ovary. These cysts (see Figure 3-4) are a result of inflamed endometrial tissue implants on the ovary surface that develop scar tissue (to wall off the implants like a pimple). But this dense, firm scarring causes the endometriosis implants (lesions) to take the path of least resistance — into the *stroma* (the relatively softer ovarian tissue).

Over time these cysts fill with endometrial tissue and old blood. A more appetizing name for these cysts is *chocolate cyst* because their dark brown fluid looks like liquid chocolate. If the cysts burst, the contents spill out into the pelvic cavity and can cause severe pain. In this case, because the fluid is highly inflammatory, scar tissue can also form in the pelvic cavity. Other structures or organs in contact with the fluid can also stick to it. The results can be dramatic and severe.

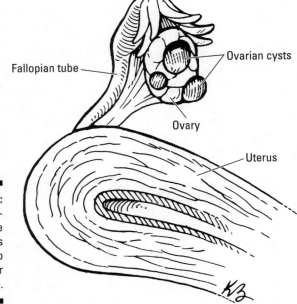

Fallopian tube

Ovarian cysts

Ovary

Uterus

Figure 3-4:
Endometri-
osis in the
ovaries
leads to
cysts over
time.

These cysts continue to grow each month because their endometrial tissue, which responds to menstrual cycle hormones, deposits more and more tissue implants and blood into the cysts each month. As these cysts enlarge, they put pressure, literally, on normal ovary tissue, distorting it and often making the tissue unrecognizable. Worse yet, the ever-increasing pressure actually destroys the normal tissue of the ovary. This loss of functioning ovarian tissue significantly decreases the number and function of *primordial follicles,* or future eggs (we cover the menstrual cycle in detail in Chapter 5), causing infertility and early menopause.

Resulting in LUF

Endometriosis may also result in *luteinized unruptured follicle syndrome* (LUF). With LUF, an egg has developed inside the *follicle* (the fluid-filled sac that the egg develops in) to supposed maturity and is ready to be released into the world (so to speak!). But for some reason, the egg never leaves the ovary. Obviously, an egg that stays in its follicle can't be fertilized, so LUF leads to infertility. But what causes this failure of the egg to leave its home? Doctors don't really know. Again, the body is wonderfully complex, and the series of events leading to follicle rupture are many. Any one of the following processes may cause LUF:

- ✔ Scar tissue from endometriosis surrounding the ovary can physically prevent release of the egg.

- ✔ The presence of endometriosis can interfere with the surface of the ovary in the usual cascade of events that leads to ovulation.

- ✔ Some women are prone to endometriosis; LUF may be a marker of the defect that causes endometriosis.

Doctors really aren't sure what causes LUF. It's the chicken-and-egg story. That is, do some women have a problem that causes LUF *and* endometriosis, or does the endometriosis cause the LUF? (See Chapter 7 for more on LUF and how the menstrual cycle works.)

Endometriosis and your pelvic cavity

Endometriosis that implants on the peritoneum in the pelvic cavity (see Figure 3-5) can cause severe inflammation that leads to adhesions or scar tissue. These adhesions can then cause all these organs and tissues — the uterus, ovaries, tubes, intestines, and bladder — to stick to each other so they don't move in the usual manner. This restriction of movement and the inflammation due to endometriosis cause the pain or discomfort. In addition, these same adhesions can make the intestines, bladder, and reproductive organs malfunction.

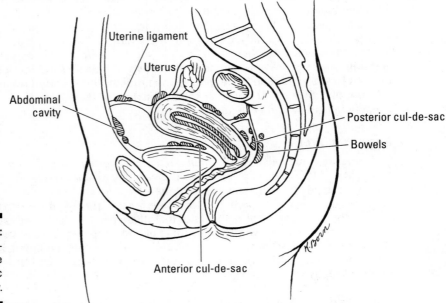

Figure 3-5:
Endometri-
osis in the
pelvic
cavity.

Labels in figure: Uterine ligament · Uterus · Abdominal cavity · Posterior cul-de-sac · Bowels · Anterior cul-de-sac

Looking closer at the pain

Endometrial implants in the pelvic cavity can result in scar tissue, which binds organs and tissue together. When the tissues and organs stick together, movement (such as occurs during sexual intercourse) results in pain. The eventual result may be a *frozen pelvis,* which is as bad as it sounds.

The local inflammation produces irritating chemicals, which also cause pain. Likewise, stretching of the lining and irritation of the nerves are painful.

Endometriosis in the pelvic cavity can cause pain in several ways:

- Nerve endings on the surface of the peritoneum can be stimulated by endometrial tissue to cause discomfort. As the endometrial implants grow into deeper tissue, they may affect larger, more significant nerve fibers that course through the pelvic cavity toward the vulva, buttock, and legs.

- Endometriosis may simply irritate these nerves or actually entrap them, causing even more bizarre symptoms, such as back and leg pain, loss of feeling in the legs, vulvar discomfort, and other lower extremity symptoms. (Check out Chapter 2 for more information on the symptoms of endometriosis.)

✔ Pelvic wall endometrial lesions can rupture. The fluid released contains many irritants that lead to pelvic pain.

✔ Fluid entering the pelvis from a ruptured endometrioma can lead to pain. This fluid is very caustic to the surrounding structures.

✔ Endometrial tissue at menstruation can cause pain. Because endometriosis has the same tissue, it causes chemical changes and affects the peritoneum to cause pain.

✔ Enlargement of endometrial implants on organs and the peritoneum can cause swelling, stretching, and pressure.

✔ Scar tissue causes pain when structures stick together in unnatural ways. (Chapter 13 shows you how you can manage the physical pain associated with endometriosis in the pelvic cavity — and everywhere else!)

Endometriosis and your uterine ligaments

Because endometriosis tends to fall into the bottom of the pelvic cavity, the uterine ligaments are a common spot for endometriosis to implant (check out "The uterine ligaments: The stabilizers" earlier in this chapter for more about these ligaments). When endometriosis implants on the ligaments (refer to Figure 3-5), it grows into the peritoneal covering and then into the ligament fibers. This invasion causes the same inflammatory response doctors see in other organs and tissues, such as in arthritis or strained muscles and ligaments.

Usually the endometriosis becomes firm and feels like nodules. In fact, the uterus can feel *fixed* (without its usual mobility) on exam because the ligaments have lost their small amount of elasticity. The nodules can also cause pain when touched because they're inflamed. So the firm feeling of the nodules, along with pain and the decrease in uterine movement, may suggest endometriosis to your doctor.

Endometriosis causes a variety of reactions in the tissues. One response is inflammation, which may scar and eventually shorten the ligament. This inflammation also irritates ligament nerves, so even normal movement of the uterus during sex or routine activity is painful. In contrast, healthy uterosacral ligaments normally stretch a little and keep the uterus in position without pain during these activities.

Endometriosis and the cul-de-sacs

This section heading may sound more like a catchy name for a 1960s singing group than a discussion about endometriosis! Of the two cul-de-sacs in the pelvis, endometriosis is more common in the posterior than in the anterior, but both locations have their share of problems. Check out Figure 3-5 for a clear picture of how endometriosis affects your posterior and anterior cul-de-sacs.

A prime location: The posterior cul-de-sac

The posterior cul-de-sac, often referred to as the *dead end* of the pelvis, is at the very bottom of the pelvis. Due to gravity (assuming a woman is walking upright), all the fluids and tissue from retrograde menstruation and anything else (such as blood and infection from other organs) probably end up here. And that makes the posterior cul-de-sac a prime location for endometrial implants. Because the ovaries hang down into the cul-de-sac, everything in the posterior cul-de-sac (including the end of the fallopian tubes, the back of the uterus, and the intestines) can also have contact with the disease.

The posterior cul-de-sac is also a common site for *deep endometriosis,* where the endometrial implants have grown through the peritoneum (covering) of the structures (the ligaments, intestines, ovaries, tubes, and uterus) and started to grow in the underlying, deeper tissues. The endometriosis can grow into the ligaments and become inflammatory nodules (see Chapter 1) that then irritate the intestines or the back of the uterus, causing all of them to stick together. Endometriosis can also become nodules that stretch the tissue or put pressure on nearby structures. The implants can even grow into the vagina (remember, the top of the vagina is at the bottom of the cul-de-sac).

In the most severe case, this inflammation actually completely closes off the cul-de-sac. That is, the whole space behind the uterus becomes one large (and very painful) mess, with the intestines, ligaments, uterus, ovaries, and tubes all stuck together in a frozen pelvis.

A less popular location: The anterior cul-de-sac

Endometriosis occurs less often in the anterior cul-de-sac than in the posterior cul-de-sac (see the previous section). This fact makes sense because the ends of the fallopian tubes are in the posterior cul-de-sac, so the regurgitated endometrial tissue goes into the posterior cul-de-sac area most of the time. (See "Endometriosis and your fallopian tubes" for more info on endometrial tissue and fallopian tubes.) Only in abnormal cases are tubes in front of the uterus in the anterior cul-de-sac.

But endometriosis in the anterior cul-de-sac isn't rare, and although this area has fewer organs, they can still stick together, just like structures in the posterior cul-de-sac. The bladder is in the anterior cul-de-sac and is the most common site for endometriosis in the anterior cul-de-sac. The bladder can stick to the front of the uterus. If the adhesions are bad, the uterus may even stick to the anterior abdominal wall (the front surface of the peritoneal cavity) compressing the bladder between these structures.

In very severe cases, the tubes, ovaries, and even the small intestine stick to the front surface of the uterus, bladder, or abdominal wall. This result isn't common, but it can cause severe pain and bowel and bladder dysfunction. Although much rarer than the posterior cul-de-sac's frozen pelvis, the anterior cul-de-sac may also be obliterated so that no space, only a mass of tissue, remains.

Endometriosis and your bladder

The bladder is the most common anterior cul-de-sac site for endometriosis, and the condition can be painful. Because it's constantly filling and emptying, the bladder is stretching several times a day, which can cause pain in itself. But the bladder is also a muscle, and inflamed muscles hurt when used — just ask someone with a muscle strain!

In addition, because the bladder muscle isn't very thick, the endometriosis can work its way through the muscle and cause bleeding in the urine. In some cases the bladder sticks to the front of the uterus or to the intestines.

Endometriosis in your bladder can cause

- Painful urination
- Bladder spasms
- Urinary urgency (when you "gotta go right now!")
- Blood in the urine

We discuss endometriosis and your bladder more in Chapter 6.

Endometriosis and your intestines

Endometriosis is quite common in the intestines and in the appendix. In fact, the intestines are the most common site for endometriosis outside of the reproductive organs (which isn't surprising because they're in the neighborhood). Endometriosis can appear in your intestines in several ways, including scar tissue and invading the walls. Resulting symptoms may be

- Painful sex
- Right- or left-sided pain
- Generalized pelvic or abdominal pain
- Bloating and cramping after eating
- Blockages in the small intestine
- Bleeding with bowel movement
- Change in stool color or consistency

We talk about endometriosis and your intestines in detail in Chapter 6.

Endometriosis and your cervix and vagina

Endometriosis of the cervix is quite rare. Why would endometriosis even develop there, because menstrual flow normally passes through these places? That question is the great mystery of endometriosis, but possible causes are an altered immune response, metaplasia, or genetic defects of the endometrium (see Chapter 4 for more info on the possible causes).

Two symptoms of endometriosis of the cervix are

- ✔ Pain during sex
- ✔ Irregular bleeding, especially after sex

The cervix is often contacted during sex, and endometriosis can make the cervix tender to touch. As a result, women with endometriosis of the cervix often have pain with deep penetration and then bleeding after, or even during, sexual intercourse. These endometriosis lesions on the cervix can also cause irregular spotting or heavy bleeding at any time during the cycle.

Even more unusual is endometriosis of the vagina, which occurs mostly in the top third of the vagina. This occurrence may be due to the fact that section of the vagina develops from the same embryologic tissues as the cervix and uterus. The symptoms are the same as those of the cervix: pain with sex and irregular bleeding.

Chapter 4

Determining What Causes Endometriosis

*E*ndometriosis isn't an unknown disease, but it's still a mysterious one. The tissue that behaves normally in the *endometrium* (the layer of tissue that lines the uterus) causes all kinds of pain and dysfunction when it hits the road and travels through the reproductive tract and beyond. One of the toughest questions is: What sets the events into motion that move endometrium from the endometrial cavity into other parts of the body to become endometriosis?

Researchers have been studying endometriosis, trying to answer this question. This chapter looks at all the most common current theories as well as some other theories that attempt to explain the development of endometriosis.

Speculating on How Endometriosis Develops: The Most Common Theories

Several prevalent theories exist as to why endometriosis develops in some women and not in others. Some days you may not really care how it got there; you just want it to go away! But understanding how a disease works is the first step to overcoming the problems it can bring. In this section, we review the most common theories.

Migrating out the tubes: Retrograde menstruation

Every woman with a uterus has *endometrial cells* (cells that line the inside of the uterus and support a pregnancy). Studies have shown that most, if not all, women also have retrograde menstruation.

What exactly is *retrograde menstruation?* Most of the shed endometrial lining during your period follows the route of gravity; it flows through the cervix, into the vagina, and then out into the world for you to deal with (check out Figure 4-1). The cramps you feel with your period are tiny contractions of the uterine muscle as it tries to push the blood out. However, some menstrual flow can take a wrong turn, so it ends up in the fallopian tubes and spills onto the ovaries and into the *peritoneum* (the membrane lining of the abdominal cavity). This process is called *retrograde menstruation.*

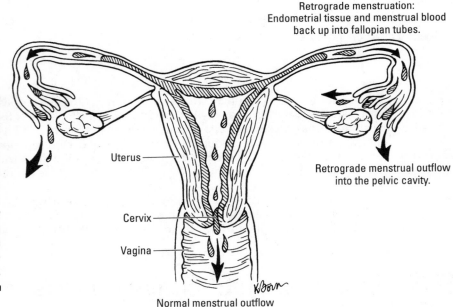

Retrograde menstruation:
Endometrial tissue and menstrual blood
back up into fallopian tubes.

Retrograde menstrual outflow
into the pelvic cavity.

Uterus

Cervix

Vagina

Normal menstrual outflow

Figure 4-1: Endometrial tissue and menstrual blood outflow into the pelvic cavity during retrograde menstruation.

Retrograde menstruation is one of the oldest theories describing the possible development of endometriosis. In the 1920s, Dr. John Sampson first identified retrograde menstruation as a possible explanation for endometriosis. But this theory can't be the only explanation of how endometriosis develops, because of these problems:

✔ This theory doesn't explain how endometriosis ends up in places far from the pelvic cavity.

✔ This theory doesn't explain why all women don't have endometriosis, because more than 90 percent have retrograde menstruation.

The following two sections look more closely at how a woman's body, combined with retrograde menstruation, can lead to endometriosis.

Pelvic abnormalities and endometriosis

Women with pelvic abnormalities (such as in Figure 4-2) are more prone to endometriosis, mostly due to mechanical factors. This fact supports the retrograde menstruation theory because these abnormalities lead to more backflow out the tubes.

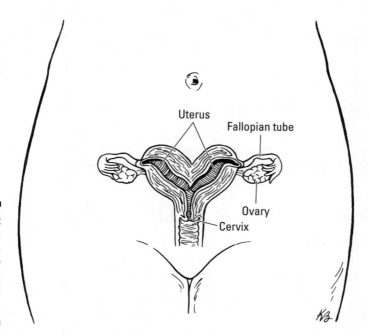

Uterus

Fallopian tube

Ovary

Cervix

Figure 4-2:
Pelvic abnormalities may lead to more menstrual backflow.

The following are some of the more common abnormalities that may cause endometriosis:

✔ **Cervical stenosis:** The cervix is more tightly closed than normal. This condition can cause a greater degree of retrograde menstruation. Because blood and debris can't escape through the cervix as quickly and easily as normal, it backs up so more of it flows backwards. Studies show that around 80 percent of women with cervical stenosis develop endometriosis.

> ✔ **Longer menstrual periods with heavier than normal flow:** These periods can increase the chance of endometriosis in the same way as cervical stenosis. Because more than 99 percent of all menstrual flow should flow out of the vagina, only 1 percent normally goes backward, or in retrograde direction. But, if your periods are closer together, heavier, or longer lasting, you have more flow than normal. As a result, your 1 percent retrograde flow is also more than normal.
>
> ✔ **Uterine anomalies:** These anomalies can be malformations of the shape of the uterus and can also contribute to endometriosis. Approximately 2 to 4 percent of all women have some sort of uterine anomaly. Uterine anomalies that are *congenital* (present from birth) often arise from problems with the Mullerian ducts. (Check out the next section.)

Malformed Mullerian ducts

The top third of the vagina, cervix, uterus, and fallopian tubes develops from two tubular structures in the fetus called the Mullerian ducts. Abnormalities of this system can cause a higher risk of endometriosis. Mullerian ducts normally begin on the sides of the pelvic area and fuse in the middle, beginning at the cervix. At the top of the new uterus, these ducts separate and form the fallopian tubes that go out to the sides of the pelvis.

The most common Mullerian abnormality is a failed fusion somewhere along the way. The most likely location for the problem is the top of the uterus, where a partial separation of the body of the uterus can occur. In very rare cases, a woman can have two of everything, including a cervix, a uterus, and a tube on each side.

Blaming Mom: Is endometriosis hereditary?

Research shows that endometriosis has a family link because it tends to cluster in families. If you have a first-degree relative (a mother or sister with endometriosis), your risk of having endometriosis is seven to ten times higher than your friend who has no endometriosis in her family. Not only are you more likely to have endometriosis if it runs in your family, but your disease is also likely to be more severe than endometriosis found in women without a family history of the disease. Aren't genetics grand?

This section looks more closely at the possible connections between genetics and endometriosis. This section also helps you check out your own family tree to see whether endometriosis is prevalent.

Understanding genetics

So why does endometriosis run in families? Today's researchers seek answers to this question. Great leaps in the study of *molecular genetics* (looking at chromosomes and individual genes) have given researchers new insight into the inheritance of the disease. As with many other diseases, such as cystic fibrosis and diabetes, many subtle changes in the building blocks of the chromosomes can have profound effects.

Researchers have observed and identified the following conditions in endometriosis patients that strengthen the hereditary theory:

- ✔ **Gene mutations:** Some of these mutations affect the survival of *detached cells* (cells that aren't part of the basic structure of the endometrium and that should die when removed, but don't).

  Scientists are finding significant evidence that the endometrial cells in endometriosis have abnormal *expression* (how they work and perform) of gene products that are responsible for survival, invasion, blood vessel growth, and the like.

  Endometrial cells from endometriosis implants show resistance to the normal, programmed cell death *(apoptosis)* that's found in these cells in the uterus. This resistance, which may be genetic, can improve their survival and allow them to implant.

- ✔ **Abnormal cell adhesion molecules:** These abnormalities may allow cells to grow on surfaces that don't normally accept them. Other enzymes help these cells invade and get a foothold where they don't belong. Progesterone usually suppresses these enzymes, but, for some reason, women with endometriosis don't have this suppressive process. An inherited mutation may be the cause for this change.

  Although estrogen is essential for endometrial growth, one enzyme, *aromatase,* converts other steroid hormones into estrogen. Normal endometrial tissue has no detectable aromatase, but endometriosis implants contain this enzyme and show high levels of activity. A genetic abnormality may allow this enzyme and its high activity to exist, leading to high local levels of estrogen that may help the cells grow, invade, and cause the disease.

  Another enzyme, 17BHSD type 2, is found in normal endometrial tissue and is activated by progesterone. This enzyme lowers *estradiol* (the main estrogen produced by the ovary) levels. Because this enzyme isn't in endometriosis glands, higher levels of estradiol and subsequent development of endometriosis can go unchecked.

These findings and additional research point to a genetic or inherited aspect of the disease. Although science can't cure bad genes, knowing the root cause may lead to better treatments.

Carrying migrant endometrial cells from birth

One twist on the hereditary theory of endometriosis states that some women have a hereditary tendency to produce cells predisposed to becoming endometrial cells. This predisposition makes sense because a fetus begins with one cell with the potential to become any and all cells in a human. These *stem cells* (multipotential cells) can become any part of the body, so the cells of the pelvic cavity (and other places) could possibly transform into endometrial cells and develop glands and stroma.

But does this only happen with endometrial cells? Does that mean an eyeball could grow in the pelvis? These questions are difficult to answer, and the answers may reside in the way the human body differentiates as it grows from one cell to embryo to fetus to full-term baby. There are other disease states where certain tissues develop in an unusual place (for example, *dermoid* cysts may have skin, teeth, thyroid tissue, and hair).

These differentiating factors may mistakenly signal cells in the pelvis to become endometrium. After all, this area is close to the uterus and normal endometrium. Unfortunately this signal to an adjacent area doesn't explain the distant forms of endometriosis in the lungs, brain, and even umbilicus — that's a bit far out.

Other possible genetic misfires include

- ✔ Faulty cells that react to the local stimulus in the wrong way
- ✔ Incorrect signals that cause predisposed cells to become endometrium rather than brain

The bottom line: Abnormalities exist and genetic predispositions to these abnormalities are certainly possible.

Checking your family tree

Trying to figure out if your family has a history of endometriosis can be hard, particularly if female family members have already gone through menopause. They may not remember all their menstrual symptoms — they're too busy thinking about their current health issues to remember what happened 30 years ago. And many women grew up believing that menstrual pain was just part of life, so they didn't dwell on it.

Of course, anything to do with menstruation, pregnancy, or reproduction wasn't polite dinner conversation, so your questions may turn your mother into a stone face who has no intentions of talking about such topics — especially not with you!

Some inherited traits can definitely signal a tendency to develop endometriosis, though, including your inherited body type. For example, you're more likely to have endometriosis if

- ✔ **You're tall and thin.** Tall, thin women frequently have shorter menstrual cycles, meaning that they bleed more frequently. They're also more likely to have cervical stenosis, another increased risk for endometriosis.

- ✔ **You have red hair.** Several studies have shown an association between red hair and endometriosis, although a recent Harvard study showed that only fertile women with red hair were more likely to have endometriosis; infertile redheads weren't.

- ✔ **You have certain types of *nevi*, or moles.** Several studies have shown an association between *dysplastic* (abnormal or unusual) nevi and endometriosis.

- ✔ **You're an identical twin, and your twin has endometriosis.** An identical twin is more likely than a fraternal twin to have endometriosis if her twin has it.

Exploring Other (Not-So-Common) Theories

A number of theories related to who gets endometriosis and why have popped up over the years; some are widely believed by laypersons even though scientific studies have proven them to be incorrect. In the next section, we sort out the fact from the fiction.

Using tampons

Many women use tampons during their periods for their convenience, but some women fear that convenience comes at a price — a higher risk of developing endometriosis. Does research support the theory that using tampons increases your chance of developing endometriosis? We take a look at the controversy of tampon use in endometriosis in the next sections.

Do tampons cause or protect against endometriosis?

For many years, some experts have been convinced that using tampons during your menstrual flow can increase your chance of developing endometriosis. Some of the factors contributing to this belief were

✔ The possibility that tampons increased retrograde menstruation

✔ The possibility that tampons still contain small amounts of dioxin, a chemical toxin in tampons until the late 1980s (see the nearby sidebar, "Understanding dioxin exposure")

Most tampons consist of *rayon,* a highly absorbent material. Because the rayon is bleached with chlorine for a white appearance, some people believe the process leaves small amounts of dioxin in tampons. Tampon makers have denied any significant amount of dioxin present in tampons, certainly not enough to cause any harmful effects.

However, a recent study of more than 2,000 women concluded that women who use tampons may actually have lower rates of endometriosis than women who use only pads during their periods. ***Note:*** This study may not have considered the many women with endometriosis who don't use tampons because the insertion is too painful. In any event, this study showed no evidence that tampon use increases your risk of endometriosis.

The most publicized study that showed a link between endometriosis and dioxin involved 24 rhesus monkeys in the 1970s. Although the focus of the study was the effect of dioxin on the monkeys' fertility, additional results showed

✔ Endometriosis does develop spontaneously in rhesus monkeys.

✔ One-third of the control group (who didn't receive dioxin) developed the disease.

✔ The two groups who received dioxin had a 71 percent and 86 percent rate of endometriosis.

✔ The higher-dosage group had the higher percentage of the disease.

The tampon battle wages on

Because of the controversy over this topic, *The Tampon Safety and Research Act of 1997* was introduced to the United States Congress. This bill asks for research on the risks of dioxin, synthetic fibers, and other additives in tampons and similar products. Unfortunately, as of this writing, this bill is still sitting in Congress.

Dioxin-free tampons with natural, unbleached, chlorine-free cotton are available. Some brands include Natracare and Terra Femme. A silk reusable tampon is also available. You can purchase these products from the following sources, among others:

www.mothernature.com

www.naturalfempro.com

Understanding dioxin exposure

Dioxins are chemical-compound byproducts from burning fuels (such as wood, coal, and oil) or from waste incineration. Dioxins can form from the bleaching of pulp and paper during paper manufacturing and from other types of chemical manufacturing. Small amounts of dioxins are in cigarette smoke, and they occur naturally in forest fires.

Environmental Protection Agency (EPA) standards have become much more rigid in the past few decades and dioxin levels have been decreasing. Industrial levels of dioxins are 90 percent lower than 20 years ago. But because dioxins break down very slowly, today's dioxin exposure can come from compounds released many years ago. For example, dioxins produced years ago can still be polluting the soil today. Today, considerable controversy continues over whether or not tampon use exposes women to dioxin.

Dioxins deposited on plants become part of the food chain, and animal fat has a high concentration of dioxins. In fact, although you can absorb small amounts of dioxin from the air, soil, and water, most dioxin exposure (more than 95 percent) comes from eating animal fats. You can reduce your dioxin exposure by eating lean meat and reducing your intake of saturated fats.

Testing for dioxin levels isn't routinely available, because the tests are very expensive and results are difficult to interpret.

Having a tubal ligation

Studies show that some women may develop endometriosis after having a *tubal ligation* (having your tubes tied to prevent pregnancy). But, you ask, if the retrograde menstruation theory is correct (refer to the section, "Migrating out the tubes: Retrograde menstruation," earlier in this chapter), how can blood back up through the top of blocked tubes?

One possibility is that some small, unseen islands of endometrial tissue were present before the surgery. These microscopic implants can then eventually grow, cause symptoms, and become endometriosis.

No matter what process causes the problem after tubal ligation, studies don't show that the surgery is actually responsible for the disease. In fact, studies haven't ever shown a relationship between a tubal ligation and *increased risk* of endometriosis.

Women who opt for this procedure have most likely had children. In reality, these women may very well have had endometriosis all their lives, but the pregnancy(s) kept it at bay (see the section "Does pregnancy help prevent endometriosis?" later in this chapter) masking the signs and symptoms. These symptoms appear then, only after long, pregnancy-free periods of time.

Scientists can find no logical reason for tubal ligation, a minor procedure, to cause endometriosis. **Note:** Historically, people have blamed this surgery for many other problems (irregular and heavy periods, pelvic congestion syndrome, and so on). But none of these connections has ever panned out either. Most women who undergo this surgery are in their late 30s to early 40s, an age group where these problems naturally increase.

If surgeries *could* increase the risk of endometriosis, then many other gynecologic procedures (hysteroscopy, hysterosalpingogram [HSG], saline infusion sonohysterogram [SIS], and the like — check out Chapter 9 for more info on these procedures) would have a more profound effect than tubal ligations because these other procedures can actually force cells out the tube and into the pelvis. But these procedures don't cause endometriosis either.

Answering some of the unanswered questions: The metaplasia theory

Most theories on endometriosis can't answer some nagging questions. For example, why is endometriosis in girls who haven't gone through puberty yet, and also (though rarely) in men? And why does the tissue in endometriosis not exactly resemble that of the endometrium? These questions have led to other theories, the current leading one being the *metaplasia theory*.

Metaplasia is the changing of a certain type of cell into a different type of cell. Recent research on tissue-typing and molecular studies suggests this theory over retrograde menstruation for the following reasons:

- The peritoneal cavity, Mullerian system, and *pleura* (lung tissue in general) all develop from the same embryologic layer of tissue, the *mesothelium*. (Check out Chapter 3 for peritoneal cavity and pleura info and the section "Malformed Mullerian ducts" earlier in this chapter.)

- Ovarian surface cells and stromal cells grow glands and stroma when cultured with estrogen.

- Endometrial tissue from the uterus is functionally different and looks different under the microscope from endometriosis tissue.

- Girls who haven't reached puberty, women with few and light periods, women with tied tubes, and even men can all have endometriosis, even though none of them can have retrograde menstruation.

The metaplasia theory suggests that when the *mesodermal* cells in the pelvis, abdomen, and lungs are exposed to some stimulus from the menstrual flow *or* an outside source, the cells *morph* (change) into endometrial cells. Back in the 1950s, Dr. John Sampson, the first proponent of the retrograde menstruation theory, noted that endometriosis may be "due to a specific irritant."

Asthma, allergies, and autoimmune issues in endometriosis

There's growing evidence that endometriosis is an autoimmune disease. There's also growing evidence that people who have one autoimmune disease are more likely to have additional autoimmune problems. One large study of more than 3,000 women with endometriosis showed the following:

✔ Sixty-one percent had allergies compared to 18 percent of the U.S. general population.

✔ Twelve percent had asthma compared to 5 percent of the general population.

✔ Chronic fatigue syndrome was more than a hundred times more common than in the female U.S. population overall.

✔ Hypothyroidism was seven times more common.

✔ Fibromyalgia was twice as common.

Understanding your immune system's role in endometriosis

Most women have the components (such as retrograde menstruation) that would make endometriosis development possible. So why does only a small percentage of women ever develop endometriosis? Why do the endometrial cells take root and grow in some women and not in others?

The answer may lie in the immune system. The study of the immune system and its relation to endometriosis and other immune-related diseases (such as lupus, fibromyalgia, and chronic fatigue syndrome) has rapidly progressed in the last decade. The immune system does seem to play a role in endometriosis.

New research sheds more and more light onto the inner workings of the immune system, but at the same time that research makes the waters murky. Endometriosis isn't immune (forgive the play on words) to this confusion. In the next sections, we highlight and try to simplify the immune system's involvement in endometriosis.

Meeting the immune cells

Normally your immune system gets rid of bad tissue and debris from injury or other problems. However, that process doesn't seem to work normally in women who develop endometriosis. The main question is, "Why does the body tolerate endometrial cells that develop in the wrong place or why do lymph nodes or blood vessels deposit them in strange areas of the body?"

In order to get a basic understanding of how your immune system affects endometriosis, you first need to understand the different types of immune cells. In this section, we introduce these cells and describe their different functions. Don't worry if you can't remember all the names — or pronounce them — there won't be a test on this!

Marauding macrophages

Macrophages, a type of white blood cell, are the body's scavenger cells. They aren't activated by *antigens* (foreign substances in the body that stimulate antibodies) and they don't rely on memory (like vaccines). These cells work by recognizing intruders and then eating or swallowing them (called *phagocytosis*). In this way they scavenge the body and rid it of dead cells, cellular debris, and some invading pathogens.

Macrophages secrete many proteins that help them do their job. The proteins include the following:

- **Cytokines:** They act as chemical messengers between cells, and can stimulate or inhibit the growth and activity of various immune cells.
- **Growth factors:** Proteins that stimulate cell growth.
- **Enzymes:** Enzymes trigger specific activity in cells.
- **Prostaglandins:** Hormonelike chemicals that, when released in the uterus, cause cramping.

Macrophages are normally in peritoneal fluid, but their numbers are higher in women with endometriosis. In addition, their secretions seem to promote the disease instead of scavenging the wayward endometrial cells.

Dodging Natural Killer (NK) cells

Natural Killer (NK) cells are another kind of white blood cell in the immune system. These cells attack cells that have antibodies stuck on them.

These NK cells also have receptors on their surface that regulate their activity by either *killer-activating* or *killer-inhibiting* the cells. The numbers of NK cells in the peritoneal fluid varies, but women with endometriosis have less cell-killing activity. The reason for this decrease seems to be that their NK cells have many more killer-inhibitory receptors than normal.

Looking at lymphocytes

Another group of immune cells are *lymphocytes,* another type of white blood cell. These cells

✔ Mature in the bone marrow and then enter the blood stream

✔ Are more prevalent in the peritoneal fluid of endometriosis victims

✔ Come in two basic flavors:

- **B lymphocytes:** Secrete immunoglobulins that are specific for certain microorganisms (this is how your body fights colds and other diseases).

- **T lymphocytes:** Help the B-cells make antibodies. They can also activate macrophages, get rid of *intra-cellular* (those within the cell itself) microbes, and kill cancer cells.

Dealing with immune cell secretions

Lymphocytes, *monocytes* (another type of white blood cell), macrophages, and other cells, including the endometrial cells themselves, secrete proteins that can have profound effects on the body. These proteins serve as messengers for

✔ *Chemotaxis* (cell movement due to chemical attraction)

✔ *Mitosis* (cell division)

✔ *Differentiation* (the reason everyone has different kinds of cells)

✔ *Formation* (of new blood vessels)

The following proteins are important (but not the only ones) in endometriosis:

✔ **Interleukin-1 (I-1)** can enhance the development of endometriosis by causing the release of factors for blood vessel growth and a molecule from the endometrial cells that hide endometrial cells from the immune system so they're not destroyed.

✔ **Interleukin-8** is released under the influence of I-1. This is a powerful stimulus of new vessel growth that also increases the ability of the endometrial stromal cells to adhere where they land. The number of these interleukins is higher in the peritoneal fluid of women with endometriosis, and the amount correlates with the severity of the disease.

✔ **Monocyte chemotactic protein-1 and RANTES** (you don't want to know what it stands for!) help macrophages get to the peritoneal cavity. I-1 and estrogen promote the production of these cells and help endometriosis to develop. Their numbers are higher in endometriosis.

✔ **Tumor necrosis factor – Alpha (TNF-a)** may help endometrial cells adhere to a cellular matrix and promote attachment of these cells and formation of endometriosis. I-1 increases its production. The number of TNF-a is higher in women with endometriosis.

✔ **Vascular Endothelial Growth Factor (VEGF for short)** helps the endometrial cells establish new blood vessels to promote development of endometriosis. Early endometriosis lesions have high levels of VEGF, and *powder burn* lesions (older, burned out disease) have lower levels. This difference in levels makes sense because the early lesions are most active metabolically.

All these factors (the immune cells and their secretions, the proteins produced from the lining of the pelvis and the endometrial cells, and so forth) can have a profound effect on the development of endometriosis. In theory, women with endometriosis have an abnormality that allows endometrial cells to survive outside the endometrium, stick to surfaces where it shouldn't be found, grow, and cause damage. But, does the immune system have an inherent defect or do the endometrial cells of these women cause the immune system to respond abnormally? This is the question for future research.

Exploring the autoimmune connection

As the previous section explains, the immune system is very complex — errors can occur. One error is when the body fails to recognize itself so it attacks its own proteins as if they were the invaders. This is called an *autoimmune disease,* and some evidence shows that endometriosis may be an autoimmune disease.

Autoimmune diseases have the following characteristics:

✔ **Hormonal element:** Because autoimmune diseases are more common in women than in men, a hormonal component is likely.

✔ **Numbers of autoimmune diseases:** Autoimmune diseases also like to travel together; after a patient has one, she's more likely to develop other autoimmune disorders. A study from the recent World Congress on Endometriosis showed 12 percent had an autoimmune disease (even though only about 2 percent of all women have such problems).

Consider the following statistics from another study on women with endometriosis:

• Almost 30 percent have fibromyalgia or chronic fatigue syndrome

• More than 10 percent have asthma

• More than 60 percent have allergies

This study concluded that these numbers suggest an association between endometriosis and autoimmune diseases.

✔ **Genetics:** Although an identical twin has a 30 percent chance of having a disorder if her twin has one, nonidentical twins or other siblings have less than a 3 percent risk of having the same disorder. Even if genetics don't exactly cause the problem, bad genes may make you more susceptible to irritants and stimulants.

✔ **Immune system abnormalities:** These abnormalities are consistent with the findings in autoimmune diseases. The same culprits — macrophages, lymphocytes, NK cells, cytokines, and other substances they produce — are all in both endometriosis and autoimmune disorders. (See the previous part of this section for a discussion of these conditions.)

These similarities and the association of these diseases with each other strongly suggest that endometriosis has an autoimmune component. Researchers haven't been able to prove it, but research continues to support this relationship.

Relating allergies to endometriosis

As the previous section notes, women with endometriosis also seem to have a higher rate of allergies than other women. (Check out the nearby sidebar, "Asthma, allergies, and autoimmune issues in endometriosis," for some interesting related statistics.) This connection makes sense because of the likely immune system component in endometriosis. Allergies are another example of an altered, or abnormal, immune response.

What happens during an allergic reaction and what is its relationship to endometriosis? In allergies and asthma, just like endometriosis, the immune system either over-responds or abnormally reacts to normal proteins or minor exposure to harmless antigens causing damage to the body. The following shows how your immune system responds during an allergic reaction:

1. **The immune system protects the body when the body is exposed to foreign material, such as _allergens_ (tissue, debris, germs, pollen, and so on).**

2. **B and T lymphocytes work together to form antibodies that attack the allergens, which the B and T lymphocytes see as a threat.**

   (See "Looking at lymphocytes" earlier in this section.)

3. **When exposed to this threat, T lymphocytes release cytokines that stimulate the B lymphocytes to multiply and make the specific antibody.**

4. **This antibody attaches to the antigen (and to the foreign material), and prepares to remove it from the body.**

   The T suppressor cells help regulate the response and help turn the response off when the job is done.

Gesundheit and g'night: The multiple responses to allergies

Some cells in the immune system cause the release of *histamines,* chemicals that cause the sneezing, runny nose, hives, itching, fatigue, and other symptoms of allergies. Histamines can also cause constriction of the *bronchials* (tubes that feed air into the lungs) that lead to the wheezing in asthma. In severe reactions, this tightening of the breathing tubes can be life-threatening.

Fatigue (chronic tiredness and loss of energy) is one of the most common signs of histamine release — and all immune diseases and abnormal inflammatory responses, for that matter. In fact, fatigue is the most common symptom of immune processes and can be debilitating.

---

5. **This immune response causes inflammation in the area because blood flow increases and blood vessels become more permeable.**

   In addition to the redness, warmth, and swelling in the area, the cytokines and pressure on the nerve endings in the tissue cause pain. Check out the sidebar, "Gesundheit and g'night: The multiple responses to allergies," for more symptoms of allergies.

If allergies and the body's response to them sounds just like the immune system and endometriosis, you're right! In both cases the immune system is responding to seemingly harmless foreign matter (endometrial cells or irritants such as pollen) in a way that wreaks havoc on the body. The association is strong: Many women with endometriosis also have multiple allergies, and both conditions run in families, indicating a genetic predisposition.

Recurring yeast infections and endometriosis

A fungus called *candida albicans* causes yeast infections in the mucus membranes, mouth, throat, intestines and genito-urinary tracts. A very common form of candida disease, vaginal yeast infection, may drive you to distraction by the itching and cheesy white coating it produces. Although this vaginal yeast is common and annoying, most healthcare providers don't consider it serious.

Candida's primary purpose is to destroy harmful bacteria in the intestines. Under normal circumstances, the following conditions control candida's growth:

- ✔ Good bacteria
- ✔ The body's *pH balance* (acidity and alkalinity); candida doesn't like acid
- ✔ A healthy immune system

So what causes a vaginal or vulvar yeast infection and how does it relate to endometriosis? The following are the main culprits:

- **Irritated skin:** This irritation can be from moisture (wet bathing suit), sprays, perfumes, laundry-detergent residue, douching, exposure to chemicals (such as chlorine), and even semen. These irritations to the vagina may alter the critical pH balance of the area. When imbalances occur, disease can follow.

- **Antibiotics:** Antibiotics kill off the *lactobacillus* (good bacteria that make lactic acid and lower the pH of the vagina). Other substances, such as douches, perfumed soaps, and feminine hygiene products, can also directly affect the pH of the vulva and vagina, making the pH less acidic and allowing the yeast to flourish. The yeast can

  - Cause an inflammatory response

  - Directly break down the protective barriers that the skin and mucous membranes of the body use.

    Once these barriers have been breached, candida can enter the body and cause infection and other problems.

- **Environmental toxins:** Dioxin, PCBs, and the usual suspects, such as too much alcohol, overindulgence in simple sugars, and cigarette smoke, compromise the skin and mucus barriers, possibly allowing the yeast to penetrate the barrier in the intestine. Because hormonal changes may contribute to this breakdown, chemicals may play another role: converting intestinal substances into hormone-like chemicals.

- **Allergic reaction to candida:** Some women may be allergic to candida, so even the normal amount of yeast can be problematic. This fact may explain why endometriosis sufferers (who are more prone to allergies in the first place) tend to be more susceptible to yeast infections. Another possibility is that a woman's intolerance to candida makes her more likely to develop endometriosis. The immune system abnormalities associated with candida, along with the chromic inflammatory response to the infection, can also encourage the growth of endometriosis.

The possible relationship between candida and endometriosis is complicated — and very controversial. Candida and its relation to immune system malfunctions need more research. If you have recurrent yeast infections *and* you have endometriosis, consider treatment for candida in addition to medical therapy for endometriosis. Some case reports have suggested that lowering candida albicans levels as much as possible may minimize autoimmune problems, including endometriosis.

The Mystery of Traveling Endometriosis

You suspect you have endometriosis, or your doctor may have diagnosed you with the disease. However, you're wondering how the endometriosis you have in your pelvic area can end up in your lungs or even your brain. It didn't catch the red-eye from your uterus to your lungs, so how does endometriosis travel to different areas in your body from the pelvic area?

Animal studies show that when scientists place endometrial tissue into an animal's pelvic cavity, the tissue eventually resembles endometriosis. (The only animals that spontaneously develop endometriosis are rhesus monkeys, as far as we know.) Yet, unlike in humans, this *artificially induced* disease in the studies doesn't seem to travel anywhere.

In this section, we discuss the ways endometriosis may hitch a ride to far-off parts of the body.

Hitching a ride in the lymphatic and vascular systems

One explanation for endometriosis ending up out of the pelvis is the lymphatic and vascular spread theory. In cancer, malignant cells travel throughout the body via two routes — the lymphatic system or the blood. Both of these methods require the malignant cells to lose their attachment to other cells nearby and still survive. This is one of the mysteries of malignancy. But don't worry, endometriosis isn't cancer.

The *lymphatic system* is a collection of small channels that roughly parallel the vascular (blood vessel) system (check out Figure 4-3). Its job description includes removal of cells, debris, and excess fluid from the tissues, so the lymph system sort of acts as a filter, where the white blood cells clean up the body. You may have had infections where your lymph nodes were enlarged and tender. This symptom is an indication that the lymph system is working.

Uterine contractions quite possibly force endometrial cells into the lymph channels and blood vessels that are in and around the uterus and then ship the cells up into the pelvis or other, far off places, such as the lungs or brain. This theory makes some sense because the uterus is rich in lymph and blood vessels.

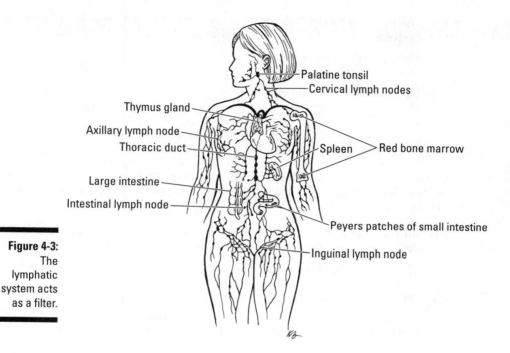

Palatine tonsil
Cervical lymph nodes
Thymus gland
Axillary lymph node
Thoracic duct
Spleen
Red bone marrow
Large intestine
Intestinal lymph node
Peyers patches of small intestine
Inguinal lymph node

Figure 4-3:
The lymphatic system acts as a filter.

But does the forced delivery really occur? Scientists have seen *apparent* endometrial cells microscopically in the lymphatic system of the uterus, but this doesn't mean the cells are viable and able to implant elsewhere. And this theory presents another question: How do the cells get out of the lymph channels? Though this is an attractive theory to explain the rare incidence of distant endometriosis, it remains unproven.

Although the lymphatic and vascular systems theory has some support, the vast majority of scientists and physicians believe this method may be secondary to other theories (see Figure 4-4). Time and research may shed light on the real cause in the near future. Endometriosis may be not one disease but several.

Spreading endometriosis through surgery

Another way endometriosis may get to distant places is through surgery. The following scenario may happen during a hysteroscopy (see Chapter 11 for more on a hysteroscopy):

1. **The surgeon forces fluid or air under high pressure into the uterine cavity.**

2. **The procedure forces endometrial tissue out of the tubes and possibly into lymph or blood vessels.**

3. **The endometrial cells may**

   - Remain in the pelvis (because this is where they first wind up)

   - Go anywhere, even to distant organs after they've entered the extensive lymph and blood systems

Endometrial cells can be dragged during surgery from the endometrial cavity or endometriosis implants in the pelvis to other areas. Two examples of this occurrence are

✔ During a cesarean section, the endometrial cavity is open and cells can spill out or be pulled out with the baby or *placenta* (afterbirth).

✔ While removing endometriosis from the pelvis, the surgeon may inadvertently plant endometrial cells into the wound opening or other parts of the abdomen.

Scientists have documented this surgical spread by observing endometriosis in old scars and other areas from previous surgery.

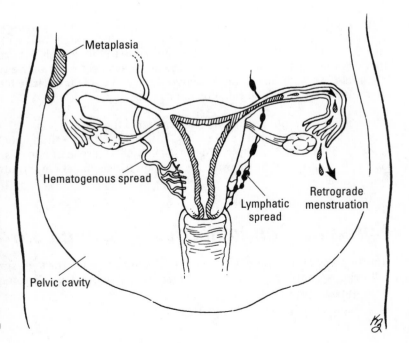

Figure 4-4: Researchers consider all of these theories as possibilities for traveling endometriosis.

Metaplasia

Hematogenous spread

Lymphatic spread

Retrograde menstruation

Pelvic cavity

Avoiding Endometriosis: Is It Possible?

If you know you have a family history of endometriosis but don't have any symptoms, is there a way to keep it from rearing its ugly head? Maybe, maybe not, but trying to avoid endometriosis can't hurt. This section looks at a couple of known risk factors for endometriosis and explains how avoiding them may decrease your chance of activating the disease or lessen its severity.

Does pregnancy help prevent endometriosis?

Evidence suggests that having children at a young age (when *you're* young, that is — *all* children are young!) can decrease your chance of having endometriosis. Likewise, most experts agree that being *nulliparous* — a fancy way of saying you've never been pregnant — increases your chance of developing endometriosis. These observations support another observable trend: Women who wait to get pregnant also tend to have a higher incidence of endometriosis.

But what causes this trend? Consider the following elements of the leading theories on endometriosis:

- ✔ The disease often occurs in women with regular, and sometimes more frequent and heavier, menstrual cycles.

- ✔ Women with years and years of uninterrupted, regular menstrual periods have much more time for regurgitation of endometrium and debris out the tubes.

- ✔ The endometrium and debris either implant on the structures of the pelvic cavity (the retrograde theory) or irritate the peritoneum to change into endometriosis (metaplasia theory).

When pregnancy stops your menstrual cycle, it also

- ✔ Stops the possible retrograde menstruation of endometrial tissue into the pelvic area

- ✔ Reduces your lifetime exposure to menstrual bleeding

- ✔ Raises levels of progesterone in your blood

  These higher progesterone levels further suppress the endometrium by preventing *mitosis* (cell division) and growth of the tissue. Without this tissue growth, endometriosis can't progress and worsen.

The lack of menstrual periods and suppression of the endometrial tissue can also minimize the symptoms of endometriosis for a long time because

- Decreased hormonal activity (over the nine months of pregnancy and several weeks to months after birth) can't stimulate endometrial implants.

- The direct effects of progesterone and the pregnancy hormones can suppress the implants.

This combination of no stimulation with increased suppression can *burn out* the endometrial implants, giving a woman long, symptom-free periods of time.

So, you may ask in an irrational moment, if pregnancy is so effective, why doesn't everyone use this method? Kids are cute and this can cure endometriosis — just stay pregnant until menopause! Ah, yes, unfortunately this logic has its problems (but you knew that!):

- Most women don't want to be pregnant for 10 to 30 years.

- This really isn't a healthy way to go. (Yes, pregnancy is normal and natural, but it's still much more risky to your health than the nonpregnant state).

- The Catch-22: Women with endometriosis often are infertile, so they can't get pregnant.

But if the timing in a woman's life is correct, if she can get pregnant (with or without help), and if she doesn't mind having a few kids, pregnancy may be an alternative to other treatments (but not exactly a cheaper one).

Watching what you eat

Good nutrition is important, no matter how healthy you are. However, it's especially important if you're trying to keep your immune system and other body systems in tip-top condition to fight off the effects of a chronic disease like endometriosis.

Can you eat away endometriosis? Probably not. Can you eat in a way that minimizes endometriosis symptoms and strengthens your immune system? Probably.

Recent studies show that

- Eating more fresh fruits and green vegetables and limiting red meat and ham may reduce your chance of developing endometriosis.

- People with diets high in polyunsaturated fats have a greater chance for developing endometriosis.

✔ Certain types of fatty acids can increase prostaglandin levels and add to the symptoms of the disease.

✔ Simple sugars that increase insulin levels may also cause a rise in prostaglandins, increasing the symptoms of endometriosis.

✔ Caffeine can stimulate cramps and contractions of intestinal and uterine muscle (common symptoms of endometriosis).

We cover these precautions in more detail in Chapter 16.

What you eat may be important, but equally important may be *how much* you eat. Studies on the effect of body mass index, or BMI, are inconclusive (check out Table 4-1 for a detailed chart of BMI), but a recent study showed a possible link between low body mass index in tall women and endometriosis. According to the study, women with endometriosis had an average BMI of 21.3 compared to an average BMI of 23.2 in a control group of women without endometriosis.

Considering environmental factors

Undoubtedly, pollution is bad for you in a number of ways. Humans produce tens of thousands of chemicals (mostly through manufacturing) that we then dump into the environment as waste or trash. Over the years, nature breaks the chemicals down, and the environment absorbs and accumulates them. In the meantime, your food (plants and animals) and water store these chemicals, and you take them in when you eat.

Endometriosis is related to environmental contamination. Dioxin, one of the first pollutants scientists studied, is an example (see the sidebar "Understanding dioxin exposure" earlier in this chapter) of an environmental effect on endometriosis. Likewise, scientists can link pollutants to multiple sclerosis, lupus, thyroid disease, chronic fatigue syndrome, fibromyalgia, and even cancer.

One of the big problems with chemicals dumped into the environment is their unknown effects on people. Researchers haven't tested many of these pollutants on humans, and, as a result, can't know safe levels of use. Also, valid studies and data don't exist regarding chemical interactions. For example, two or more harmless chemicals may combine to make a potentially lethal substance.

Be aware of your environment and avoid the obvious toxins, such as dioxin and PVCs; use the safest products and eat the healthiest foods you can. In this way you can minimize your risks of endometriosis and other environmentally-linked diseases (and you can feel better at the same time). See Chapter 16 for specific ways to decrease your exposure to chemicals in your environment.

78

Table 4-1						Body Weight in Pounds According to Height and Body Mass Index							
BMI (kg/m²)	**19**	**20**	**21**	**22**	**23**	**24**	**25**	**26**	**27**	**28**	**29**	**30**	**35**	**40**
Height (in.)						Weight (lb.)								
58	91	96	100	105	110	115	119	124	129	134	138	143	167	191
59	94	99	104	109	114	119	124	128	133	138	143	148	173	198
60	97	102	107	112	118	123	128	133	138	143	148	153	179	204
61	100	106	111	116	122	127	132	137	143	148	153	158	185	211
62	104	109	115	120	126	131	136	142	147	153	158	164	191	218
63	107	113	118	124	130	135	141	146	152	158	163	169	197	225
64	110	116	122	128	134	140	145	151	157	163	169	174	204	232
65	114	120	126	132	138	144	150	156	162	168	174	180	210	240
66	118	124	130	136	142	148	155	161	167	173	179	186	216	247
67	121	127	134	140	146	153	159	166	172	178	185	191	223	255
68	125	131	138	144	151	158	164	171	177	184	190	197	230	262
69	128	135	142	149	155	162	169	176	182	189	196	203	236	270
70	132	139	146	153	160	167	174	181	188	195	202	207	243	278
71	136	143	150	157	165	172	179	186	193	200	208	215	250	286
72	140	147	154	162	169	177	184	191	199	206	213	221	258	294
73	144	151	159	166	174	182	189	197	204	212	219	227	265	302
74	148	155	163	171	179	186	194	202	210	218	225	233	272	311
75	152	160	168	176	184	192	200	208	216	224	232	240	279	319
76	156	164	172	180	189	197	205	213	221	230	238	246	287	328

Are endometriosis and cancer related?

Having endometriosis is bad enough, but the thought that endometriosis may increase your risk of developing certain types of cancer is even worse. Even though studies are inconclusive about a definite link between certain cancers and endometriosis, research indicates that endometriosis doesn't increase the *general* risk of cancer. However, endometriosis may increase the risk of certain rare cancers.

According to a very large (64,000 women) retrospective study (researchers looked at statistics only after the study was complete) in Sweden, the cancers that are more prevalent in women with endometriosis are

✔ Ovarian cancer

✔ Non-Hodgkin's lymphoma

✔ Certain endocrine cancers

✔ Certain brain cancers

Other significant and interesting conclusions from this study are

✔ Women who had endometriosis and a hysterectomy showed no increase in ovarian cancer over the general population.

✔ Younger women who developed endometriosis between the ages of 20 and 40 had a higher risk of getting ovarian cancer than other age groups.

✔ Women with endometriosis developed cancer at a younger age than the general population.

✔ Women with endometriosis had a lower risk of cervical cancer than the general population.

The reason for this conclusion isn't clear, but a common symptom may play a role. You guessed it — painful sex! (Check out Chapter 2 for more information on this and other symptoms of endometriosis.) When you consider that cervical cancer rates are higher in women with more active sex lives (and number of partners), the symptoms of endometriosis can decrease this activity and, as a result, lower the cervical cancer rates in women with these symptoms. (This is just an unproven theory, so don't use it as an excuse for avoiding sex!)

Can endometriosis ever turn into cancer? Yes and no. Endometriosis isn't a cancer itself; it's only endometrial tissue. ***Note:*** Cancer that develops in the endometrial lining of the uterus is, oddly enough, endometrial cancer. However, this disease mainly affects postmenopausal women, the one age group that endometriosis seldom strikes!

Endometrial cancer can develop in younger women, but rarely does. These women almost always have *polycystic ovarian syndrome* (PCOS) or very infrequent periods. In other words, these women have no regular menses and, logically, no symptoms of endometriosis. One rare form of endometrial cancer (clear cell carcinoma) does occur in the implants of endometriosis. As with any other abnormality, you should have a biopsy on any suspicious area.

Dr. K., who has been active in gynecology at major teaching and referral hospitals for 30 years, has seen only one case of cancer in endometriosis in his career. Because the chances of your having this disease are extremely rare, Dr. K. doesn't recommend surgery to explore the possibility.

Part II
Digging Deeper into Endometriosis

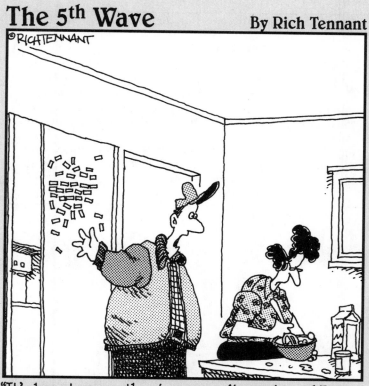

The 5th Wave   By Rich Tennant

"It's been two months since your diagnosis, and I know you're reluctant to talk about it. But we've got to start discussing it in some way other than messages left on the refrigerator with these tiny word magnets."

In this part . . .

Are you fairly familiar with endometriosis but want to discover a little more? This part delves a bit deeper into how endometriosis affects your menstrual cycle, fertility, and systems outside the reproductive tract, such as your intestines and bladder. Do you suspect you have endometriosis but want to know for sure? We tell you how a doctor makes the diagnosis; and, just as important, we help you find the right doctor to treat you.

Chapter 5

Understanding Your Menstrual Cycle (And Its Relationship to Endometriosis)

....

....

*Y*our menstrual cycle is complex. Hormones and complicated feedback systems orchestrate your reproductive system's march each month toward a single goal — the production of a healthy egg that can grow in a properly prepared uterine cavity. In other words, all your body cares about each month is making sure you can get pregnant.

Endometriosis can disrupt the normal march of your menstrual cycle by interfering with your hormones, your egg's production and release, the fertilization of the egg, and the egg's ability to travel to the uterus. In addition, endometriosis can cause pain throughout your menstrual cycle, especially around your period.

This chapter looks more closely at your menstrual cycle and the ways endometriosis can mess it up. We uncover the relationship between your period and endometriosis by first looking at a normal period and then comparing it to a period with endometriosis.

We also tell you how to know whether your pain is endometriosis or another gynecologic problem. Next we discuss medical and surgical treatments to regulate your menstrual cycle and decrease pain and irregular bleeding. Finally, we take a brief look at menopause and its effect on endometriosis

Your Period and Endometriosis: Why Are They Connected?

Fact: Endometriosis and your menstrual cycle are closely related. Because endometriosis derives from endometrial tissue, it functions in much the same way; it grows like your uterine lining does during the first part of your menstrual cycle and bleeds when your uterine endometrial lining sheds during your period. For this reason, many women experience more pain from endometriosis around the time of menses than any other time. (See Chapter 3 for more background on endometrial tissue.)

To understand the symptoms of endometriosis, you need to first understand the inner workings of the menstrual system. In the next sections, we tell you how your menstrual system works when it's in perfect order and then give you the lowdown on how endometriosis can throw your menstrual cycle out of synch.

Looking at a healthy cycle

A normal menstrual cycle is like a complex work of art (check out Figure 5-1). Okay, you may not think that when you're changing pads or dealing with cramps, but your reproductive system really is amazing. And yet many women understand little of the menstrual cycle. When you understand all the intricate workings, you have a much better grasp of how endometriosis can gum up the works, so to speak.

What exactly is the menstrual cycle anyway? Is it just the time you're actively bleeding, or is it the time between bleeds, too? When your doctor starts asking questions about your cycle, you may not be sure exactly what he's asking. Our goal is to translate that jargon into regular talk for you.

How long is the cycle?

When your doctor asks you how long your cycles are, he wants to know the number of days between Day 1 of one period and Day 1 of the next. Menstrual cycles are traditionally 28 days. However, only one in ten women actually experience regular 28-day cycles. Cycles are usually 21 to 35 days apart.

Day 1 of your period is the first day of full flow. If you spot on and off for a few days before breaking out the pads and tampons, you haven't started your new cycle yet. Even when you start a full flow period just before bedtime, it's still Day 1 of your new cycle.

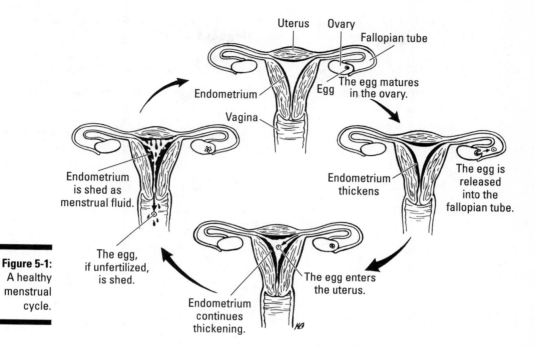

Uterus Ovary

Fallopian tube

The egg matures
in the ovary.

Endometrium

Egg

Vagina

Endometrium
is shed as
menstrual fluid.

The egg is
released
into the
fallopian tube.

Endometrium
thickens

Figure 5-1:
A healthy
menstrual
cycle.

The egg,
if unfertilized,
is shed.

The egg enters
the uterus.

Endometrium
continues
thickening.

The most consistent element of the menstrual cycle is that periods start 13 to
14 days after ovulation. (Check out Chapter 7 for more about ovulation.) If
you ovulate early (before day 14), your cycles are shorter than normal. If
you ovulate later than 14 days into your cycle, your cycles are longer than
28 days.

When your doctor asks how long your period lasts, he wants to know how
many days your bleeding lasts. Menstrual flow normally lasts two to seven
days, with an average of four days.

How do hormones orchestrate your cycle?

So what regulates all this flow? The answer is hormones. When you're feeling
out of sorts and irritable, you may say you're feeling hormonal, but the truth
is that you're hormonal all the time. Estrogen goes up, follicle-stimulating
hormone (FSH) goes down . . . your body constantly has something happening hormonally. The three hormone-control systems that work together to
manage your cycle are

✔ The **hypothalamus** (the small structure in the middle of the brain that regulates the nervous and endocrine systems)

✔ The **pituitary** (an endocrine gland at the base of the brain below the hypothalamus that secretes several hormones)

✔ The **ovary** (the female reproductive organ that produces estrogen, progesterone, and eggs)

Right before your period starts, your hormone levels drop to their lowest levels. At this moment, the cycle starts again. (Check out Figure 5-2.)

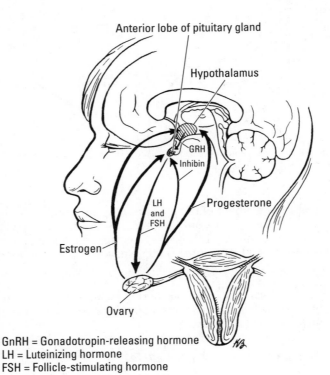

Anterior lobe of pituitary gland

Hypothalamus

GRH

Inhibin

LH and FSH

Progesterone

Estrogen

Ovary

Figure 5-2: The rise and fall of hormones during your menstrual cycle.

GnRH = Gonadotropin-releasing hormone
LH = Luteinizing hormone
FSH = Follicle-stimulating hormone

What are the steps in a normal cycle?

The following list describes the menstrual cycle:

1. **The hypothalamus, the master gland, produces a gonadotropin-releasing hormone (GnRH).**

   This production tells the pituitary gland to start making follicle-stimulating hormone (FSH).

2. **FSH travels through the bloodstream to the ovaries.**

3. **Anywhere from 1 to 15 eggs containing follicles start to grow in the ovary.**

   One egg — sometimes two — grows faster than the others and becomes the dominant follicle or follicles. The rest stop growing and fade away, never to be seen again.

4. **FSH stimulates the ovaries to produce estrogen, one of the main female hormones.**

   Estrogen helps the eggs mature and starts to thicken the uterine endometrial lining, which is very thin right after your period.

5. **As estrogen rises, FSH is suppressed and then rises again in conjunction with the release of a luteinizing hormone (LH) from the pituitary gland.**

   This process occurs mid-cycle as the egg nears maturity.

6. **LH causes the dominant follicle to enlarge and the egg to fully mature, weakening the follicle wall.**

   This causes the egg to burst out of its follicle in the process called *ovulation*.

7. **The follicle that was home to the released eggs collapses.**

   Under the influence of the pituitary hormone LH, the collapsed follicle becomes the corpus luteum that produces progesterone. This progesterone then changes the composition of your endometrial lining, making it denser and more receptive to a potential embryo. Your basal body temperature rises one half to one degree when your progesterone rises.

8. **The pituitary gland stops producing FSH so that no more eggs mature.**

9. **If no embryo implants, your estrogen and progesterone levels begin to drop ten days or so after you ovulate.**

   The uterine endometrium produces prostaglandins (see Chapter 3 for more about prostaglandins) that change the blood supply to the uterus and stimulate uterine contractions. The thickened lining now sheds as your menstrual period — a combination of blood, cells, and debris.

Normally, your endometrium is approximately 10 millimeters thick at the end of your cycle. The shedding, along with blood from the torn blood vessels, cervical mucus, endometrial tissue, and cellular debris, add up to a little more than 30 milliliters (an ounce) of discharge, although it certainly seems like a lot more! More than 80 milliliters (a little less than 3 ounces) of discharge is abnormal.

Menstrual blood normally doesn't clot, unless your flow is very heavy. Sometimes the lining is shed in large fragments (sometimes called *decidual casts*) that can look like an early miscarriage.

Understanding how endometriosis affects your period

Endometriosis can interfere with your menstrual cycle in a number of ways. Starting right from Day 1 of your cycle, endometriosis on or around your ovary can interfere with your egg production. If you're not planning on getting pregnant, you may say, "So what?" But the whole purpose of the menstrual cycle is the maturation, release, and implantation of an egg. Disrupting the process in any way impacts your periods.

Although the exact reasons aren't clear, endometriosis in and around the ovaries can interfere with your period by

- **Keeping a maturing egg from producing enough hormones, specifically estrogen and progesterone.** When hormone levels are lower than they should be, your periods may be shorter than normal.

- **Destroying part of or the entire ovary, leading to early menopause, a lack of ovulation, long cycles (more than 35 days apart), or irregular bleeding.**

- **Causing inflammation that produces toxins that interfere with egg growth and maturation.**

What do short menstrual cycles mean?

What's worse than having periods every four weeks? Having periods every three weeks! When cycles are less than 21 days, a woman is said to have *polymenorrhea*. Short cycles are more than an inconvenience; they can be a sign of *luteal phase defect*, or early ovulation. (See the sidebar "Luteal phase defect: Running out of progesterone" and Chapter 7 for more on this condition and pregnancy.)

Women with short menstrual cycles may also be more likely to develop endometriosis if they don't already have it. This connection may exist because of the retrograde menstruation theory (see Chapter 4 for more about this theory). Bleeding more frequently means that more blood spills into the pelvis, giving endometriosis more chances to grow where it doesn't belong.

An occasional short cycle is nothing to worry about, but you may want to be tested if your cycles are repeatedly short (less than 25 days apart). When periods start less than 14 days after ovulation, you have luteal phase defect, which can affect your ability to get pregnant.

Luteal phase defect: Running out of progesterone

Whether or not endometriosis can cause luteal phase defect is somewhat controversial, because studies have shown some evidence for and some evidence against the connection.

As soon as the egg has matured and released, the luteinizing hormone (LH) causes the cells of the follicle to produce the hormone progesterone. At this point, the follicle is called a *corpus luteum,* or yellow body, because the molecular changes give these cells a yellow color.

You can think of progesterone as the opposite of estrogen. While estrogen causes the endometrium to proliferate (grow) and the glands of the breast to develop, progesterone stops the growth and cell division in these tissues. At that point, progesterone prompts the endometrium to become more complex with the development of glands, *vacuoles* (pockets of energy), and *spiral arterioles* (coiled blood vessels). All these changes make the endometrium ready for the embryo to implant and grow.

However, when the ovary (the corpus luteum) fails to produce enough progesterone, the normal changes in the endometrium inside the uterus may not happen. Or, the changes may not be in the correct sequence, or the timing may be off. Your period comes earlier than normal because you're not making enough progesterone to keep your period from starting for a full two weeks — you're running out of progesterone early.

The lack of adequate progesterone is called a luteal phase defect because the time between egg release and menstruation is the luteal phase. This condition can happen in women without endometriosis, but it's common in women with the disease.

Early ovulation

Even though your period may start 14 days on the dot after ovulation, your cycle may still be short because you're ovulating very early, before Day 10 of your cycle. Endometriosis can cause short cycles by destroying part of your ovary, resulting in decreased ovarian reserve.

Why do some women ovulate early? The answer may be that

- It's a normal variant (that is, it's just how you are!).
- It's a sign of *perimenopause,* the years leading up to menopause.
- You have decreased ovarian reserve because endometriosis has destroyed part of your ovary.
- You have another endocrine problem.

Dealing with abnormal uterine bleeding (AUB)

If endometriosis has damaged your ovary to the point where you're not ovulating regularly, you may have irregular bleeding. Sometimes you bleed too much because the uterine lining grows too thick before being shed, and sometimes you bleed in the middle of your cycle, usually at times when you least expect it. *Adenomyosis* (endometriosis that infiltrates the uterine wall) can also cause irregular bleeding.

Few women complain about bleeding too little with their periods — bleeding too much is a far more common complaint! However, bleeding too much may be in the eye of the beholder. Some studies show that approximately 50 percent of the women who *think* they have heavier than normal periods actually don't.

Bleeding that doesn't fit the norm — either in timing or amount — is called *abnormal uterine bleeding* (AUB). About 20 percent of women with endometriosis have AUB. The primary cause of AUB in women with endometriosis is *anovulation* (lack of ovulation), although adenomyosis can also cause AUB. Abnormal bleeding has some unpronounceable names:

✔ **Menorrhagia:** Bleeding too heavily every month or for too many days

✔ **Metrorrhagia:** Bleeding at odd times

✔ **Polymenorrhea:** Periods occurring less than 21 days apart

✔ **Oligomenorrhea:** Periods occurring more than 35 days apart

✔ **Menometrorrhagia:** Excessive bleeding at irregular intervals

The best way to deal with AUB depends on your age and desire for future fertility (check out Chapter 7 for more on other fertility issues). At one end of the spectrum is *benign neglect* (do nothing but have your pads and tampons ready). At the complete other end is the ultimate way to stop bleeding, a hysterectomy. However, most of the time your options include medication to regulate your cycles (see "Regulating Your Menstrual Cycle to Reduce the Pain" later in this chapter) or surgical treatments less final than hysterectomy.

Never choose *Ignore It* as an option for dealing with AUB. You and your doctor must consider the possibility of cancer in cases of repeated AUB.

Are long cycles harmful?

Although having periods a few times a year doesn't seem like such a bad thing, it can be harmful. Endometriosis growing on your ovary can cause infrequent periods by destroying part of the ovarian tissue. When this happens, your periods come much less frequently than normal. In fact, you may ovulate and have periods only a few times a year. (See Chapter 3 for more on the effects of endometriosis on your ovaries.)

Cycles that occur more than 40 days apart are called *oligomenorrhea*. Women with oligomenorrhea often have problems getting pregnant and are at risk for very heavy periods. Even worse, over time, oligomenorrhea can increase the risk of overgrowth of the endometrium (called *hyperplasia*) and, in some cases, endometrial cancer.

A Pain by Any Other Name Is Still a Pain, But Is It Endometriosis?

Do you experience monthly pain with your period? Occasional, mild pain isn't unusual. However, for recurrent and/or severe pain during your menstrual cycle, you need to see your doctor so he can determine whether you have endometriosis. Although the only way to definitely diagnose endometriosis is through surgery, the pattern and type of pain you feel each month may lead your doctor to a presumptive diagnosis of endometriosis. Pain during or around your period is a classic sign of endometriosis. (Check out Chapter 9 for more on how your doctor makes a presumptive diagnosis.)

Identifying the pain

Women with endometriosis tend to have pain that begins right before their periods and lasts for several days. The pain of endometriosis may

- ✔ Be severe
- ✔ Worsen over time
- ✔ Be accompanied by nausea
- ✔ Be accompanied by diarrhea
- ✔ Be accompanied by back pain or leg pain

Don't ignore painful periods. Consult your doctor right away if

- ✔ You have more severe pain than usual.
- ✔ The pain is different than usual.
- ✔ You run a fever.
- ✔ You have foul-smelling discharge (you could have an infection).
- ✔ You have an IUD that was placed less than three months ago.
- ✔ Your period was very light, you have pain, and you're sexually active (you could have an ectopic pregnancy; see Chapter 7 for more info).

What causes the pain?

You may feel powerless when you're in pain during your period. Knowing the cause of your pain may not make you feel better, but at least you can know why you're feeling so lousy.

Generally classifying menstrual pain

General pain with your period is formally called *dysmenorrhea,* pronounced dis-men-or-*ee*-ah. This pain usually lasts for the first two to three days of your period. Painful periods are the number one symptom described by women with endometriosis.

Dysmenorrhea can be primary or secondary. Primary dysmenorrhea has the following characteristics:

- ✔ Primary dysmenorrhea is unrelated to any other disease process (such as endometriosis). In other words, women with primary dysmenorrhea *don't* have endometriosis.

- ✔ Ninety percent of women with painful periods have primary dysmenorrhea.

- ✔ Primary dysmenorrhea usually starts within the first three years after you start menstruating.

- ✔ Primary dysmenorrhea doesn't usually start in the first six months of a young woman's periods; ovulation may not occur for a few months after her periods start. Painful periods in the first six months of menstruation can be due to cervical or uterine problems and should be checked out by a doctor.

Secondary dysmenorrhea has the following characteristics:

- ✔ Secondary dysmenorrhea is usually caused by physical disease.

- ✔ Endometriosis is the most common cause of secondary dysmenorrhea.

- ✔ A number of other causes for secondary dysmenorrhea are also possible. So having secondary dysmenorrhea doesn't mean you definitely have endometriosis.

The following are some of the causes of a painful period:

- ✔ **Uterine cramping** from high levels of prostaglandins

    Prostaglandins (hormones released by the uterus) cause the cramping that helps the uterus squeeze off the uterine lining and push it (along with the blood) out of the uterus. Prostaglandin levels appear to be much higher in women with painful periods than in women who experience few menstrual symptoms.

- ✔ **Inflammation in your pelvis** from the toxic chemical produced by endometriosis implants

- ✔ **Adhesions,** or scar tissue, pulling on organs and tissues

- ✔ **Irritation of nerves** due to endometriosis implants

- ✔ **Direct effect of endometriosis** on the uterus, ovaries, or other organs

You can reduce much of the pain related to endometriosis by regulating your menstrual cycle (see "Regulating your Menstrual Cycle to Reduce the Pain" later in this chapter). Medication to prevent egg development and ovulation can keep pain from showing up on a monthly basis. Obviously, these medications aren't a good choice if you plan to get pregnant in the near future.

What's with the mid-cycle pain?

Many women spend a day or two a month wondering whether they have appendicitis because mittelschmerz (German for *mid-cycle pain*) on your right side can mimic the symptoms of appendicitis. But you can experience mittelschmerz without having endometriosis.

Mittelschmerz appears at the time of ovulation. Twenty percent of women feel mid-cycle pain at some time in their lives. The pain can be so precise that many women know the exact moment that they ovulate.

The rupture of the follicle housing the egg causes mid-cycle pain. When the follicle ruptures, a small amount of follicular fluid and blood escapes into the abdomen and can irritate the abdominal lining, causing pain.

Mid-cycle pain has characteristics that are unlike other pelvic pain:

✔ It's recurrent each month.

✔ It's one-sided.

✔ It lasts from a few minutes to one or two days.

✔ It switches from one side to another, depending on which ovary is ovulating.

✔ It's usually a sharp, crampy pain.

✔ Women don't usually have fever or other organ-system symptoms.

Mittelschmerz is somewhat of a misnomer because it doesn't always occur in the middle of your menstrual cycle. It actually occurs approximately 14 days before the start of your next period. So, if you have short cycles (around 23 days), mid-cycle pain occurs on Day 9. If your cycles are long (around 35 days), mittelschmerz occurs around Day 21.

Regulating Your Menstrual Cycle to Reduce the Pain

To reduce the pain, you basically have two choices: medication and surgery. This section briefly looks at your options. Chapter 10 looks more in-depth at medication to treat endometriosis, while Chapter 11 discusses your surgical options.

Using medication

One way to reduce the pain of endometriosis during your period is to regulate your menstrual cycle through the use of medication. These same medications can help if you also have irregular bleeding (AUB) (check out the sidebar "Dealing with abnormal uterine bleeding [AUB]" earlier in this chapter). Most of these medications stop the normal menstrual cycle of egg development, ovulation, and progesterone production.

Without the normal hormonal stimulation to the endometrial tissue, the endometrium doesn't bleed off, which means that endometriosis tissue doesn't bleed either! The following hormonal medications are very effective and may be all you need to get pain or irregular bleeding under control:

- **Birth control pills:** Both estrogen and a progestin in a convenient pack.

- **Progestins:** Two examples include medroxyprogesterone acetate (better known by the more pronounceable name Provera) and norithindrone acetate (Agyestin).

- **Estrogen and progestin separately**

- **Hormone-impregnated IUD:** Levonorgestrel intrauterine device.

- **Gonadotrophin Releasing Hormone agonist:** Lupron or Zoladex are two examples.

(These are, not surprisingly, the same medications we talk about in detail in Chapter 10 as treatments for endometriosis!)

In most cases, your physician starts with hormonal therapy, unless you're planning on getting pregnant immediately. The exact treatment varies from woman to woman. You and your doctor can decide on which therapy or therapy combination is best for you.

Your doctor may first suggest you start taking ibuprofen before your period begins as a treatment to control heavy bleeding. Obviously, this treatment won't help if your bleeding comes at odd times or isn't predictable. Ibuprofen is also very helpful in controlling menstrual pain.

Considering surgery

You can also consider surgery to regulate your painful period. Irregular bleeding from endometriosis can be just a nuisance or it can become troublesome enough to look for a remedy. When bleeding is very heavy, you can become anemic (that is, have a low iron count). If medical therapy doesn't work or you can't tolerate the hormones, your doctor may suggest a surgical option to control irregular bleeding and to decrease pain. These options may be

- Dilation and curettage (D&C)

- Hysteroscopy

- Uterine artery embolization (UAE)

- Endometrial ablation (EA)

- Partial or total hysterectomy (all or part of the uterus)

Which procedure you choose depends on your desires. If pregnancy is in your future plans, then the only approved options are a D&C and hysteroscopy. Most surgeons combine these procedures during one operation. Some doctors feel that uterine artery embolization is appropriate for women seeking future pregnancy, but these doctors are in the minority. The data is controversial at best, and the UAE isn't approved by the Food and Drug Administration (FDA) for women who plan to have children. (Check out Chapter 11 for more specifics about these procedures.)

Hello Menopause: Goodbye Endometriosis?

For many women with endometriosis, there's an end in sight; it's called *menopause,* the cessation of menstrual periods. Normally women stop having periods between the ages of 45 and 55 because the ovaries produce less estrogen and progesterone. At menopause, all (or almost all) primordial follicles are used up so eggs can't form. With no follicles or eggs, a woman's body doesn't produce estrogen. As a result, the tissues that normally respond to estrogen (like the endometrium and breast) no longer grow.

Because hormones are responsible for the symptoms of endometriosis and because artificially induced menopause (with hormone therapy) often reduces the pain of endometriosis, we can expect menopause to end endometriosis. Although the pain of endometriosis continues into menopause for a small percentage of women, the end of menstrual periods is the end of pain for many women.

This change may not happen all at once, but, after months without hormonal stimulation, the endometrial tissue — no matter where it is — shrivels up and, in a sense, dies. After the endometrial tissue dies, the endometrial cells can no longer respond to estrogen. Even when the body continues to produce estrogen or a woman takes estrogen for menopausal symptoms, at some point the endometrium isn't able to respond.

Unfortunately, a few women don't follow the rules. They may be taking estrogen for hormone replacement or making some estrogen themselves, so the endometrium (in the uterus or pelvis) continues to react to it. These women may still have symptoms of endometriosis after menopause. But for many (if not most) women, the end of periods is — fanfare, please — the end of endometriosis.

Chapter 6

Looking Closer at How Endometriosis Also Affects Other Body Parts

*F*ocusing on endometriosis and its effect on your period and your fertility may not be that difficult. However, you may not realize that endometriosis can affect other body systems as well. In fact, in very rare cases, endometriosis has been found *only* outside the pelvis.

In this chapter, we look at how endometriosis can affect areas outside the reproductive tract, from your intestines and urinary tract to your lungs and even your head.

What a Gas! Endometriosis and Your Intestines

If they're not out of order, you probably take your intestines (the interchangeable term for *bowels*) for granted. When it's working right, intestinal plumbing is fairly predictable, reasonably painless, and only occasionally inconvenient. But for many women with endometriosis, their intestines are truly in an uproar much of the time.

That winding path of intestines is more complex than you may realize. For starters, that path is much longer than it first appears — your large intestine is 5 feet long and your small intestine is 20 feet— not exactly a short jaunt for the food you swallow.

If you suspect that endometriosis is affecting your intestines, then this section is for you. This section looks at how endometriosis can affect your intestines, what you can do if you suspect you have endometriosis there, what symptoms you need to look for, how your doctor diagnoses endometriosis at this site, and what your treatment options are.

Twisting through your intestines

Before you can clearly understand the relationship between endometriosis and your intestines, you need to understand what your intestines entail. (Refer to Chapter 3 for more information on the intestines.) The intestines literally start at your mouth and esophagus and continue to the anus. The small intestine is narrower and more coiled than the large intestine and has three sections:

- ✔ Upper intestine (stomach and duodenum)
- ✔ Jejunum
- ✔ Ileum

Most digestion occurs in the small intestine. (The large intestine absorbs water and solidifies waste that is excreted as stool, and that's about it — a dirty job, but something has to do it!)

The intestinal wall, both large and small, has three separate layers:

- ✔ The *serosa,* the thin, outside layer that's also the continuation of the peritoneum
- ✔ The muscle, which makes up most of the intestinal wall
- ✔ The *mucosa,* the thin, inside layer where absorption and secretion occur

The location of endometriosis on the intestines has a lot to do with your symptoms. When the endometriosis is on the serosa, you likely have bloating, nausea, and loose stools during your period. If the endometriosis has grown through the serosa and muscle layers to the mucosa, you may have rectal bleeding during your period. Endometriosis on the intestines is more common on the serosa and muscle layers and less common on the mucosa. (Check out the next section for the different symptoms you may encounter if endometriosis has invaded your intestines.)

Suspecting intestinal endometriosis

Intestinal problems are common in endometriosis — at least 30 percent of patients, probably more, have some intestinal symptoms. But endometriosis isn't the first problem doctors think of when they hear patients complain about intestinal issues. In fact, endometriosis may be the last diagnosis they consider. Despite this fact, endometriosis in the intestines, not the pelvic area, is the most common site for post-menopausal women.

You don't have to have endometriosis on your intestines to have intestinal symptoms; in fact, most people with symptoms don't have endometriosis on their intestines. Most symptoms are due to irritation from endometrial implants in adjacent areas (such as the ligaments) and adhesions from other areas to the intestines. In addition, inflammatory factors can affect intestinal function just as they can affect other organs.

Endometriosis can cause the following intestinal issues:

- Abdominal bloating
- Abdominal pain
- Alternating constipation and diarrhea
- Constipation
- Diarrhea
- Intestinal cramping
- Nausea and/or vomiting
- Painful bowel movements
- Rectal bleeding
- Rectal pain

When patients do have endometriosis on their intestines, the implants are usually *superficial,* which means they're found just on the surface of the intestine, and may be easy to remove. But, because most symptoms come from inflammatory issues and not from the endometriosis implants themselves, removal of the implants on the intestines may not cure the pain and cramping.

Sometimes endometriosis in areas right next to the intestines can cause intestinal symptoms. This effect is most common near the uterosacral ligaments or rectovaginal septum (see Chapter 3 for more on these areas) because the intestine is in contact with these areas. The inflammatory process around these other areas can cause intestinal symptoms as well. Adhesions that attach intestines to nearby organs can also cause intestinal symptoms.

Endometriosis may even cause intestinal contractions and hypoglycemia

A study by Baylor University looked at a group of women with endometriosis and found they had increased frequency of contractions within the muscle layer of the intestine, which can be related to the production of prostaglandins and other substances by the endometrial implants. (Prostaglandins are produced in the endometriosis and then released into the surrounding tissues, blood vessels, and lymphatic tissue.) This occurrence may also account for cramping and intestinal symptoms in women who have endometriosis in places besides the intestines.

Furthermore, the same study had another odd conclusion: Women with endometriosis also had *reactive hypoglycemia* (a drop in blood sugar) during a glucose tolerance test, even though the women had normal insulin levels.

Two possible reasons for this conclusion are

✔ Women with endometriosis may be more sensitive to the actions of insulin than women without endometriosis.

✔ Nerves that help control the actions of the intestines may overreact to the amount of insulin present.

Eying where endometriosis attacks the large intestine

Endometriosis is more common in the large intestine and can show up there in many different ways. The following list shows the areas where endometriosis can invade your large intestines and the symptoms it causes.

✔ **The pelvic portion.** Endometriosis most often affects the pelvic portion, including the *sigmoid colon* (last section of the large intestine) and the rectum. Meanwhile, the *retroperitoneal* (the length of intestine that passes under the abdominal cavity covering, or peritoneum) part of the large intestine can be shielded from endometriosis by this peritoneum.

The definition of true large intestine endometriosis is the presence of deeply infiltrating endometrial-like glands and stroma more than 5 millimeters under the peritoneum. However, shallower endometriosis on the intestine can still cause symptoms as severe as the deeper disease.

✔ **The nerves.** Some studies have shown that *deep endometriosis* most often affects the area along the nerves in the large intestine, which may be the reason for the common symptoms of cramping and contractions of the intestines. These cramps and contractions are the cause of constipation and diarrhea that often accompany a patient's period.

✔ **The lumen.** When endometriosis penetrates deep into the intestine, it can bleed into the *lumen* (the open, interior area of the intestine that leads to the outside of your body) and cause bleeding with bowel movements. This bleeding can be bright red or darker in color, depending on the location of the endometriosis.

✔ **Near the uterus and cervix.** Pain during sex can also be a characteristic of large intestine endometriosis due to the proximity of the uterus and cervix to the large intestine (these organs actually touch each other). The movement of these organs during intercourse can cause irritation and stretching of adhesions between them. (Refer to Chapter 3 for more about the relationship of the intestine to the uterus and cervix.)

✔ **The junction with the small intestines.** Endometriosis near the junction of the small and large intestines can result in right-side pain that can imitate appendicitis. In fact, you can have endometriosis inside your appendix! Because the appendix is a relatively common place to find endometriosis and the symptoms are similar, some women have had an appendectomy because of the confusion. Adhesions can also attach the intestines to other nearby structures and cause pain there as well.

Differentiating between IBS and intestinal endometriosis

Two diseases that people easily confuse and doctors misdiagnose are *intestinal endometriosis* and *irritable bowel syndrome,* or IBS. A lot of people — up to one in five — have some symptoms of IBS, and one in ten doctor visits relates to its symptoms.

IBS can come and go, or it can become a chronic condition. The symptoms — bloating, cramping, diarrhea, and constipation — are similar to the symptoms of intestinal endometriosis, so you may not realize which problem you have.

IBS symptoms are more common in women and are more annoying during menses. Changes in the nerves that control the contractions of the intestinal wall may cause IBS. Endometriosis has these same problems, making the diagnosis between the two conditions difficult.

If you or your healthcare provider can't differentiate between the two problems, you may need a gastroenterology consult. Tests like a barium enema, colonoscopy, and upper-GI series with follow-through may give you a clue to the problem. A CAT scan or MRI may help to determine the cause of the problem, but are expensive and really don't add much information. Blood tests may not help either. Many of the same findings are present in both diseases.

If you don't have a diagnosis of endometriosis but do have symptoms that seem like IBS, your doctor may treat you for IBS through diet, stress reduction, and medications. No rule says you can't have more than one disease. If you already have endometriosis and then develop IBS-like symptoms, you may have both diseases (aren't you lucky!). The endometriosis may make your IBS worse, so do whatever you can (such as dietary and lifestyle changes) to control the IBS while dealing with your endometriosis.

Recognizing a different plan of attack in the small intestine

Small intestine endometriosis causes different symptoms than in the large intestine. The primary reason? The two parts of the intestine function in completely different ways. Although both are part of waste elimination, there are differences in what they do, how they do it, and even in their physical structure, nerves, and enzymes.

The main concern you have with endometriosis in the small intestine is bowel obstruction, which results in bloating and the inability to eat much food at one time. These symptoms may be due to the fact that the small intestine is, well, smaller. (Makes sense, doesn't it?) Because of these logistics, the small intestine has a greater chance for partial or complete obstruction of the lumen. This obstruction can cause very serious problems.

A lot of the large intestine is *fixed,* or immobile, behind the peritoneum. However, the small intestine isn't as *bound down,* or immobile. Because the small intestine is very long and freer to move around, the adhesive bands of endometriosis can restrict its movement, making it kink and bend around, much like a garden hose can be obstructed by bending on itself.

Diagnosing (and treating) intestinal endometriosis

Because endometriosis may not invade as deep as the mucosa, it's almost impossible to find during diagnostic tests, such as a barium enema or a colonoscopy. As a result, the best way to diagnose intestinal endometriosis is the best way to diagnose any endometriosis — surgically. But endometriosis on the intestine may be difficult to see during either *laparotomy* or *laparoscopy.* Both types of surgery have their advantages and disadvantages.

What are the main differences between the two surgeries in terms of diagnosing endometriosis in the intestines?

- **Laparotomy,** a more invasive surgery, involves a large incision through the abdomen. It has the advantage that the surgeon can *run the intestine,* or examine the entire length, and check all areas by sight and by touch. Sometimes the surgeon can't see a deeper disease but can feel it with trained hands. Also, the surgeon can do more extensive surgery at the same time if he determines the patient needs it.

- **Laparoscopy** is less invasive and generally has an easier recovery. Another advantage is that the scope magnifies the view by 1.5 to 2 times, so your surgeon can find a more subtle disease. But, seeing all the small intestine through the laparoscope is difficult, and feeling anything through the laparoscope is impossible. Another problem is that very few skilled surgeons can remove endometriosis from the intestine via laparoscopy, so a second surgery may be necessary.

Getting ready for a bowel prep

The phrase "This too shall pass" probably has no greater significance than when you're doing a bowel prep (a cleansing of the intestines) to reduce the risk of complications after the surgery. (And remember the dual meaning to this: It's going to pass physically *and* mentally.) So put your positive attitude hat on as we answer your questions about a bowel prep.

1. **Why do I have to do this?** Bowel preps empty your intestines of fecal material. Why? Not just to keep the surgeon clean during the procedure, although that's part of it. Stool can obscure the doctor's view during the procedure, it can increase the chance of infection after the procedure, and it can make a mess during the procedure. These are three darn good reasons for the bowel prep.

2. **How can I make this easier on myself beforehand?** Eat lightly for a few days before your prep, and avoid foods that are greasy and bulky. What's greasy and bulky? Foods like fried chicken. Eat less meat and dairy and more fruits and veggies. Also, don't plan any major events for the day of the prep. You won't be able to do much of anything — unless you can do it in the bathroom.

3. **What do I have to actually do?** Starting one or two days before surgery, you need to be on a liquid diet. You also need to drink a preparation that removes (via the usual route) every last bit of stool from your intestine.

4. **How do I drink this (awful) stuff?!?** Some people find the preparation easier to drink when it's chilled. Other people find they can get the taste out of their mouths with liquids, gum, or hard candy. (Make sure your doctor gives you the okay to use these "chasers.") Having a pleasant scent nearby may also help. If you have to, spray a whiff of a favorite scent on a handkerchief and hold the handkerchief under your nose while you drink.

5. **How can I make the bathroom a fun place?** You spend a lot of time in there for a day or two, so make it enjoyable. Scented candles, lots of books if you're a reader, and music can all help. Put out your best towels so you have something pretty to look at, and clean up the cobwebs and clutter so they don't drive you crazy every time you're in there.

Still, most of the time laparoscopy is the preferred method for diagnosis and treatment. Surgeons perform laparotomies only for special or troublesome cases. (We deal with surgical issues in more depth in Chapter 11, including answering the question whether you really need surgery.) If the endometriosis is only on the intestine's serosa (surface), your doctor can *excise* or *ablate* it (destroying the lesion by vaporizing, burning, denaturing, or otherwise destroying the abnormal tissue). Discuss these approaches with your doctor to be sure you're both comfortable with the choice you make.

If the endometriosis is deep and the surgeon can't simply remove or destroy only the abnormal tissue, the surgery involves entering the intestine. If your doctor thinks you have a real chance for endometriosis of the intestine and that he may have to operate on the large or small intestines, you have to do a *bowel prep,* a cleansing of the intestines, to reduce the risk of complications after the surgery. (Check out Chapter 11 for more on surgery and the nearby sidebar "Getting ready for a bowel prep" for more info.)

Removing damaged intestine when your deep intestine endometriosis is severe

If you have deep intestinal endometriosis or the intestine is injured while removing superficial disease, the surgeon may have to remove a part of the intestines. This is a fairly routine procedure in a controlled situation, and a bowel prep can make the surgery and your recovery much simpler. (Fortunately, only about 1 to 2 percent of women with endometriosis on the intestines need this type of surgery.)

When the surgeon anticipates and plans the removal of intestinal parts, he can perform a *primary anastomosis* (reattaching of the new intestinal ends with suture or staples) without a *colostomy* (an opening through the abdominal wall to remove waste) in most cases. And often a surgeon can repair small insults to the intestine wall (inadvertent or intentional) without removing sections of intestine and without need of a colostomy. These procedures, however, depend on the location of the involved intestine, blood supply, and healthiness of the tissue.

If the endometriosis has caused extensive scarring and/or inflammation of the intestinal wall, the best choice may be to remove this piece of intestine because the surgeon may not be able to determine the extent of tissue damage. But attempting reattachment at the same time in an unhealthy area may cause the intestine to break down, leading to leakage and severe complications. So even though you had a bowel prep, the surgeon may prefer to let the fresh ends of the intestine mature and heal before putting them back together.

In this case, the surgeon performs an interim procedure, a *diverting colostomy,* where the surgeon brings the end of the intestine (or a loop of intestine) up through the abdominal wall and sutures it in place. A bag is placed over the opening on the outside of the abdomen to collect the stool. Later, after the damaged section of intestine has had a chance to heal and be rid of the inflammation and compromised tissues, the surgeon can reverse the colostomy and reattach the intestine. Yes, doing so involves another surgery, but it prevents multiple surgeries and *peritonitis* (infection of the abdominal cavity) that can be life threatening. In most of these cases, a general surgeon may help your gynecologist.

Although the procedure of entering the intestines may sound simple, it's actually very involved, and the surgeon must be very careful. He must repair any compromised areas immediately and expertly. In many cases, he must remove whole sections of the intestine to insure that damaged and weakened areas don't cause future problems, including *necrosis* (essentially death) of remaining sections due to subsequent breakdown, infections, leakage of stool, and dysfunction of the intestine. When the surgeon must remove sections of the intestine, he also may perform a *temporary colostomy* (see the nearby sidebar, "Removing damaged intestine when your deep intestine endometriosis is severe"). Fortunately, only a small percent (1 to 2 percent) of patients with endometriosis on the intestine need extensive surgery with removal of part of the intestine.

In any event, when the surgeon removes endometriosis of the intestine, even when it's superficial, he must take great care to be sure not to compromise the integrity of the intestine, being very careful and meticulous to avoid severe complications. Be sure to discuss this procedure and its possible complications with your doctor.

Endometriosis and Your Urinary Tract: More Than Just Another Infection

Although the bladder is relatively near other organs in the pelvis, endometriosis in the urinary tract itself is fairly rare. (Check out Chapter 3 for a full discussion of these organs.) However, if you or your doctor suspects you have endometriosis in your urinary tract, then this section is for you. In this section, we take a closer look at endometriosis in the urinary tract by identifying some of the common symptoms, figuring out how to diagnose it, and naming the best treatment options.

Naming the main symptoms

Endometriosis is more likely to appear in the bladder than in the *ureters* (the tubes that take urine from the kidney to the bladder) or the kidneys, and the lower ureters are a more common site than the upper ureters. Symptoms for endometriosis in the urinary tract can include any of the following:

Painful urination

Pain with urination isn't unique to endometriosis; many problems, including bladder infection and *interstitial cystitis* (chronic bladder inflammation) can cause bladder pain. Furthermore, all bladder pains aren't alike. For example, bladder pain can feel like any or all of the following:

- ✔ Burning pain when you first start to urinate
- ✔ Pain at the end of urination, which can be sharp and knifelike
- ✔ Pain even when you're not urinating; a constant feeling of spasm or pressure in your bladder
- ✔ Feeling like you have to "go" all the time, even when you just went
- ✔ Tenderness over your pubic area related to your bladder
- ✔ Pain radiating up your back to your kidney

Endometriosis of the bladder can cause any of these preceding symptoms, which is why it can be hard to diagnose and treat. You may mistake many of your symptoms for urinary tract infections and may think your doctor can just prescribe an antibiotic.

However, you need a urine sample. Having a urine analysis and culture to check your urine for bacteria and other abnormalities is important, especially if you have seemingly endless urinary tract infections. Cultures will be negative for bacteria when you have endometriosis or interstitial cystitis — and antibiotics can do nothing to cure your symptoms. Unnecessary antibiotics can do more harm than good.

Blood in the urine during your period

Endometriosis in your bladder can cause blood in your urine. Blood in the urine isn't always visible to the naked eye. A large amount of blood can make your urine look cloudy or a shade of red, but you may only see small clots of blood in the bowl or on toilet paper after you wipe. If you have just a small or moderate amount of blood in your urine, you may not be able to see it (especially if you use colored toilet paper and your toilet bowl water is blue from the toilet bowl cleaner!). Here, a urine analysis can help find it.

Any time you have cloudy, dark, bloody, or scant urine, you should see your doctor for a urine test to provide a *clean catch* specimen. First clean the *urethra* (the tube leading from the bladder to the outside) and vaginal opening carefully with an antiseptic before urinating, and then let a small amount of urine out and catch the midstream urine in a cup. A simple dipstick urine analysis test can find pus, blood, sugar, bacteria, and other stuff in your urine.

If your doctor has any doubt about whether your urine sample is contaminated by improper cleaning, she may do a bladder catheterization. This procedure involves cleaning the urethra and vaginal opening with an antiseptic and then inserting a small tube called a catheter directly into your bladder, which prevents the bacteria in the vagina or on the skin from contaminating the urine specimen.

After obtaining your specimen, your doctor can order a urine culture, which tests for bacteria growth over a period of several days.

Other urinary symptoms

Endometriosis on the bladder can cause other urinary symptoms including the following:

- **Urinary frequency:** Endometriosis on the bladder can irritate the organ and cause you to urinate frequently. This symptom is unrelated to infection or IC but may be due to the inflammation caused by the endometriosis. You urinate more often than normal even though your bladder isn't full.

- **Urinary urgency:** Endometriosis can also cause you to feel a sudden need to urinate (and even to lose your urine). This is due to spasms that come suddenly and uncontrollably.

- **Urethral obstruction:** Endometriosis can grow around the urethra and compress it, much like running over your garden hose with a tire. This can lead to retention of urine or incomplete emptying.

Understanding a cystoscopy

The only way to diagnose the problems with your bladder may be with a *cystoscopy,* a procedure that allows a specialist to look inside your bladder and urethra. The procedure, which uses a very thin, lighted tube to examine and, sometimes, treat problems inside your urinary tract, can take place in the doctor's office, at a free-standing surgical center, or at the hospital. The location depends on how extensive your doctor expects the procedure to be and the anesthesia you'll need.

What should I expect during a cystoscopy?

Generally, you need no special preparation for a cystoscopy, unless you're having general anesthesia. In this case, you need to follow your anesthesiologist's instructions about not eating or drinking before the surgery. You'll have local anesthetic and/or intravenous sedation to make the procedure more comfortable. Usually you don't have to stay in the hospital overnight.

The lab will check your urine before the procedure to make sure you don't have an infection at the time. The procedure follows these easy steps:

1. **You lie on your back with your knees apart and your feet in footrests.**

2. **The doctor inserts the tip of the cystoscope into the urethra and then advances it up into the bladder.**

3. **The doctor first fills your bladder with saline or sterile water through a sterile catheter so he can examine all areas of the bladder.**

   This expansion can cause a feeling of urgency, which can be somewhat uncomfortable. Deep breathing and relaxing your pelvic muscles can help you through this part of the exam.

4. **You can empty your bladder as soon as the exam is over.**

   The whole exam usually takes less than 20 minutes. Afterwards you may feel slight stinging when you urinate, and you may notice a small amount of blood in your urine. These symptoms are normal.

However, you need to tell you doctor immediately if you have any of the following:

- Chills and/or fever
- Cloudy or foul smelling urine
- Dribbling of urine
- A lot of blood or clots in your urine
- Inability to urinate 8 hours after the procedure
- Mild symptoms lasting longer than 24 hours
- Severe pain

Try to drink enough liquids to urinate well every two hours after the procedure. A warm, moist washcloth over the urethra may feel soothing when you have pain. Ask your doctor about when you can take a warm bath. You may need to take an antibiotic for a few days to ward off infection. If your urethra is very swollen, you may need a catheter to drain your urine until the swelling subsides.

Why may I need a biopsy during cystoscopy?

Your doctor may decide to biopsy any suspicious-looking tissue inside the bladder or urethra. This involves removing a small piece of tissue from the bladder wall during the cystoscopy and then examining it under the microscope for evidence of endometriosis or other disease processes, like interstitial cystitis (see the nearby sidebar "Differentiating between interstitial cystitis and endometriosis in the bladder" in this chapter). The biopsy is relatively painless and can be very useful in the diagnosis. Afterwards, you may have some slight bleeding as with a regular cystoscopy.

Treating urinary tract endometriosis

Unfortunately, as with so many types of endometriosis, curing the disease in the urinary tract isn't possible. The goal of treatment is to decrease symptoms and prevent worsening of the disease. Your doctor tries to accomplish this with a nonsurgical approach, such as hormonal treatment and other medications, in most cases (see Chapter 10 for more info).

In severe cases of endometriosis of the bladder, your doctor can perform surgery to remove part of the bladder (called a *partial cystectomy*) or other involved areas. But, the implants are usually superficial inside the bladder or on the pelvic surface of it, so this procedure is rare. The endometriosis doesn't affect the bladder nearly as often as the intestines, and medical therapy seems to work well.

Differentiating between interstitial cystitis and endometriosis in the bladder

Interstitial cystitis (IC) is a complicated disease — many doctors feel it may actually be several diseases that can cause symptoms identical to those of endometriosis. IC is a chronic inflammation of the bladder affecting mostly women. Symptoms occur when the immune system allows the protective coating of the bladder to wear away in small areas, exposing the bladder wall to irritants. So, like endometriosis, IC may have an autoimmune component.

The protective coating, with the really long technical name *glycosaminoglycanmucus-mucin layer,* normally allows the urine to sit in the bladder for hours without causing any symptoms.

When this layer is missing, the underlying cells can become irritated. Although the bladder has no infection, the symptoms of painful urination with urgency and frequency are the same symptoms you may feel if you have a urinary tract infection.

The best way to differentiate between the two conditions is through a cystoscopy. If you have IC, your doctor can see pinpoint hemorrhages on the bladder wall during the cystoscopy. The effectiveness of treatment is still controversial, but medications and minor procedures are available.

More common is disease that has scarred the tissues around the ureter. This scar tissue can retract and actually kink and obstruct the ureter. This can lead to kidney problems and even loss of the kidney. In this extreme case, your doctor may advise the careful removal of the scar tissue to prevent any long-term kidney complications. This surgery is delicate and difficult, and your gynecologist may have a urologist assist.

Most people automatically assume that bladder pain or pain on urination is an infection. You may be tempted to treat yourself when you have bladder symptoms by taking any old antibiotics you have lying around the house. Doing so is a bad idea for a couple of reasons. First of all, you may not have a urinary tract infection at all. Second, even if you do have an infection, the antibiotic you're taking may not cure the specific bacteria that normally infect the bladder. The antibiotic may suppress symptoms just enough to make you think you're cured, but treating with the wrong antibiotic can actually escalate a bladder infection into a kidney infection by allowing the bacteria to continue to multiply.

Endometriosis in Your Lungs: Coughing, Chest Pain, and Breathing Problems

Endometriosis in your lungs isn't common, and it can be really hard to diagnose because your doctor won't think of it when you come in coughing up blood. You may not even think to tell him you're having your period, and he's unlikely to ask.

Diagnosing endometriosis in the lungs, or *thoracic endometriosis,* requires an inquiring mind. Even if you know you have endometriosis elsewhere, you may think that relating it to your lung problems is too far fetched. Thoracic endometriosis can cause many different symptoms, all seemingly unrelated to your pelvis. But suspecting thoracic endometriosis is the first step to diagnosing it, and you may be more likely to make the connection than your doctor, especially after reading this book.

Thoracic endometriosis causes different symptoms, depending on the location of the lesions. Endometriosis can be either in the lung tissue (the *parenchymal* tissue), or in the lining of the lung (the *pleural* tissue). Endometriosis is about five times more common in the pleura than in the parenchymal tissue.

This section looks at how endometriosis manifests itself in the different lung tissues and how your doctor can diagnose endometriosis in your lungs.

Endometriosis in the lining of the lung (pleura)

More than 90 percent of cases of pleural endometriosis are on the right side. Often small holes are in the *diaphragm,* the muscular membrane that separates the abdominal and thoracic cavities. Most patients with pleural endometriosis also have pelvic endometriosis. One theory is that endometriosis travels through the small holes in the diaphragm. When endometriosis is in the pleural tissue, the most common symptoms are

✔ Difficulty breathing

✔ Pain

✔ Pain with breathing motions

✔ *Pneumothorax* (collapsed lung)

✔ Pleural effusion (fluid on the lung)

✔ Shortness of breath

Endometriosis in the lung tissue (parenchyma)

Parenchymal endometriosis, an uncommon disease, has a completely different course and probably a different way of spreading than pleural endometriosis. Most patients with parenchymal endometriosis cough up blood during their period but don't have pain or trouble breathing.

Also, patients with parenchymal endometriosis often don't have pelvic endometriosis but do have a history of pelvic surgery or vaginal delivery. *Note:* One theory of how endometriosis arrives in the lung tissue is that the endometrial cells spread through the blood vessels as *emboli* (small clots that travel through the blood stream). (You may have heard about these clots from varicose veins in the legs causing severe problems!)

Diagnosing thoracic endometriosis

The key to diagnosis of thoracic endometriosis is suspicion that it's there. A chest X-ray, CAT scan, or MRI may help visualize the lesions. A bronchoscopy or thoracoscopy with biopsy may help to differentiate between endometriosis and other diseases, including malignancy. These procedures are usually performed on an outpatient basis, depending on how extensive the surgery becomes. A pulmonologist or thoracic surgeon performs these tests for you.

Treating thoracic endometriosis

Thoracic endometriosis can be treated with hormonal suppression or with surgical removal of scar tissue and endometrial lesions via thorascopy (laparoscopy of the pleural space and thorax). (Check out Chapters 10 and 11 for more info about drugs and surgical treatments.)

Endometriosis in Your Brain: Rare, but Possible

The idea of endometriosis ending up in the place farthest from its initial source may sound impossible, but it's true — endometriosis can, in rare cases, end up in your brain. (So no matter what some people think, endometriosis is definitely *not* just in your head.) Obviously, more than retrograde menstruation must send endometrial tissue all the way up to your head, so endometrial tissue must arrive there via one of the other theories of endometriosis transmission. (See Chapter 4 for the theories on how endometriosis travels all over your body.)

Cerebellar endometriosis, or endometriosis in your brain, can cause headaches, seizures, or, in very rare cases, bleeding in the brain. The diagnosis may be aided by CAT scan or MRI. A *spinal tap* (placing a small needle into your back to get spinal fluid out) may show blood or endometrial cells. Cases of endometriosis in the brain are rare, so standard treatments don't exist. Brain removal usually isn't an option! Most of the time, doctors prescribe medical treatments, such as hormone-suppressing drugs (see Chapter 10) to decrease symptoms.

Chapter 7

Endometriosis and Infertility: Having a Baby (Or Trying To)

· ·

In This Chapter

▶ Understanding the link between endometriosis and infertility

▶ Overcoming ovarian challenges

▶ Utilizing the uterus

▶ Following up on fallopian tube problems

▶ Taking advantage of diagnostic testing

▶ Deciding to take the first steps to treat infertility

▶ Contemplating surgery

▶ Making the big decision: In vitro fertilization

▶ Tying miscarriages to endometriosis

· ·

*I*f you have endometriosis, you may already know that many women with endometriosis have trouble getting pregnant. But take heart; although up to 40 percent of women with endometriosis have trouble getting pregnant, many techniques, from medication to surgery to in vitro fertilization, are available to help you have the baby you want.

In this chapter, we discuss how endometriosis can affect your fertility, from preventing ovulation to blocking your tubes. We then look at how you can get a diagnosis for infertility and what your treatment options are, including whether in vitro fertilization is a reasonable option. Finally we talk about ways endometriosis increases the risk of miscarriage and what you can do about it.

Figuring Out Why Endometriosis Is a Major Cause of Infertility

Many women find out they have endometriosis *because* they've been unsuccessful at trying to get pregnant. They never mentioned the menstrual cramps, diarrhea, and pain that come with every period to their doctor (probably because their mom told them those symptoms were just part of being a woman). But now, after six months of trying to have a baby, they're beginning to suspect that mom's advice ("Just relax and you'll get pregnant!") may not be all that accurate.

How big a deal is endometriosis when you're trying to have a baby? Endometriosis can be a very big deal, depending on where it is and how much you have. Are there ways to overcome endometriosis and have that bundle of joy you dream of? Yes, but it's not always easy — or cheap. But, first we give you a quick review of the normal steps to pregnancy so our discussion of endometriosis and infertility is easy to understand. We also look at the number of women with fertility problems due to endometriosis — you'll see that you're not alone!

A quick overview: The steps to pregnancy

Pregnancy may seem like a sure bet each month you try, but even when you have everything in place, you may not get pregnant because Mother Nature isn't as efficient as people think. The fact is, even with the proper ingredients and timing, women under age 35 have only a 17 percent chance of becoming pregnant each month. That means the average woman will conceive less than one out of five cycles. If you're older, your chances each month are even less; eventually you reach menopause, where the chance is zero.

The following steps show the normal path leading to pregnancy:

1. **A woman's menstrual cycle begins each month on the first day the outer layer of the endometrium is shed as menstrual flow.**

2. **This occurrence signals the start of the first phase of the cycle, the *proliferative* or *follicular* phase.**

    The hormone estrogen (the most active one being 17-beta-estradiol) causes the growth or proliferation of eggs containing follicles (check out the sidebar in this chapter, "Creating a good egg," for more info).

3. **The ovaries start to form many early eggs, or *antral follicles*.**

   One antral follicle becomes dominant (more than one is rare, but twins do happen!), and this dominant follicle produces more and more estrogen.

4. **The endometrium starts to thicken in preparation to house a future embryo.**

5. **As soon as the dominant follicle grows enough to become a mature egg, a woman ovulates — that is, the ovary releases the egg to be fertilized — and this egg is picked up by the fallopian tube.**

   This is an essential step to getting pregnant because you can't get pregnant if your egg never gets out of the starting gate and into the fallopian tubes to meet the sperm of its dreams!

6. **The egg enters the fallopian tube and gets fertilized by a friendly sperm.**

7. **The fertilized egg floats gently all the way down the fallopian tube without getting stuck or otherwise sidetracked.**

   Although embryos can — and, unfortunately, do — implant in the fallopian tube, this is never a workable arrangement (the tube is so narrow that a six-pound baby will never fit!). The tube can rupture if the pregnancy grows too long there, with life-threatening consequences for Mom. (We discuss ectopic pregnancy later in this chapter.)

8. **After ovulation, the uterine lining changes again under the influence of progesterone from the corpus luteum (the leftover shell of the follicle) to provide support for an embryo, should one show up.**

If anything interferes with, blocks, or prevents one of these steps, pregnancy can't occur or early miscarriage may occur. And if no embryo arrives, hormone levels drop, and the lining begins to shed again as in Day 1 of the cycle. Unfortunately, endometriosis can interfere with the perfect progression of these steps in many ways.

Each stage of endometriosis (usually noted as Stage I through IV, with IV the most severe) can affect different aspects of fertility. These variables make it very difficult to accurately predict your fertility. (Check out Chapter 9 for more on what the different stages mean.)

(If you're chomping at the bit to read more about fertility and all aspects of reproduction, check out *Fertility For Dummies* by Jackie Meyers-Thompson and Sharon Perkins, RN, [Wiley].)

Whose fertility is affected by endometriosis?

Although you may feel like you're the only one in the world not able to get pregnant, you're not alone. Having trouble getting pregnant is a major concern for women with endometriosis. The following statistics show the widespread effects of this disease on infertility:

✔ About one in six couples suffers from infertility. That's a lot of people — about 6 million people (2 to 3 million couples) in the United States alone.

✔ Endometriosis is responsible for around 30 percent of these infertility cases.

✔ Thirty percent of laparoscopic surgeries for unexplained infertility result in a diagnosis of endometriosis.

✔ About 40 percent of women with endometriosis have some degree of infertility.

How long should I try to get pregnant on my own?

Most people start trying to get pregnant with the attitude that it will occur quickly, like five minutes after they consider the idea! Unfortunately, becoming pregnant isn't easy for many women with endometriosis — although, if your endometriosis is mild, you may get pregnant just as fast as the next guy (or girl, in this case). How long you should try before seeing your doctor depends somewhat on your age and circumstances, but the following guidelines may be helpful:

✔ **Under age 35:** After one year. (This assumes you have the patience to wait a year. We don't know many people who can wait this long!)

✔ **Over age 35:** After six months. (Ditto the above.)

✔ **Over age 40:** Make an appointment before you start trying, or as soon as possible. You don't have as much time to lose, and you may want to discuss other considerations with your doctor.

If you know you have mild endometriosis, see your doctor sooner than the guidelines suggest. And, if you have moderate or severe endometriosis or suspect you have, see your doctor before you start trying because

✔ You may need help getting pregnant.

✔ Your risk of problems (such as an ectopic pregnancy) is significant.

However, the news on pregnancy and endometriosis isn't all bad. Consider that

- As many as 70 percent of women with minimal or mild endometriosis and infertility do conceive within three years without any therapy.
- Studies show that surgical treatment of minimal or mild endometriosis increases pregnancy rates even more.
- In one study, more than 40 percent of women with moderate or severe endometriosis became pregnant after surgery.
- In vitro fertilization (IVF) has helped many women conceive, even in previously hopeless cases. (Check out "Is In Vitro Fertilization [IVF] Necessary?" later in this chapter for more info about IVF.)

Endometriosis In, Around, and On Your Ovaries

Ovaries are one of the most common sites for endometriosis. Endometriosis here can gum up the works, so to speak, and interfere with pregnancy by

- Keeping an egg from developing normally
- Destroying much of the ovary, which also destroys eggs
- Preventing an egg from releasing by
  - Encasing it with endometrial tissue and scar tissue
  - Interfering with the normal mechanism of egg release
- Causing an immune response that's detrimental to fertilization

Ovarian endometriosis was the first endometriosis to be seen microscopically, and it can develop on the surface of the ovary or bury itself deep inside. This section looks more closely at how endometriosis affects the ovaries and causes infertility.

Creating a good egg

The first step in pregnancy is the development of a mature egg that's capable of becoming a baby. This step seems simple enough, considering the number of people on this earth, but it's an extremely complex process that begins when *you're* a fetus in your mother's womb. Consider the following:

- All the eggs you'll ever have are present and accounted for by Week 20 gestation (about halfway through a normal pregnancy). Unlike men, you will never produce any more *gametes* (eggs in you, sperm in him) and you will lose all of them by menopause.

- The eggs live in early shells called *primordial follicles.* The eggs are in a sort of suspended animation and don't change until puberty and the call to ovulation.

- Nature is never perfect. In fact, it's far from perfect, and makes up for this imperfection by sheer numbers. So men produce millions of sperm over and over to get a few good men. But women never make more eggs — you're stuck with the ones you have (which is one of the reasons only about one in five ovulations results in a pregnancy).

- When you begin menstruating, a number of hormonal changes happen in the ovary to stimulate a bunch of primordial follicles to develop. Early in your reproductive life, hundreds of primordial follicles appear, and, as you near menopause, you have fewer and fewer to choose from. But, no matter how many of these follicles begin each cycle, only one (with a few exceptions, as in fraternal twins) continues to develop past the first few days. The rest die off, never to be seen again.

- Each month, the dominant follicle interacts with the surrounding ovarian tissue until it is ready to be fertilized. On the final steps toward maturation

  The egg has the correct number of chromosomes.

  The *cytoplasm* (the liquid around the nucleus) is capable of orchestrating the penetration of the sperm and the first few cell divisions.

In menopause, no eggs remain (or at least no more that can function normally), and a woman stops producing estrogen and progesterone. There's no turning back; the chances of releasing a good egg (or any egg) are over — or extremely slim.

Understanding the link between endometriosis and egg development

Endometriosis has four classifications of severity, from Stage I to Stage IV (see Chapter 9 for more on endometriosis staging), and different stages impact egg development in different ways.

Early-stage endometriosis and your ovaries

Early-stage disease, Stage I (minimal) and Stage II (mild) endometriosis, seems to cause different problems related to egg production:

- ✔ Even with in vitro fertilization (IVF), implantation rates are lower than normal.

- ✔ Early-stage endometriosis seems to cause poor embryo quality, which is related to either poor egg quality or poor sperm quality.

Stage I and II endometriosis appear to have a worse effect on egg development than Stage III and IV disease. But this theory doesn't make sense! Why are the earlier stages worse on the eggs? The following explanations are possible:

- ✔ The early stages are very active with growth of the endometrial tissue and production of destructive proteins, enzymes, and cells. These toxic substances and cells may have a detrimental effect on the development of the egg.

- ✔ The toxic substances may damage the egg after it's released into the pelvic cavity, before or after fertilization.

- ✔ The later stages of endometriosis are mostly *burnt out* (no longer growing) and are much less metabolically active than the earlier stages.

This situation isn't hopeless, however. One of the basic treatments for infertility is *superovulation,* stimulating drugs to help the follicles produce more/better eggs. (Check out "Starting with Simple Treatments" later in this chapter for more info.)

Severe endometriosis and your ovaries

Endometriosis is classified as *severe* depending on the amount of endometriosis you have, where it's located, and how far it's advanced (see Chapter 9 for how endometriosis is staged). Severe endometriosis, typically Stages III (moderate) and Stage IV (severe), decreases your chance of getting pregnant in the following ways:

- ✔ Distortion of the anatomy (blocking tubes, causing scar tissue)
- ✔ Loss of *fimbriae,* the fingerlike projections that guide the egg into the fallopian tubes
- ✔ Loss of ovarian volume (which decreases the number of eggs)

These problems don't mean pregnancy is impossible. Studies have shown that an *embryo* (fertilized egg) implanted via IVF into the uterus (thereby bypassing the fallopian tubes and fimbriae) of a woman with severe disease has the same chance of pregnancy as in women without endometriosis.

Processing how endometriosis destroys ovarian tissue

Researchers and doctors know that endometriosis can hinder egg development, especially in early stages of the disease. But when a woman has the late-stage disease (which is metabolically less active), why is achieving pregnancy still hard?

One major reason for this problem is the loss of *ovarian reserve* (the medical term for decreased number of eggs). You only have a finite number of eggs to last your whole reproductive life (check out the sidebar "Creating a good egg" in this chapter). If that number decreases for any reason, you may run out earlier than usual and have premature menopause. This decreased ovarian reserve leaves you with fewer good eggs — possibly no good eggs — for a pregnancy.

How does endometriosis decrease ovarian reserve, causing you to lose eggs? In simple terms, the advancing process of endometriosis destroys the ovarian tissue. The following steps indicate this process:

1. **Endometriosis implants on the surface of the ovary (not inside).**

2. **The misplaced endometrial tissue begins its monthly growth and shedding.**

The repeated growth and bleeding on the surface of the ovary causes an inflammatory response that releases toxins and irritants that begin to produce scar tissue around the endometrial implants.

3. **The endometrial implants are encased in this scar tissue.**

   The implants follow the path of least resistance and grow into the ovary instead of spreading over the surface.

4. **The destructive process literally eats away the area of the ovary that houses the primordial follicles, leaving you with less ovarian tissue (and thus fewer follicles).**

Encountering endometriomas (chocolate cysts)

Scar tissue that covers the surface of endometrial implants on the ovary is tough and fibrous. As this endometriosis spreads across the ovary, it takes the path of least resistance by growing into the softer *stroma* (the inside) of the ovary. As a result, chocolate cysts, or *endometriomas,* form from the surface of the ovary inwards. (The term *chocolate* refers to the brown-colored liquid made of old blood and tissue that's inside the cyst.)

These cysts of endometriosis aren't true cysts. ***Note:*** A normal cyst is filled with fluid from the lining of a structure. The walls of an endometrioma, however, are different because they consist of fibrous tissue, inflammatory material, and endometrial tissue — none of which produce fluid.

As the endometrioma expands, the following process occurs:

1. **The endometrioma squeezes out and compresses nearby normal ovarian tissue.**

2. **Because the normal ovarian tissue has nowhere to go, it stops functioning and may eventually die.**

3. **When ovarian tissue stops functioning, it disrupts the normal hormonal environment of the ovary, which can then affect the menstrual cycle and cause an early menopause.**

Dr. K had a young patient with problems of infertility but no other complaints. On examination, he discovered huge endometriomas on each ovary. These cysts were so large that this 28-year-old woman had only a thin layer of ovary with virtually no ovarian tissue. She never did get pregnant.

Losing ovarian tissue during surgery

Ovarian tissue can also be lost as a result of surgery. Any time a surgeon tries to remove endometriosis or the consequences of the disease (adhesions and other scarring), the surgery can harm the ovary.

When a surgeon attempts to remove adhesions that glue the ovary to the intestines, fallopian tube, or uterus, he must take great care to protect all of these structures. Unfortunately, if a structure has to be sacrificed, it's usually the ovary because injury to the ovary doesn't cause dire results to your health. On the other hand, injury to the other structures can lead to bleeding, life-threatening infection, or ectopic pregnancy. The prudent surgeon is usually conservative and doesn't risk intestinal, bladder, or tubal damage.

No matter how careful a doctor is, the ovary inevitably loses some pieces along with the chocolate cyst because just the process of cutting into the ovary to remove the cyst wall and its contents invariably damages some of the ovary. And even in the best scenario (when the surgeon removes no tissue), suturing the ovary back together destroys some of the ovary.

Losing even a small amount of ovarian tissue results in decreased ovarian reserve and possible infertility. Ask your doctor what method he prefers to use in surgery and why (check out Chapter 11 for different surgical methods). Let him explain to you the pros and cons of all the options. In the end, it's your body and you have the final say.

Looking at luteinized unruptured follicle syndrome (LUF)

For whatever reason, women with endometriosis are more likely to have a problem with egg release and infertility due to luteinized unruptured follicle syndrome (LUF).

An egg that never leaves the ovary can never be fertilized and find its way to the uterus. Some women with endometriosis may not release the egg from the ovary, even though everything may be going swimmingly (no, wait, that's sperm). In other words,

1. **The egg develops to maturity (on its own or with the help of fertility drugs).**

2. **The levels of estrogen rise appropriately, the luteinizing hormone (LH) surges (again, either naturally or with help), and progesterone rises.**

3. **Just when everything's looking great, nothing happens!**

   The egg stays right where it is, in the ovary.

If your doctor doesn't do an ultrasound after you ovulate, he may miss the egg's lack of movement. Because doctors usually monitor estrogen and progesterone, these hormones may still rise appropriately, fooling your doctor into thinking all systems are *go*. An ultrasound may even show a normal-size follicle, but a follow-up test a few days later still shows that the follicle hasn't shrunk as it should.

The reason for LUF is unclear. However, the following are possible causes:

✔ The scarring and adhesions on and around the ovary can make it impossible for the egg to get out of its follicle, as if it's encased in concrete.

Normally follicle cells near the ovary's surface dissolve the layers surrounding the egg so the egg can flow out with the follicular fluid. Hormonally everything happens just as it should — but the egg can't escape.

Surgery to clear these adhesions and scar tissue may help in these cases. IVF, which removes the egg from the follicle with a needle, may also be successful.

✔ Endometriosis may interfere with the complicated processes in the surface of the ovary that allow the egg to rupture and escape.

✔ Inflammatory reactions may interfere with the interaction of all the above complicated processes.

Interfering with a Good Uterine Environment

Developing a good egg, having it fertilize, and making sure it journeys down the tube to the uterus is only half the battle. As soon as the fertilized egg gets to the uterus, it has to successfully implant and grow. Endometriosis has several ways of preventing an embryo from implanting after it reaches the uterus. This section takes a closer look at those ways.

Checking out other hormonal problems: Luteal phase defect

Your menstrual period usually arrives 14 days after ovulation, unless you're pregnant. A condition called *luteal phase defect* (LPD, *luteal* referring to the time after ovulation) can cause your period to arrive sooner than 14 days. This shortened luteal phase means the embryo doesn't have time to implant well and results in an early miscarriage.

A shortage of progesterone can cause LPD. Ideally, the leftover follicle shell (the *corpus luteum*) from the developed egg generates progesterone after you ovulate. But, when the follicle generates too little progesterone, the result is a shorter time between ovulation and the start of your next period.

Progesterone plays important roles in helping a new pregnancy take root:

✓ It changes your uterine lining to make it into a nourishing place for an embryo to implant.

✓ It affects the appearance of receptors for implantation of the embryo. (These receptors make it possible for the embryo to attach to the endometrium and burrow in for the long haul, so to speak.)

The receptors are present for only a short time and must be there when the embryo floats by. If they're not present or the embryo's timing is off, pregnancy can't occur.

Why doesn't a corpus luteum make enough progesterone? A couple of possibilities are

✓ Endometriosis may affect the ovary's ability to produce normal amounts of both estrogen and progesterone, just as it affects the egg's maturation. (See "Understanding the link between endometriosis and egg development" in this chapter for additional information on egg maturation and endometriosis.)

✓ Endometriosis can somehow decrease the corpus luteum's ability to make enough progesterone at the right time.

Noting the chemical effects of endometriosis

Endometriosis can have serious chemical effects on *peritoneal fluid* (the fluid that accumulates in the abdominal cavity) and other parts of the reproductive tract. These chemical changes can make fertilization and implantation difficult. Because the peritoneal fluid is in constant contact with the ovaries and fallopian tubes, any toxic chemicals from the fluid can affect the ovaries and tubes, as well as the eggs, sperm, and embryo.

Some of the possible effects from toxic chemicals include

✓ Peritoneal fluid that interferes with sperm motility or movement.

✓ An overproduction of prostaglandins, especially Prostaglandin E2.

An excess of prostaglandins may interfere with their assistance in the fertilization and implantation of the embryo. Prostaglandins also cause uterine contractions that may interfere with embryo transport and implantation.

> ✔ An overproduction of white blood cells and immunoglobulins in the peritoneal fluid.
>
> Although your body's white cells make *immunoglobulins* to help protect you from infection and other diseases, an excess of these immunologically active cells and proteins may damage normal tissue.

Evaluating enzyme abnormalities

Women with endometriosis appear to have a number of genetic enzyme abnormalities that may allow endometriosis to develop and attach more easily where it doesn't belong (see Chapter 4 for more about genes and endometriosis).

One recent study found that some women with endometriosis-related infertility lack an enzyme necessary for an embryo to implant. The enzyme holds a molecule called *L-selectin* to the uterine wall. Without L-selectin in place at the proper time of the menstrual cycle, an embryo can't attach to the uterus and grow.

Messing with Your Fallopian Tubes

A blocked fallopian tube is like a dead-end road; your egg isn't going anywhere. Fallopian tubes are, unfortunately, common sites for endometriosis; the disease can block the tubes anywhere from the opening at the top to the bottom near the uterus. And blocking an egg from the uterus or the sperm from the egg pretty much prevents a healthy pregnancy.

In this section, we focus on the fallopian tubes to see how endometriosis can block the tubes and cause infertility. We also discuss a serious concern that endometriosis can cause — the ectopic pregnancy.

Adhesions tangle your fallopian tubes

A body's inflammatory response to endometrial implants can cause *adhesions,* or scar tissue, that really snarl up your fallopian tubes. Common sites for *paratubal* (around the tube) adhesions to form and, as a result, interfere with fertilization or egg/embryo transport are

✔ By the fimbriae (at the ovarian end of the tube). When the fimbriae become entangled in adhesions, the tube has trouble picking up the egg after ovulation.

✔ Around the outside of the tube (causing the tubes to stick to the uterus, pelvic wall, or intestine).

✔ Inside the tube itself, making it difficult for an egg to get through the tube to the uterus or the sperm to get to the egg.

Blocked tubes can cause ectopic pregnancy

The word *ectopic* means *outside*. So an ectopic pregnancy is outside the uterus and usually, but not always, inside the fallopian tube. Very rarely, ectopic pregnancies can implant in the abdomen or in the ovary itself, although approximately 95 percent implant in the fallopian tubes.

The damage that endometriosis does to the fimbriae and the tubes in general greatly increases the risk of ectopic pregnancy. Damage to the fimbriae or tubes can cause the following potentially dangerous scenarios:

✔ The disease can inhibit egg pick-up so the egg never gets into the tube.

If the egg doesn't get into the tube, it can't get to the uterus. If sperm manage to reach the egg, the fertilized egg can implant in the abdominal cavity or even in the ovary. These cases are very rare, but they do happen.

✔ Adhesions around the tube can cause kinking. This kinking may cause partial obstruction somewhere in the tube so that the fertilized egg gets stuck in the tube. *Note:* The sperm are a thousand times smaller than an egg so they can get through these narrowed areas.

If you have a blocked tube, you may end up with an ectopic pregnancy in any of the locations shown in Figure 7-1.

Your uterus is the only part of your body that's capable of carrying a pregnancy. No other area has the supporting structures to allow the fetus to draw nutrients from you without doing you harm. When a pregnancy implants somewhere other than the uterus, it almost invariably results in a rupture of the structure and hemorrhage, which can be fatal. Ectopic pregnancies always require medical or surgical removal.

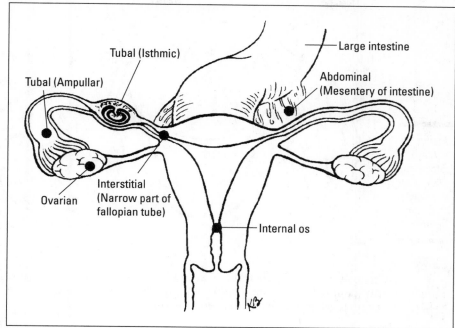

Figure 7-1:
Endometriosis can cause ectopic pregnancies in these possible sites.

Labels in figure:
Tubal (Isthmic)
Tubal (Ampullar)
Large intestine
Abdominal (Mesentery of intestine)
Ovarian
Interstitial (Narrow part of fallopian tube)
Internal os

Partially blocking tubes are bad too

Sometimes endometriosis doesn't block the tube altogether; it may create a *hydrosalpinx* (a chronically dilated, swollen tube). See Figure 7-2.

The *hydrosalpinx* can fill with fluid that is toxic to embryos. (The fluid is a result of endometriosis's inflammatory process and is full of *endotoxins,* that is, inflammatory proteins, white blood cells, and other harmful substances.) If the end of the tube that connects with the uterus is open, even a little, the fluid from the tubes can drip down into the uterus. (See Chapter 2 for more about hydrosalpinx.)

This toxic fluid makes embryo implantation difficult, even if an embryo does reach the uterus. Even if the embryo does implant, this poisonous fluid can increase the risk of miscarriage. (Check out "Miscarriage and Endometriosis: Is There a Connection?" later in this chapter.)

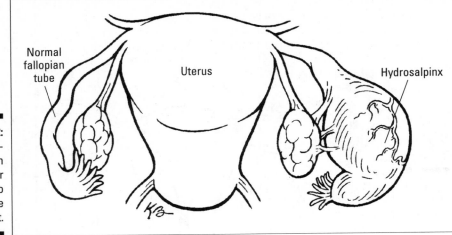

Normal fallopian tube

Uterus

Hydrosalpinx

Figure 7-2:
A hydro-salpinx can affect your ability to become pregnant.

Because these fluid-filled tubes aren't likely to be useful for getting pregnant, your doctor may recommend removing them altogether. Of course, your only option to get pregnant at that point is IVF — or a miracle.

Diagnosing Infertility Caused by Endometriosis

Infertility for any reason can make the road to pregnancy rocky — emotionally, physically, and financially. Before embarking on that road, you want to know all you can about the landmines along the way. Finding the right person to help you is your first step.

This section first identifies the importance of seeing a specialist in order to get a correct diagnosis (see Chapter 9 for more on tests used to diagnose endometriosis). This section also looks at the different tests you may undergo in order to reach a diagnosis of infertility.

Seeing an infertility specialist

If you haven't become pregnant within a reasonable time (see the sidebar, "How long should I try to get pregnant on my own?" in this chapter to find out what a reasonable time is), you need to make an appointment with a doctor. Most people start with their gynecologist (GYN) or their family doctor.

Is it absolutely necessary to see a specialist? That depends on your age, degree of endometriosis, pregnancy history, and personal preference. (Many women under the age of 45 don't have a GYN, although they should.) Some women want to go right to the big guns — the specialist. Even though consulting with a specialist may not be necessary, this decision may help a woman feel like she's doing all she can. If you feel this way, by all means, see a specialist.

Your GYN may be able to help you with the initial diagnosis and treatment. (See Chapter 8 for tips on finding a doctor you can work with.) No matter what type of doctor you decide to see, she'll most likely suggest doing some diagnostic tests. The following sections describe these diagnostic tests (some overlap with tests in Chapter 9, but the tests in this chapter measure infertility). Although some of the tests may be simple blood tests or imaging studies, like ultrasounds or fluoroscopy, other tests are more invasive and uncomfortable. But all of them help ascertain the reason for infertility and guide your doctor toward the most direct treatment and the shortest road to a pregnancy.

Drawing and testing blood

Nobody likes to have blood tests. (But usually men are the ones who turn pale and fall over.) Your family physician or GYN may suggest some blood work early in your treatment. Or, she may defer to a specialist and only do Pap smears and cultures.

However, one of your doctors should look for clues in your blood. You doctor may order a blood test that checks for the following:

- ✔ **Elevated sedimentation rates,** which indicate infection or inflammation
- ✔ **Ca-125,** a protein, which possibly comes from endometriosis
- ✔ **Abnormal thyroid results,** which may lead to a search for related, possibly autoimmune, problems, such as endometriosis
- ✔ **A mature egg and progesterone** via estradiol and progesterone testing at various times of the cycle
- ✔ **Ovaries damaged from endometriosis and your ovarian reserve** via an FSH and estradiol draw early in your cycle
- ✔ **Luteinizing (producing progesterone as a result of changes in the follicle cells) too early or indications of LUF** via LH and progesterone testing (see "Checking out other hormonal problems: Luteal phase defect" in this chapter)

Whatever the findings of your tests, blood work is a mainstay of fertility diagnosis and treatment. Your doctor will order repeat tests until she's sure your treatments are appropriate for your problem.

Debating the endometrial biopsy

An endometrial biopsy can be an uncomfortable but easy test. The doctor slides a small tube through the cervix that, by gentle suction or scraping, removes a small piece of the endometrium. This test takes place near the end of your menstrual cycle to see whether your endometrial lining has developed normally.

Abnormalities can suggest a luteal phase defect or other rarer problems. The value of endometrial biopsies remains controversial, so some doctors no longer do this test. But, because the debate continues, listen to your doctor's recommendations. (Check out Chapter 9 for more on biopsies.)

Having a hysterosalpingogram (HSG)

Don't let this long medical word scare you away from this test. This mouthful of letters refers to an X-ray test of your uterus and fallopian tubes with dye injected into your uterus. If the dye exits the top of the fallopian tubes, the tubes are open (see Figure 7-3). However, your tubes may not be blocked even if the dye doesn't spill out — sometimes the tubes can go into a spasm from the dye and only appear to be blocked.

If the uterus contains fibroids, adhesions, polyps, or anything else that shouldn't be there, the dye can't go to those spots, so they're visible on the X-ray. In addition, a tube with hydrosalpinx will appear dilated and swollen. The HSG, however, can't evaluate your ovaries or other parts of your pelvis and can't see adhesions or endometriosis.

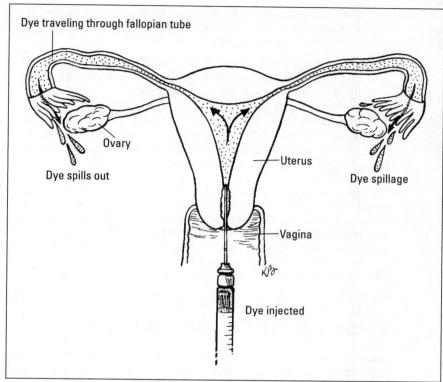

Dye traveling through fallopian tube

Ovary

Dye spills out

Uterus

Dye spillage

Vagina

Dye injected

Figure 7-3:
Dye injected into the uterus spills out of the fallopian tubes during an HSG if there are no uterine or tubal abnormalities.

If your doctor orders an HSG, you can expect the following to happen:

1. **You lie down on an exam table in the *lithotomy* position (legs up in stirrups).**

2. **Your doctor places a speculum in your vagina.**

3. **Your doctor gently cleans your cervix with betadine or another sterile solution.**

4. **Your doctor places a *cannula* (a small tube) in the opening of the cervix to inject the dye into the uterus.**

The dye may have an iodine base, so if you're allergic to iodine, you should avoid this test; your doctor may perform a *sonohysterogram* in its place (see the next section).

5. **Your doctor injects the dye and takes a photograph that shows the outline of the uterus and the fallopian tubes, including the spill of the dye into the pelvis if the tubes are open.**

Schedule an HSG after your period has ended but before you ovulate to avoid interfering with a possible pregnancy. HSG takes 30 to 60 minutes and is an outpatient procedure, usually without any anesthetic. HSGs generally take place in a surgery center or in the hospital.

Your doctor may recommend you take an NSAID, such as ibuprofen, an hour before the procedure because cramping during and immediately after the HSG is normal. You may also have a small amount of bleeding for a day or two, but report any heavy bleeding, fever, or extreme weakness to your doctor right away. Infection is the main complication of HSG, but it occurs in less than 1 percent of cases. You can go back to your normal activities after an HSG, although some doctors recommend avoiding sex for a few days afterward.

Opting for a sonohysterogram

Your doctor may choose a *sonohysterogram* or *saline infusion sonohysterogram* (SIS — an ultrasound that tracks normal saline that is injected into the uterus) over an HSG (if you're allergic to iodine dye, these are safer). Sonohysterograms may not give enough information about the fallopian tubes, but they're excellent for diagnosing problems in the uterus. If your doctor has scheduled a laparoscopy (check Chapter 11 for more info), the SIS may be all you need. You may have this test in your doctor's office, and side effects are similar to those for the HSG.

Doing a hysteroscopy

If your doctor wants to look directly into your uterus, he may suggest a hysteroscopy. Many doctors can perform these in their office. In this procedure, the doctor passes a small telescope through the cervix. Your uterus is distended with saline or carbon dioxide so that the entire uterus is clearly visible. You may have a local anesthetic and a sedative, such as valium, for the procedure.

If the doctor sees adhesions or other problems, she may be able to remove them with small instruments that she inserts through the scope. For more extensive work, you'll need to go to a hospital.

Probing with ultrasounds

Doctors use pelvic ultrasounds to evaluate infertility. Ultrasound, which uses sound waves to bounce off internal structures, can be vaginal or abdominal to evaluate the pelvis and observe the following structures:

- ✔ Ovarian cysts (and follicle size)
- ✔ Endometriomas
- ✔ *Paratubal* cysts (benign, fluid-filled remnants from fetal development)
- ✔ Dilated tubes *(hydrosalpinx)*
- ✔ *Fibroids* (common, benign tumors in the uterus)
- ✔ Other uterine abnormalities
- ✔ Other pelvic pathology (for example, a pelvic kidney)

Starting with Simple Treatments

After conducting the appropriate diagnostic tests (see the preceding section), you doctor can determine what is causing your infertility.

The good news: Infertility caused by endometriosis is treatable.

If you have mild, Stage I or Stage II endometriosis, you may not need to jump right into the big guns of infertility treatment, such as IVF. Most fertility experts recommend treating infertility from mild endometriosis as if it were unexplained. In other words, start with treatments that don't require you to remortgage your house. This section looks at some of the simple treatments available.

Ovulation Induction (OI)

If you're not ovulating at all, your doctor may suggest ovulation induction (OI) to get you to produce an egg. If you're already ovulating but not getting pregnant, he may suggest OI to produce more than one egg, on the theory that producing more than one egg is more likely to result in pregnancy.

Ovulation induction (OI) can do the following:

✔ Increase your chance of developing one or more viable egg

✔ Help insure that a mature egg will ovulate

✔ Help cure a luteal phase defect or LUF (For more information on these two conditions, check out "Checking out other hormonal problems: Luteal phase defect" and "Looking at luteinized unruptured follicle syndrome [LUF]" earlier in this chapter.)

Some doctors prescribe medications to help egg development. Clomiphene citrate (Clomid) may be the first drug your doctor recommends for OI because it's

✔ Cheap

✔ Taken by mouth

✔ Has fewer side effects than injected medications

Clomid has some negative effects; it can decrease cervical mucus and interfere with your uterine lining. These adverse effects (a Catch-22 where the treatment to help may hurt) aren't common, but they can decrease the chance for pregnancy. If these problems arise, your doctor can bypass the cervical mucous by putting the sperm into the uterus or have you take estrogen to make the mucous and lining better.

If Clomid doesn't help you get pregnant within a few months, then your doctor may recommend injectible hormones, FSH or LH, as the next step in OI. You usually start these injections early in your menstrual cycle, as early as Day 2 or 3, and continue them each day until a mature egg has developed. Doctors often prescribe another injected hormone, human chorionic gonadotropin, or HCG, to take after an egg has matured to be sure the egg releases. This hormone is usually taken only one time.

A woman can use these medications until a good egg forms, and these treatments don't have the potential bad effects on cervical mucous and the endometrium that Clomid can have. But nothing's perfect; these injectible medications are

✔ More potent than Clomid

✔ Not cheap; many times more expensive than Clomid

✔ Injected once or twice a day for several days

✔ Riskier for overstimulation and multiple births (twins or more!)

Intrauterine Insemination (IUI)

Intrauterine Insemination (IUI) may help you get pregnant more easily by putting the sperm a little closer to the egg. The journey for sperm is long and arduous, and sperm aren't particularly bright. Only 50 percent of a good sperm sample knows how to swim forward. Most sperm in any sample are imperfect and have serious problems; they may

- ✔ Lack tails
- ✔ Swim in circles
- ✔ Have funny-shaped heads
- ✔ Not ask for directions (typical male trait!)
- ✔ Not be able to take a joke

IUI may offer an advantage in infertility because it weeds out the poorer sperm and, ideally, puts only the best swimmers much closer to the target. With any luck, all the bad stuff around the tubes and ovary (endotoxins, white blood cells, and the like) won't affect these macho sperm.

IUI often takes place in conjunction with OI or *controlled ovarian hyperstimulation.* (See "What's involved with IVF?" later in this chapter for more information on this treatment.) Egg-stimulating medications help multiple eggs to

- ✔ Grow and stimulate an egg to mature properly
- ✔ Overcome some of the negative effects that endometriosis has on egg development

Progesterone supplements

Progesterone therapy is another simple treatment that may help you achieve pregnancy. Because a lack of adequate progesterone can cause infertility in several ways, including luteal phase defect, your doctor may recommend additional progesterone after ovulation to be sure your levels are sufficiently high.

Your doctor may give you progesterone after you ovulate on an OI or IUI cycle. Though exact dosage depends on the situation, too much progesterone doesn't seem to cause problems. You may take progesterone as a suppository, injections (ouch!), or caplet.

Be careful — not all *progestogens* are *progesterone.* Only the real progesterone — like your ovaries make — is safe in pregnancy. Other progestogens (like Provera, Agystin, and the like) may increase the risk of birth defects.

Considering alternative treatments for infertility

Many of the same methods for overcoming the pain of endometriosis (see Chapter 12) may be used to help you get pregnant. Traditional Chinese Medicine (TCM) using herbs or acupuncture have been utilized by many women, although success rates are hard to verify. Several years ago, the medical journal *Fertility and Sterility* published an article suggesting that acupuncture could improve pregnancy rates when used in conjunction with IVF. (See Chapter 12 for more on choosing an acupuncturist.)

Taking the Next Step: Surgery to Treat Infertility

If patience or medical therapy hasn't helped to get you pregnant and if male problems have been eliminated, you may want to consider surgery. Fortunately, surgery is much easier and safer today than it was a couple of decades ago, even safer than a few years ago because of advances in anesthesia and tremendous development in technology and instrumentation for minimally invasive surgery.

Your doctor may suggest surgery to help you get pregnant because

- You've had no success with simple treatments.
- You've had long-standing, unexplained infertility.
- You're older than 35, more so if you're older than 40.
- Your doctor strongly suspects endometriosis.
- Other factors, like pelvic inflammatory disease, blocked tubes, fibroids, and adhesions may be present (suggested by your history or tests).

The vast majority of women can have outpatient surgery, although some cases require a hospital stay, especially if extensive adhesions, bowel involvement, or previous surgeries indicate a greater risk. Discuss the risks and benefits of any surgery with your doctor.

This section looks at the different surgical options to help you get pregnant. You can also check out Chapter 11, which gives you much more in-depth info about your surgical options and removing your endometriosis.

Removing adhesions

A surgeon can remove adhesions caused by endometriosis, but one result of this surgery is — you guessed it — more adhesions. Between 60 and 90 percent of surgeries create more adhesions. What to do!?

If your surgery is primarily for infertility, your surgeon may need to disregard your other symptoms to maximize your potential for achieving a pregnancy. As a result, he may ignore adhesions that don't directly affect your chance at pregnancy.

For example, if your large intestine sticks to your pelvic wall and you have some pain there (but not enough to drive you crazy) or if you have some mild symptoms with bowel movements, your doctor may leave the adhesions alone. Why? Because the risk of bleeding, tearing the intestine open, injuring other vital organs, or creating more adhesions that *will* affect your shot at pregnancy may be too great. Sometimes — even many times — prudence is better than attempted heroics.

In light of this information, why does any woman have surgery for adhesions? Some of the best reasons are

- ✔ The most common places for endometriosis to develop are on the tubes and ovaries.
- ✔ Adhesions around these important structures hinder fertility, so removing this scar tissue can increase the chance of pregnancy.
- ✔ Freeing up the ovaries from dense adhesions can also increase the chances of pregnancy with IVF.

You're most likely to get pregnant in the first six months after surgery to remove adhesions. The longer the time after surgery, the greater the chance for adhesions to start forming again.

Taking out endometrial implants or not?

Removing endometrial growths may improve your chance for pregnancy. Success may depend on their location, but implants around the tubes and ovaries (and possibly anywhere) can affect fertility. Most experts agree, however, that surgeons should remove an endometrioma found during surgery because it can compress and destroy ovarian tissue. These cysts may also

✔ Interfere with development of a follicle

✔ Contribute to an inaccurate ultrasound reading because the cyst looks like a developing follicle

✔ Hinder normal follicular rupture

✔ Prevent egg pick-up by the fimbriae and tube

But, deciding what to do with endometriosis implants on other organs can be more challenging. Removing or destroying the implants when the surgeon finds them makes perfect sense. But, by doing so the surgeon may actually do more harm than good. Experts have not been able to prove that removing endometriosis from another organ, say the bladder, has any effect on fertility. Pain, yes — infertility, no.

In fact, removing endometriosis lesions from areas other than the tubes or ovaries may cause more scar tissue and adhesions that can lead to more problems, especially when these structures had no adhesions to begin with. These adhesions from the surgery can then interfere with sperm, egg, and embryo transport.

So, what about the other effects of endometriosis on fertility, such as ovulation problems, immune issues, and the like? Does surgery to remove endometriosis improve these conditions when the disease isn't on the ovary or tube? Well, who knows! Two problems with its removal are

✔ Surgeons can't see all the endometriosis because microscopic disease undoubtedly remains.

✔ Microscopic early disease, Stage I or II, is very active metabolically and can still disrupt fertility in these same ways as the removed endometriosis did.

So the question remains: Remove all visible endometriosis or not? Again, discuss this with your doctor to get his opinion.

Other than endometriomas (which most doctors agree should be removed), the treatment of endometriosis on the surface of the ovary is problematical. If endometriosis covers extensive areas of the ovarian surface, surgery may cause more damage by destroying primordial follicles along with the lesions.

Removing adhesions doesn't damage the surface of the ovary. But removing or destroying implants on the surface may involve

✔ Extreme heat (cautery and some types of laser)

✔ Vaporization (laser)

✔ Coagulation of proteins

All these forms of energy can harm normal ovarian tissue. Even when removing adhesions with a scalpel or scissor, the surgeon must remove a margin of normal tissue to insure no endometrial tissue remains.

All these methods diminish active ovarian tissue and can reduce the number of primordial follicles (the finite number of eggs) in the ovary. This reduction, of course, can lead to infertility itself — not a good idea when you're trying to solve the problem! So doctors are in a quandary with no consensus about the proper procedure.

Going for the Big Guns: Is In Vitro Fertilization (IVF) Necessary?

If your fallopian tubes are completely blocked, in vitro fertilization (IVF — the removal of eggs from your ovaries by a surgical procedure and fertilizing them with sperm in a Petri dish and then putting the embryos into the uterus) is not only the best way to become pregnant, it's the only way. (For much more information on getting pregnant with IVF, check out *Fertility For Dummies* by Jackie Meyers-Thompson and Sharon Perkins [Wiley].)

And if the tubes have partial closure, the risk of ectopic pregnancy also makes IVF the best way to go. ***Note:*** In some cases of severe endometriosis, the tubes may be open but the rest of the anatomy is so distorted that pregnancy may never happen without IVF.

If mild endometriosis seems to be your only problem and you've tried and tried to become pregnant but haven't been successful, your doctor may tell you IVF is the next step. Even though the exact reason for infertility isn't clear in this case, IVF may be the only way to achieve your goal.

Two unique advantages to IVF are

- ✔ It may also help overcome poor egg quality by stimulating more than one follicle to grow to maturity.

- ✔ Removing eggs from their follicles when they mature means that you're bypassing possible problems of LUF. (See the earlier section "Looking at luteinized unruptured follicle syndrome [LUF]" for more about LUF.)

This section looks more closely at IVF, how it helps you get pregnant, and its advantages and disadvantages so you can determine whether you want to take this step.

What's involved with IVF?

IVF is a complex process that can eat up your time, money, and sanity! Before you lose any of the three, you may want to know what IVF involves.

IVF includes the following steps:

1. **Stimulation of your ovaries** with high-powered hormonal drugs to help you produce more than one egg.

2. **Removal of eggs directly from ovarian follicles** through a minor procedure.

3. **Fertilization with sperm in a laboratory.**

4. **Implantation of embryos into your uterus** through the cervix, bypassing the fallopian tubes altogether.

IVF also involves *ovarian hyperstimulation,* that is, you take drugs (primarily through an injection) that stimulate your body to produce more eggs than normal.

How does IVF bypass the problems of endometriosis?

No one does IVF for fun; your doctor will only suggest it if he thinks it will help overcome your fertility problems. IVF bypasses several of the inhibiting factors of endometriosis. For example, it

- Removes eggs from their follicles and bypasses the problems of LUF, adhesions, and scar tissue around the ovary

- Stimulates the ovaries until the eggs are mature (eliminating the effect of endometriosis on maturation)

- Protects the eggs from the potentially toxic peritoneal fluid

- Allows manipulation of the endometrial lining to assure maturity for implantation

- Fertilizes the eggs in the laboratory, decreasing the chance of sperm damage from toxins in the tubes

- Bypasses the fallopian tubes for embryo transport, placing embryos directly into the uterus

What's the downside of IVF?

So, you're thinking IVF is the perfect way to get pregnant, right? Unfortunately, IVF isn't a bed of roses leading you to dirty diapers, empty bottles, and bundles of joy. You do need to consider the following cons before deciding if IVF is right for you:

- ✔ **Cost:** IVF is very expensive, and not all insurance companies cover the cost.

- ✔ **No guarantee of success:** Your chances of pregnancy may be 50 percent or less.

- ✔ **Emotional strain:** Undergoing IVF can be stressful and frustrating, particularly if you have to do more than one cycle.

- ✔ **Time consuming:** Frequent doctor's visits and tests can take a tremendous amount of time away from work and family.

- ✔ **Possible ethical and religious questions:** Many people have ethical concerns about the manipulation of eggs and sperm in a laboratory.

The bottom line on IVF is that some women can't get pregnant without it. If you're one of them, it's worth every penny and all the emotional turmoil. Unfortunately, not even IVF can get everyone pregnant, which can be devastating after such a huge emotional and financial outlay.

Miscarriage and Endometriosis: Is There a Connection?

Experts continue to debate whether endometriosis increases the risk of miscarriage after you become pregnant. Many pregnancies end in miscarriage before women even realize they're pregnant. Sometimes a period that's especially heavy or arrives a day or two late is actually a very early miscarriage (sometimes called a *chemical* pregnancy).

Endometriosis may cause miscarriage by interfering with the chemical support necessary to maintain pregnancy by

- ✔ Lowering progesterone levels or increasing prolactin levels.

- ✔ Creating the immune issues that many women with endometriosis face.

Women who don't have endometriosis but do have an autoimmune disease (like lupus or rheumatoid arthritis) also have an increased risk of miscarriage and failed implantation. So, given the possible association of the immune system and endometriosis, it's understandable that women with endometriosis are also more likely to have a miscarriage.

Likewise, if you believe the molecular genetic explanation of endometriosis (see Chapter 4), then this defect may make it more difficult for an embryo to implant or continue to grow. These abnormalities can affect receptors and other factors that make implantation and continued development possible. The embryo and endometrium may not work well together. Either way, this defect can also explain the increased risk of miscarriage.

The following facts about miscarriage may surprise you:

- More than 50 percent of all embryos stop growing before they develop a heartbeat.
- One in four women has a miscarriage in her lifetime.
- Eighty percent of miscarriages occur in the first 12 weeks of pregnancy.
- A chromosomally abnormal embryo causes at least 50 percent of all miscarriages.

Of course, knowing these facts does nothing to ease the pain and heartache of miscarriage. Some studies have shown, however, that the treatment of endometriosis does reduce miscarriage rates in women with endometriosis.

Chapter 8

Finding the Right Doctor

. . . .

. . . .

Finding a doctor you love these days isn't easy. For starters, your doctor has to be conveniently located, unless you're prepared to spend large chunks of time (not to mention gas money) driving back and forth to appointments. Second, he has to have privileges at a hospital that's acceptable to you. Third, he needs to be taking new patients. Last of all (but certainly not least), your doctor has to be in your insurance network, unless you're independently wealthy. No wonder so many women don't even have a gynecologist!

In this chapter, we talk about how to find a competent doctor, how to avoid doctors who never heard of the Hippocratic Oath, which states, "First, do no harm," and how to establish a good working relationship with your doctor. Finally, we show you how to gracefully part ways from a doctor, if the need arises.

Finding a Gynecologist

When I (coauthor Sharon) first started working in an infertility clinic, I was amazed at how many women didn't have a regular gynecologist (or GYN — a specialist in women's health issues). Some GYNs are also obstetricians, or OBs — doctors who deliver babies. (See the sidebar "Gynecologist or obstetrician: What's the difference?" in this chapter.) Some women had their family practice doctor do Pap smears and breast exams, which can be just fine, but many women weren't having any screenings. They didn't want their family doctor to do the tests, and they didn't have a GYN, so these women were skipping a crucial part of their health care. But these same women were coming to our clinic to find out why they weren't getting pregnant.

Are you a woman who doesn't have a GYN? Have you considered seeing one but just didn't know where to start? Or are you wondering why you really need to see a gynecologist? If you suspect you have a health problem related to your reproductive organs, the best person to see is a gynecologist, because they have extensive training in diagnosing and treating women's disease.

This section can help you by showing you how to look for a gynecologist appropriate for you, how to narrow the search, and what to expect from your first appointment.

Looking for the right doc

You may think some women don't have routine GYN checkups because they lack the health coverage. However, most health insurance plans cover at least one yearly visit to the gynecologist. And even if a woman has no health insurance, some clinics charge fees on a sliding scale. So really, the insurance issue isn't a good excuse for not having a gynecologist.

If you know — or suspect — that you have endometriosis, finding the right GYN becomes even more complicated. Now you need a GYN that specializes in endometriosis. You may think that all GYNS would be competent to treat endometriosis, and for basic treatment of endometriosis, they probably are. But some GYNs are especially interested in one area of women's health more than another, and specialize in it. GYNs with a special interest in endometriosis are most likely to have kept up with the latest surgical techniques and advances in endometriosis.

Overcoming the fear factors

Most women don't avoid the GYN altogether; only 3 percent of the women in one large study said they'd never been to the gynecologist. However, although 75 percent had yearly exams, another 20 percent saw their gynecologist only every two to five years.

Why do women avoid the gynecologist?

✔ Fear of the exam itself

✔ Embarrassment — many women avoid going to a GYN, for example, if they're overweight

✔ Fear of what the doctor may find

It's your doctor's job to help you solve health problems, not to make you feel more uncomfortable about them, so if you're avoiding the GYN because you're afraid she's going to yell at you for something, it may be time to change GYNs!

But what's the best way to find a gynecologist who specializes in endometriosis? You can look to the following for a recommendation:

- **Your insurance company:** If your insurance company issued you a large book with doctors who participate in its plan, you probably need to start there, unless you're willing to pay extra to see the doctor of your choice.

- **A nurse:** You can check with a nurse who works in that specialty at the hospital where you want to go for treatment. She may not tell you who is a bad GYN — but she may tell you who *she* goes to!

- **Your family doctor:** Asking your doctor may be a good starting point for finding a GYN, but you need to take this information with a grain of salt. Doctors tend to recommend other doctors they know maybe because they went to medical school together, or they're on the same medical staff, or they go to the same health club. Your doctor's golf buddy isn't necessarily the best choice for you.

- **Your current gynecologist:** You may already have a gynecologist, so you can ask her for a referral to a specialist who deals with endometriosis issues. She probably knows and can suggest other doctors in the field.

  But what if your gynecologist is hesitant to refer you to another physician for care? She may feel that she knows everything about your problem and that you don't need another opinion. Or perhaps you're not comfortable with the way she's handling your problem with endometriosis (or other concerns). If she refuses to give a referral, ask her why. She may not refer you to someone because she doesn't know of anyone within a reasonable distance, especially if you live in a rural area. In that case, ask your primary care physician (PCP) or refer to Web sites dedicated to endometriosis (check out Appendix B for some Web sites).

- **Your friends and family:** Your friends and family can recommend a new GYN, but try to remain objective. Not all patients really know how to judge whether or not a doctor is *good*. Your friends may base their perceptions on whether the doctor treated them kindly, listened to them, and best of all, cured them. But, even though all these qualifications are important, they don't really define a good doctor. Some people can't be cured, and people's perceptions of good treatment may vary considerably.

- **The phone book:** Despite the ease and one-stop-shopping convenience of the phone book, letting your fingers do the walking isn't the best way to find a GYN — or any other doctor, for that matter. Nonetheless, you can find GYNs in any phone book under "Obstetricians and Gynecologists" or "Women's Health Center."

If you're still not able to find a referral in your general location, then you may have to stick with your doctor and work together, or you may have to travel some distance for care. But, when you do get a referral (and we hope this process has been painless for you and your present doctor), you still want to do some of your own research. Just because your PCP or GYN refers a specialist, she still may not be the best for you.

Gynecologist or obstetrician? What's the difference?

You may wonder why some doctors have the title of *gynecologist* and some are *obstetricians*; this distinction is mostly about the focus of their practices. All *board-certified* obstetrician/gynecologists have been residency trained and then tested to practice in both fields. Some doctors with the specialization focus on obstetrics — delivering babies. If you're considering becoming pregnant in the future, you may want to select a gynecologist who also does obstetrics, so you don't have to start the whole search again if you become pregnant.

But some specialists don't want the uncertain hours of obstetrics, the risk of lawsuits, and the high malpractice costs, so they decide to keep their focus on gynecology.

Some gynecologists narrow their focus even more, choosing to treat mostly patients for infertility or for issues related to *urology* (study of the urinary tract). However, these doctors may also see general gynecology patients.

Narrowing your search

To make good choices as you look for possible GYNs, you want to find a doctor that meets your specific needs and other criteria. This checklist may help you narrow your search for the gynecologist of your dreams:

❑ **Do you want to see a man or a woman GYN?** Many women have strong preferences for one or the other. If you're more comfortable with a woman, or a man, focus your search in that direction.

❑ **Is the doctor board-certified in gynecology?** Board certification assures that the doctor has met certain standards and maintains certification by keeping up with new information. Doctors who are just out of school may be listed as *board eligible*. This classification means they have the education and are working toward the certification exam, which requires doctors to have a certain number of surgeries under their belts. You can find out if a doctor is board certified by asking whoever answers the office phone; if that person doesn't know, ask him or her to look at the doctor's certificates hanging on the walls! You can also look on www.acog.org for board-certified doctors.

❑ **Is the doctor an MD (Medical Doctor) or a DO (Doctor of Osteopathy)?** (You can notice this distinction by the initials after the doctor's name.) These two routes through medical school used to be quite different, with the DO putting more emphasis on holistic medicine and manipulation of the spine to cure disease, but today the programs are very similar.

❏ **How far do you want to travel?** Having a chronic disease like endometriosis may mean frequent visits to the office. Although you're willing to travel an hour or more to see a specialist once, are you willing to make this trip on a weekly or monthly basis?

❏ **Do you care where the GYN has hospital privileges?** Doctors can't just walk into the nearest hospital and start performing surgeries; they have to be on staff at that hospital. If you have strong preferences about local hospitals, make sure your GYN is on staff where you want to go. Most hospital Web sites have a list of doctors on staff, or you can ask the person who answers the phone at the office where the doctor practices.

Scheduling your first appointment

After you narrow down your list of choices (if you live in a rural area, your list may be one name long), you can call the doctor's office to find out the following:

✔ Is the GYN·taking new patients?

✔ Does she still take your insurance? (Doctors start and stop taking insurances at regular intervals.)

✔ How far out are the new patient appointments? (The office may be scheduling months in advance.)

Calling an office can be very illuminating. For example, you can get a good idea of how you'd be treated as a patient by the office phone etiquette. Is the person who answers your call abrupt, putting you on hold without even asking if it's okay? Or does she ask the question, but then not listen to the answer? Can you even reach a live person, or do you get a maze of recordings that tell you to "Press 1, press 2, press 7 . . ." until you forget what you called for?

Prepping for the call

Before you actually call the doctor, prepare yourself. Make sure you have all the important information before you pick up the phone so you don't have to run into the other room for more documents.

The following tips can help you prepare for phoning a doctor's office:

✔ **Have your insurance card ready so you can give the correct information.** "It's a blue card . . . blue something" isn't very helpful in determining whether that office takes your insurance.

✔ **Have your appointment book out.** You're calling for an appointment, so have your calendar handy when the scheduler gives you times and dates.

✔ **Know the reason for your appointment.** Different appointments may require different time slots. For example, a first appointment may take more schedule time than a surgical follow-up.

Making the call

You can help your first contact by being a good potential patient. If you're ready to make the call, remember the following pointers when talking to the scheduler:

✔ **Call at a time when you can pay attention to the conversation.** In other words, don't call when you're driving, trying to make dinner, or working where you may have many interruptions.

✔ **Ask how long you can expect to be at the office, especially for a new patient appointment.** Your potential doctor may want to do blood work, ultrasounds, or other testing on your first visit. If you're worrying about picking up your son from school half an hour after your appointment time, your stress level is probably going to rise considerably.

Note: Obviously, if you're seeing more than one potential GYN, they all can't do testings like Pap smears or mammograms. Your insurance company won't pay for more than one. You can make your first appointment a "getting to know you" event, with more talk than action. (See Chapter 9 for more on what to expect during your first exam.)

✔ **Ask what information you should bring with you.** If you have your medical history or any type of medical records, you can bring them with you. But, unless you're sure this is Doctor Right, don't have all your medical records transferred to him. Wait until you're sure that you want to work with this new doctor before asking another doctor to send records — most offices charge you for this service.

✔ **Tell the person you're making the appointment with that you're making the appointment to get to know the doctor without making it sound like you're "doctor shopping."** Most docs appreciate that a comfortable patient-doctor relationship is important, but they also don't want to feel that they're just one of a long list of docs that you're trying out. Saying, "I'd like to talk with Dr. Smith before she does an examination; is that possible?" sounds less harsh than "I want to talk with Dr. Smith before I let her examine me."

Navigating the First Doctor's Visit

After you've pared your list down to one (or possibly a couple) doctors and scheduled an appointment, you need to make sure you're ready for your visit. Your time is valuable — and so is your doctor's — so make sure you're all set.

During this visit, the doctor may conduct several tests (see Chapter 9 for specifics on the actual exam). However, this section focuses more on what *you* need to do.

Avoiding charlatans

In your search for your GYN, you may encounter a few bad apples. Most doctors are professionals who take their jobs very seriously. Unfortunately some doctors are out to make a quick buck off the unsuspecting public. These doctors fall into two basic categories:

✔ *Doctors* who know they're fleecing the public.

✔ *Doctors* who truly believe in what they're doing, even if no one else does.

You want to watch out for doctors whose treatments are basically worthless and whose main goal is a fatter bank account. These *pros* are pretty easy to spot.

✔ They charge a lot of money for what they're peddling, whether it's a book, a medication, or a treatment.

✔ They claim to be the *only* one who knows this secret. (If you found a miraculous cure, would you keep it to yourself?)

✔ They tell you that everyone else has done something wrong; no matter what it was, it was not what they would have done.

✔ They treat people who are desperate. (Would people be breaking down the doors for a cure to dandruff?) These doctors target people who have received no satisfaction from conventional medicine.

Doctors who truly believe in what they're doing but are somewhat unconventional in their approach are more difficult to deal with. For example, they have no trouble sounding truly sincere because they usually are. This attitude makes them quite persuasive. And these doctors may not charge much for their services, relatively speaking, because they really want to cure people and believe they have *the* answer.

Not all charlatans are medical doctors; they may be naturopaths, herbalists, or someone who just put a few initials behind his name and made up a title to fit them. Often these charlatans have practices with lofty, impressive-sounding names that, coincidentally, include the name of another well-known institution. How do you protect yourself from medical charlatans? Remember these facts:

✔ If a remedy sounds too good to be true, it probably is.

✔ If he has a true medical breakthrough, other people know about it.

✔ Legitimate medical practitioners are open to questioning and share new findings with other doctors.

✔ The Better Business Bureau may have complaints against institutions or clinics; check it out.

✔ Ask your own doctors what they think, but remember that they may pooh-pooh a doctor who has legitimate, valid, but unorthodox approaches.

Describing your symptoms

You can save the doctor's time — and your own — if you can bring a coherent list of symptoms. (See Chapter 2 for more on keeping track of your symptoms.) "What brings you here today?" is probably one of the most poorly answered questions in any doctor's office.

In order to prepare for this first visit, create a list that includes the following:

- ✔ What do you feel (severe pain, dull ache, and so forth)?
- ✔ Where do you feel pain (pelvis, right or left side, vagina, and so on)?

    Draw a picture of yourself, with an X on the pain spots. If you have any artistic ability at all, an illustration is a great way to help your doctor understand.

- ✔ When do you have symptoms (time of the month, relation to your period)?
- ✔ How long do your symptoms last?
- ✔ How often do your symptoms occur (regularly — every month, every day, every minute — or irregularly)?
- ✔ How long have you had the symptoms (a year, since yesterday, your whole life)?

In addition to your symptoms, create a list of how you've tried to deal with the pain. If you've already tried every over-the-counter, nonsteroidal anti-inflammatory drug on the shelves, write this information down. If another doctor has tried hormone replacement therapy, note this treatment too. This list saves time so your doctor can begin focusing on a more promising course of treatment.

Interviewing your doctor

Now that you and Dr. Prospective are face to face (and hopefully you're fully clothed and talking across a desk, not wearing a paper gown and lying on a table), it's time to find out how compatible you are.

On your list of questions to ask, you should have the following:

- ✔ **Do you treat many patients with endometriosis?** (The answer should be "Yes.")
- ✔ **How many patients with endometriosis do you see in a year?** (The more the better; a few or a dozen or so isn't very many.)

> ✔ **What kind of testing can you do to diagnose endometriosis?** (There aren't many tests for endometriosis; surgery is the most definitive way to identify it.)
>
> ✔ **Do you do surgery often for endometriosis?** (The answer should be "Yes, when necessary.")

If the doctor already has his prescription pad out and is writing on it before you even have your coat off, he may not be the doctor for you. Treating a chronic illness, such as endometriosis, is more than suppressing the symptoms, and rarely does a simple prescription cure your ills. Ordering medications isn't wrong, as long as the doctor has heard the whole story first and has a good idea of what he's treating.

Making your final decision

At the end of your first visit, you'll probably have a good idea of whether or not this doc is a keeper. Has he

> ✔ Answered your questions thoroughly?
>
> ✔ Encouraged you to ask questions?
>
> ✔ Really listened to what you say without trying to rush the conversation?
>
> ✔ Made recommendations based on your symptoms and not a cookie-cutter approach?

If you feel good about the visit and your personalities seem to mesh, you may want to make the relationship permanent. If you're comfortable that you've made the right choice, you can start discussing specific testing and treatments. You can schedule them for a later date, or get started the same day of your *get-acquainted* visit.

Sometimes you know immediately that this doctor isn't for you, and a brief visit is enough before saying *goodbye*. Don't feel bad about this decision; doctors know they can't please everyone.

Working with Your Doctor

After you've chosen a doctor, you need to do your part to keep the relationship a beneficial one. Your doctor will best be able to help you if you communicate honestly and work together. In the next sections, we tell you how.

Communicating your concerns

You're never going to be happy with your doctor unless you feel like he's taking your concerns seriously. But presenting those concerns in an organized, straightforward manner can help him understand your specific situation.

What can you do if he doesn't seem to take your symptoms seriously? You need to find another doctor. But if you initially felt comfortable with this doctor, you may want to try and salvage your relationship. To take another stab at developing a good relationship, try the following:

- ✔ **Restate your concerns.** Maybe you weren't clear. Try writing symptoms down and reading them to him — or just hand him the list.

- ✔ **Stay factual.** Overstatement is okay when you're telling a dramatic story to your friends, but exaggeration usually gets poor results in the doctor's office.

- ✔ **Be honest about your concerns.** Many people were taught as children not to complain. They carry that attitude into the doctor's office, minimizing their symptoms, so the poor doctor has a terrible time trying to figure out what's really wrong with them. Conversations that start with "Tell me how you've been." "Oh, not too bad, Doctor Perfect. How are your kids doing?" aren't going to help him find out what's wrong with you. A doctor's office is no place to keep a stiff upper lip.

If he still isn't taking your concerns seriously, then you may need to move on to another doctor on your list.

Keeping your expectations realistic

Sometimes people expect too much of their doctors. Your doctor isn't a member of the holy family, nor does he keep a halo hidden under his bed. He's just a person like you — only with a medical degree and possibly a house at the shore.

As much as you hope he can, your doctor can't pull cures out of thin air or make symptoms disappear with a few words. When you're dealing with a chronic disease, such as endometriosis, remember that the condition usually requires some degree of trial and error with different medications and treatments before you notice progress. Unfortunately, you'll probably never be able to say that your endometriosis is gone forever — at least not before menopause.

Blaming your doctor is easy if you're not cured quickly. But you need to remember one important point: Although endometriosis isn't curable, it is controllable in many cases. Look at endometriosis as a condition that you'll have to live with and deal with for some time, not as a disease that comes once and goes away, like the measles.

Trusting your doctor

I (coauthor Sharon) have worked in doctors' offices for ten years. I've seen far too many people on both extremes — patients who would jump off a bridge if their doctor told them to and patients who acted like their doctor was trying to kill them. Take my advice: If you've taken the time to pick the right doctor, then trust him. I don't mean blind trust; ultimately, you're the one who has to live with his recommendations. Also, try to avoid taking an adversarial stance with your doctor.

Keeping up on all the latest research is difficult unless you're a doctor. So you don't need to tell your doctor about the groundbreaking treatment that you read about in a well-known women's magazine. Most of the time, these magazines have old, incomplete, or even faulty information. Doctors generally hear about promising research in medical journals long before the news shows up at the supermarket checkout counter. After you choose a doctor, trust that he's going to keep up on all the newest treatments, that he has your best interests at heart, and that he's not trying to do you harm.

Divorcing Your Doctor Painlessly

As much as you respect and like your doctor, sometimes you need to break off the relationship and say "Goodbye." Maybe he's not listening to you, or he's not helping you, or you're just not comfortable with the progress of your treatment.

Don't worry too much about hurting your doctor's feelings if you decide to change practices, but do try and leave on good terms. When you're ready to move on, make sure you

- ✔ **Get a copy of your treatment record.** Instead of having your records sent to a new doctor, get a copy for yourself. The copy may cost about a dollar or two per page, but keeping your own records is a good idea. You can make a copy for your next doctor.

- ✔ **Say what you have to say in a letter.** If you have had serious issues with the practice that don't relate specifically to the doctor, send a letter to inform him. Maybe his front desk staff is alienating patients or his billing staff is continually messing up on insurance issues. The doctor needs to know about these problems. Of course, if the receptionist is his wife and the billing person is his daughter, writing a letter probably won't accomplish much, but the exercise can make you feel better.

✔ **Stick to your reasons for leaving.** Don't make accusations, such as "The receptionist deliberately hung up on me!" unless you can prove it. And stay away from threatening statements (even though your brother is a lawyer).

✔ **Be careful how you talk about your problems with a doctor's office with others.** You may be talking within earshot of the receptionist's best friend or the doctor's brother-in-law!

Finding a doctor if you don't have insurance

Unfortunately, many women who need medical care don't have medical insurance. The cost of medical care, and especially hospitalization, can be unbelievably high. If you're uninsured, we suggest you keep the following in mind when considering medical care:

✔ If you're married, see if your husband's insurance plan can include you.

✔ If you're partnered and your partner's company includes domestic partnership coverage, see if the plan can include you.

✔ If you're working, see if you can purchase insurance through your job.

✔ If you're not working, see if you're eligible for Medicaid or Medicare.

✔ If you live in a large town, it probably has at least one hospital clinic for the uninsured and the underinsured. The hospital may help you apply for an insurance program that you're eligible for, and the hospital may have a sliding-scale fee plan based on your income.

✔ If you live in a larger city, look for a medical school or residency training program. These teaching programs have enthusiastic, young doctors in training with close supervision by senior staff physicians. The clinics often have sliding-scale fee plans. Although the wait is often longer, the level of care is excellent.

✔ If you have to see a private physician and don't have insurance, make sure to mention to her that you're uninsured. Even if the front office personnel are aware, the doctor may not be. Many doctors reduce their fees and give discounts to patients who pay for their care at the time of service, so it never hurts to ask. If the doctor is rude about the issue, this is probably a good time to look for a new doctor!

Chapter 9

Do You Have Endometriosis? Your Initial Exam and Diagnosis

. . . .

In This Chapter

▶ Knowing what to expect during the exam

▶ Communicating with your doctor

▶ Relying on diagnostic tests

▶ Taking a close look at endometriosis

▶ Classifying the stages of endometriosis

. . . .

*H*ow do you find out whether you have endometriosis? You may suspect it, think that your symptoms match those in every book and on every Internet support board, know that your mom and six sisters all have it — but how do you know for sure? When you really want a diagnosis, you need to talk with a doctor.

But how does a doctor know you have endometriosis? In many cases, this disease isn't easy to diagnose. In this chapter, we tell you about preparing for your first diagnostic appointment, what occurs at that exam, and how you can communicate most effectively. We also tell you what's in your doctor's bag of tricks to properly diagnose endometriosis, including lab tests, imaging techniques, and the granddaddy of diagnostic gold standards — a biopsy. After you have a diagnosis, we tell you how the doctor analyzes your condition and what the different stages mean so you can understand how severe your endometriosis is.

Preparing for Your Diagnostic Exam

Your appointment is tomorrow, but how can you prepare for the exam? This section covers a few essentials that you need to do (and not do) before you show up at your doctor's office for your diagnostic exam.

Knowing what to do (and not do)

Before you arrive at your doctor's office, you need to make sure you come ready for the exam. Keep in mind the following important pointers:

- ✔ **Don't douche.** Women seem to think they need to be clean and dainty *down there*. But douching isn't good for you because it increases the chance of developing a pelvic infection. In addition, the doctor needs to see the natural conditions *down there*. Take a shower, yes. Douche, no.

- ✔ **Shave your legs and whatever else you normally shave.** Shaving really isn't required, but if you forget, you're going to look down and say, "I can't believe I forgot to shave." You'll be so embarrassed by your stubble that you won't hear a word the doctor says.

- ✔ **Come to your appointment with a full bladder.** The nurse will probably hand you a little jar to urinate in (and going on command is hard enough, but going when you just went is even harder!). If the nurse hasn't given you a jar and you need to urinate before your appointment, let her know so you don't waste a valuable sample and can complete the ritual before you go into the exam room.

Should you bring your partner to this visit? That's up to you and your partner. Your partner may be able to

- ✔ Give you support.

- ✔ Add details that you forgot to mention.

- ✔ Give a different perspective.

- ✔ Provide a second pair of ears. (You may be nervous and forget details of the discussion.)

Bringing information with you

Most important of all, bring your diary with you (see Chapter 2), the one with all your symptoms. You started the diary for this appointment — to give your doctor a concise and accurate description of your situation. So don't leave home without it.

If you have old records from other doctors, bring them along also. This step is especially helpful if you've had previous treatments or surgery for endometriosis. Past problems (medical, surgical, or gynecologic) and records (testing, findings, and treatment) are very important to your healthcare provider. Don't trust your memory on this.

And don't think that your appendectomy at age 5 isn't relevant now. All medical facts, no matter how trivial you may think they are, can help your doctor figure out which disease may be causing your symptoms. Every bit of this information can help your doctor decide on the diagnosis, testing, and treatment to try.

Understanding How Your Doctor Makes a Diagnosis

So, you're in your little paper gown and perched on the exam table when you hear that shuffling at the door that means your doctor is about to appear. Or maybe you're sitting in the chair, trying to put off climbing on the table for one more minute and in comes your doctor. He may sit and chat with you for a few minutes to help you relax before insisting that you hop up on the table, but eventually the time comes to get on up.

Many physicians have a nurse, assistant, student, or other doctor in the room for the pelvic examination. If you feel uncomfortable with someone else in the room during the exam, your doctor may allow her to leave at your request. Or, if no one is in the room with you and your doctor and you're uncomfortable with this, tell him you want someone with you.

Don't worry though. Your doctor knows his job. This section helps you understand your doctor's routine, including the general exam and the pelvic exam. This section also addresses what you can do if you experience pain during the pelvic exam.

The general exam

Because your gynecologist isn't a general practitioner or internist, she may not do a complete general exam. But she still should cover all the areas that may relate to your gynecologic problems.

As you talk, your doctor is assessing your overall appearance in the following ways:

✔ Are you over or underweight by a lot?

✔ Do you have excessive hair or an unusual pattern of hair growth or loss?

✔ What's your general body type, and have you developed normally for your age?

✔ Do you have unusual markings, rashes, or lesions of the skin?

Your doctor may also

- Check your lymph nodes and thyroid gland to be sure you have no enlargements or other abnormalities.
- Examine your face, chest, and back for acne.
- Note color and temperature changes of the hands or feet.
- Note joint pain or tenderness.
- Listen to your heart, lungs, and abdomen with a stethoscope (just to be sure you have no obvious problems).
- Examine your breasts for masses and leakage.
- Palpate your abdomen (explore with the hands) to find abnormal masses.
- Check your back for muscle spasm or tenderness.
- Check your legs for varicose veins and swelling.

All this information is important and provides clues to your diagnosis. If a detail seems different from the norm, your doctor may refer you to another specialist or to your primary doctor, or she may order other tests.

The pelvic exam

Eventually you need to get into the *lithotomy* position, which is lying on your back with your knees and hips flexed and thighs spread apart. Granted, it's not the most dignified position in the world, but your doctor can see what he needs to see, and, remember, that's what you came for. Usually the actual *pelvic* exam is done after the rest of the general exam. The following shows the different steps of a pelvic exam:

1. **Your doctor visually and tactilely examines the vulva and the opening of the vagina.**

   She looks at the skin for any rashes, color changes, lesions (such as warts, ulcers, moles, or scars), abnormalities of the structures, or discharge. She may then touch the skin to feel for firm or tender areas and the pliability of the tissues. Doing so assures your doctor that other problems (such as infections or structural abnormalities) aren't causing your problems.

2. **Your doctor places the *speculum* into the vagina.**

   The speculum is a device that looks like a duck's bill and holds the walls of the vagina apart (gently, we hope, and warmed is even better) so the doctor can see the inside of the vagina, its lining, and the cervix.

3. **The doctor can take specimens by swab, brush, or spatula (no, not the kind you flip hamburgers with!) from the vagina or cervix.**

   These swabs provide information for

   > Cervical problems (Pap smears)
   >
   > Vaginal and cervical infections
   >
   > Hormonal evaluations
   >
   > Fertility testing

4. **The doctor can take an endometrial or cervical *biopsy* (removal of a small part of tissue).**

   You may have local anesthesia to make you more comfortable.

5. **The doctor performs a *bimanual* (two hands) exam.**

   During this part of the exam, he places one hand on the lower abdomen above the pubic bone and one or two fingers of the other hand into the vagina until he reaches the cervix.

   During this very important part of the exam, your doctor can:

   - Feel lumps and irregularities of the tissues in the vagina and cervix

   - Feel the uterus, ovaries, and any other masses in the pelvis by placing the internal organs between his hands

   - Detect *fibroids* (usually benign tumors of the uterus), ovarian cysts, lesions, other pelvic masses, and irregularities of the pelvic organs

6. **Your doctor may perform a rectal exam.**

   He places one gloved and lubricated finger into your rectum and another finger in the vagina to help him feel any thickening in the area between the rectum and uterus.

   Because this area is a very common site for endometriosis, any nodules or thickening of this area can strongly suggest endometriosis.

7. **Your doctor can perform a test for blood in the stool after the rectal exam.**

   See "Checking your stool for blood" in this chapter to see how your doctor does this.

When your doctor has completed the entire exam, he may suggest more tests, such as an ultrasound and blood tests, to help make a diagnosis.

Ouch! Tenderness during the exam

The pelvic exam shouldn't be painful. It may be uncomfortable both mentally and physically, but real pain is unusual and may mean that you have an underlying problem. If you do have discomfort or pain, be sure to let your doctor know. Everyone has a different pain threshold, so don't worry about looking like a wimp — don't try to hide it and suck it up. Your doctor wants to know what you're feeling no matter how trivial you may think it is.

If you're going to the gynecologist because you have pain, your provider may try to duplicate it. For instance, if you have pain in a certain area of the pelvis during sex, he may try to push in that area or move parts around to re-create the pain. With these moves, he hopes to find the reason (a mass, nodule, or *fixed* [unmoving] structure) for the pain.

If you've been having pain at home or if you experience pain during your routine exam, discuss this symptom with your doctor now. He may not have felt or seen a problem during the exam, so telling him about the pain lets him know that he needs to investigate further and, ideally, prevent future pain.

Keeping the Lines of Communication Open

Talking honestly and opening with your doctor can be difficult, but the more medical information you give him, the better able he'll be to diagnose your problem. Some information that he needs to know may be embarrassing to discuss, and some details may be very personal. Try to remember that he is a doctor, and he's heard it all (and more!) before.

Even if you don't feel like being social during your exam, you still need to be proactive. This is no time to be a dainty wallflower. This section tells you how to talk to your doctor during the exam and how to get your doctor's diagnoses in writing for your own records.

Talking openly with your doctor

Talking to doctors is hard enough when you're fully clothed and sitting in a chair at eye level; it's even harder when one of you — and it's never the doctor! — is wearing a paper gown and has her legs up in stirrups. Some doctors choose this time to start small talk about your job, family, or whatever to help you relax.

Don't feel like you have to carry on a full-fledged conversation; this isn't a tea party, and your doctor's not grading you on your social skills. If you answer in monosyllables, he'll catch on that you don't feel like talking during the exam, or he may just carry on a monologue. If possible, talk with your doctor only when you're fully dressed and sitting across a desk from him. You'll feel more like an equal and probably retain more of his ideas. Besides, how are you going to whip out your diary if you're wearing a paper gown?

After your exam, if you feel like your doctor didn't listen to you or that you didn't feel comfortable asking him certain questions, then you need another doctor. You don't need to settle for a doctor who acts as if you shouldn't bother your little head about medical details or talks down to you. Doctors, for the most part, are aware of the plethora of information (and misinformation) on the Internet; they know that many patients have read obsessively about their condition before they ever get into the office.

Your doctor should always give you chance to ask questions at the end of the exam. Saying "Anything else bothering you?" as he walks out the door isn't good enough! A good doctor addresses all your concerns during your visit, and she wants to be sure you understand your condition, so she may provide written instructions or pamphlets for you to read.

Maintaining your own set of records

In this age of frequent moves and insurance changes, keeping your own records is very helpful to you and your future medical practitioner. But you don't need to sneak your chart out of the office to photocopy it before anonymously returning it. You don't need records of every detail.

Keeping your own records makes it easier to supply new doctors with information if you need to change or add doctors due to insurance changes or new diseases. But you don't need to lock these records in Fort Knox. Keeping them in a drawer where you can find them easily is fine. If they contain information you don't want anyone else to see, you may consider buying a safe.

Copies of all your tests or procedures and surgical reports are very handy. If you ask for a copy of a procedure or test result on the day of your visit, most doctors give it to you without a charge. If you call in and ask for a copy of your chart, you may have to pay a dollar a page.

Undergoing a Few Diagnostic Tests

"We're just going to run a few tests," your doctor says, handing you a handful of prescriptions just before he leaves the room. You look at the prescriptions (which are, of course, illegible) and wonder, "What tests? Why? Where do I go for them?" We hope your doctor is more communicative than this and actually explains the what, why, and where for you. But in case he doesn't, this section can help you make your appointments and tell you what to expect.

It's a draw — blood, that is

Few blood tests help to diagnose endometriosis. In fact, no blood test can prove or disprove the presence of endometriosis. So why is Nurse Ratchet coming at you with a needle and an evil smile on her face?

Although endometriosis has no specific blood test, one called CA125 can be a diagnostic tool because many women with endometriosis in the pelvic area have an elevated CA125 level. An elevated CA125 level is the result of irritation of the peritoneal surface by the disease. However, other diseases, such as fibroids or ovarian cancer, can also cause an elevated CA125, so the test isn't a reliable way to diagnose endometriosis by itself. In most labs, a normal CA125 level is less than 35 U/ml (units per milliliter).

Current research is focusing on the diagnosis of endometriosis by cytokines (see Chapter 4 for more on cytokines) that develop in response to the inflammation of endometriosis. Down the road, scientists may identify specific gene markers for endometriosis and then isolate those markers in a blood test.

If you're trying to get pregnant, your doctor may use a blood draw to evaluate your ovarian function by checking hormone levels such as estrogen, progesterone, and follicle-stimulating hormone (FSH). (See Chapter 7 for more about hormone levels and fertility.)

Checking your stool for blood

A *hemoccult* or *stool guaiac* test checks for blood in your stools. If blood is present, your doctor can order more specific tests to determine the source of the blood. Endometriosis on the intestines can cause blood in your stools during your period, so a positive test may suggest this problem.

Although it sounds fairly disgusting, the hemoccult isn't painful and your gynecologist may take a sample without your realizing it. He simply inserts a gloved finger into the rectum to obtain a small amount of stool and smears it on a special paper. Within a few seconds, the paper changes color to indicate the presence of blood.

Your cup runneth over: The urinalysis

Endometriosis on your bladder can cause abnormalities in your urine, so your doctor may want to do a *urinalysis,* a test of your urine (see Chapter 6 for more on endometriosis in your bladder). Urinating into a cup isn't all that difficult, unless you're klutzy or can't aim. It can also be challenging if you can't urinate on demand. Our advice: Always go to your doctor's appointments with a full bladder — that way you can minimize your anxiety and happily accommodate the request for a specimen.

A urinalysis can diagnose any number of conditions, from kidney and liver problems to urinary tract infections. Most urinalysis tests check for the following:

- Bacteria
- *Bilirubin* (a chemical excreted by the liver and stored in the gall bladder)
- Blood
- *Ketones* (chemicals that are products of tissue breakdown)
- *Nitrates* (chemicals that may signify bacterial growth)
- Protein
- Sugar
- White blood cells

Finding any of this stuff in urine is abnormal. Although urine is normally sterile (hard to believe, isn't it!), vaginal secretions and skin bacteria can contaminate it. A *clean catch* specimen (cleaning with a soapy cloth before urinating and then discarding the first part) is important to avoid contamination.

Testing, testing: Ultrasounds, X-rays, CT scans, MRIs, and more

Have you ever wished you could just look inside your body and see what's giving you trouble? Although Superman's X-ray vision was great, today's ultrasounds, X-rays, computed tomography-scan tests (CTs), and Magnetic Resonance Imaging (MRIs) are the next best thing.

Undergoing ultrasound

Ultrasound can help your doctor diagnose distorted or swollen fallopian tubes, endometriosis, other pelvic problems, and uterine anomalies. Ultrasound bounces sound waves off internal organs or tissues, detecting differences in the density of various tissues. Your doctor can then see whether organs are in the right location and have a normal density.

Two ways to do an ultrasound are

✔ **Transabdominal:** This is the most common and least invasive approach. Doctors commonly use this ultrasound for obstetrics, but it can also show fibroids, check the position of organs, and give fairly good information on the uterus and other pelvic organs.

✔ **Transvaginal:** This approach uses a probe through the vagina up to the cervix at the top of the vagina, where the abdominal cavity begins. Because the ovaries should be in this location, a transvaginal ultrasound offers a better view for various problems in the ovaries and tubes (especially for an ectopic pregnancy and endometriomas) and in the endometrial cavity.

Many times a doctor may ask for both kinds of ultrasounds to be sure he doesn't miss anything.

HSGs, SIS, X-rays, and CT scans

Your doctor may suggest a number of additional tests to get a better look at your insides, particularly if you're planning on trying to get pregnant. Some of these tests are more effective than others in diagnosing endometriosis. He may recommend the following tests:

✔ **Hysterosalpingogram (HSG):** In this test, dye is passed through the uterus and the fallopian tubes. Your doctor can tell if your tubes are blocked by adhesions or dilated by inflammation, as well as check for uterine anomalies (see Chapter 7 for more on HSGs and how they're done).

✔ **Saline Infusion Sonohysterogram (SIS):** This test may be done to get a better look at the structure of the uterus and endometrial cavity. The procedure is done with a small tube placed into the uterus (like a very thin catheter) so that saline can be infused into the endometrial cavity while the ultrasound is completed.

✔ **X-Ray:** X-rays are useful for looking at bony structures and some soft tissue, such as the lungs or parts of your abdomen. Unfortunately, an X-ray only tells you whether you have a mass or obstruction in your lungs, bladder, or bowel; it can't diagnose whether the blockage is endometriosis or some other kind of mass.

✔ **CT scan:** A computed tomography-scan (or CT), similar to X-rays, can show masses and obstructions as well as cysts, but they can't differentiate between endometriosis and other types of masses. Because they consist of multiple slices of the area, CT scans can give a more distinct image of a body part. This increased resolution can be better than a single, simple X-ray picture.

Magnetic Resonance Imaging (MRIs)

An MRI machine consists of a large tube that you slide into (or are slid into) so that the specific body part is in the exact center of the magnetic field that runs through the MRI. The tube is actually a big magnet. Your doctor can use MRIs to diagnose endometriosis if the lesions are larger than 2 centimeters (about 1 inch) and to diagnose *endometriomas* (cysts caused by endometriosis). Check out Chapters 3 and 7 for more on endometriomas.

MRIs are very expensive compared to other diagnostic tests but may be useful in distinguishing between certain abnormalities. Although the MRI can't see cysts well, this diagnostic test may help to rule out other problems, such as fibroids or pelvic abnormalities. The MRI has not supplanted the gold standard of a biopsy for endometriosis (refer to the next section).

So how do MRIs work? MRIs use magnets and radio waves to create images. A computer creates the images by sending radio waves through your body and collecting the signal that's emitted from the hydrogen atoms in your cells. An antenna collects this information and feeds it into a sophisticated computer that produces the images. MRIs can show much greater detail in soft tissues (they're not so good with bones) than CT scans. MRIs can also scan from many different angles, but CT scans can only scan horizontally.

The magnets in MRIs are extremely powerful and can attract metal even if the metal's inside you! An MRI isn't for you if you have

- A pacemaker
- A cochlear implant
- Pieces of metal in your eye
- Metal clips in your brain or elsewhere
- Dental bridges
- Braces
- Belly button rings, toe rings, a pierced tongue, or any other metal decorations or piercings

Diagnosing Endometriosis Surgically

The best and only way doctors can definitively diagnose endometriosis is through surgery. During surgery, doctors have two basic options in making the diagnosis — by taking a biopsy or by visually diagnosing the disease. This section looks more closely at these two and also looks at what endometriosis looks like under the microscope.

Biopsying endometriosis

Physicians refer to surgically removing endometriosis and identifying it microscopically as the *gold standard,* that is, the best procedure to diagnose endometriosis. Your doctor can make this diagnosis through *laparoscopy,* a minimally invasive procedure, or by a *laparotomy,* a larger incision (see Chapter 11 for descriptions of the surgeries). Biopsy of endometriosis is fairly easy, but, like all procedures, it carries some (though small) risk. Also, a biopsy may miss the endometriosis, or the endometriosis may be unrecognizable to the pathologist due to distortion of the tissues.

Because endometriosis isn't accessible from outside the body, a surgical procedure must provide the specimen. Two procedures are possible: an open procedure (laparotomy) or a less invasive procedure (laparoscopy). Although the laparoscopic approach takes more skill and experience, most surgeons can get a specimen via this route.

The easiest way to get a specimen is by peeling or wiping it off the surface of the pelvis or organ. Often, the early lesions (blebs and thin filmy areas) are hardest to see but the easiest to remove during laparoscopy with special instruments. A lab then verifies whether the pieces are endometriosis. Peeling off lesions can also be done during a laparotomy, although seeing these lesions without the magnification of the scope is more difficult.

Older, deeper, and more scarred endometriosis takes much more care and skill to remove during a biopsy. The surgeon must make a shallow incision in the surrounding tissue and remove the endometriosis (or part of it when only biopsying). The surgeon must be very careful that the lesion isn't stuck to an important structure, such as a ureter, piece of intestine, large blood vessel, or the bladder. Tearing any of these structures, especially without realizing it, can be disastrous!

A surgeon removes endometriosis on the ovary with the same procedure. However, when the disease has invaded the ovarian tissue, the surgeon must save as much normal ovarian tissue as possible and then repair any damage, which prevents adhesions. Again, only experienced surgeons should attempt such intricate surgery, especially if the patient hopes for a future pregnancy.

Diagnosing endometriosis visually

An experienced surgeon may also recognize endometriosis visually, and he may not biopsy at all if he sees obvious disease. Visual diagnosis also avoids the rare but serious complications of biopsy. Given the advantages of visual diagnosis, having an experienced surgeon who knows what he's looking at *and* is comfortable with the procedure is of utmost importance.

Keeping calm in the MRI

Many offices now tout their MRIs as being open and less likely to cause claustrophobia, but their definition of *open* and yours may differ! If you're claustrophobic, undergoing an MRI even in an open tube is a stressful experience. You need to remain as still as possible, the machine makes ominous noises, and even though the side may not be totally enclosed, you will still be surrounded by metal. How can you get through the test without trying to escape in the middle of it?

First of all, remember that someone is always within hollering distance in the room — they don't just walk away and leave you there. Just knowing someone is nearby can be comforting.

Then, to get through the procedure, keep your eyes closed to take your mind off the close walls. Earplugs also help block out noise. They may allow you to move your fingers a bit (sometimes just being able to move any part is comforting!). But always ask whether this movement will interfere with your test. And don't worry — they don't strap you in!

Many times I've seen new patients whose endometriosis was obviously missed during an earlier surgery. The previous surgeon may have not recognized the disease because he was relying on the textbook description — a classic *powder-burn* lesion appearance. We now identify that traditional appearance as *end-stage* disease (check out "Staging Endometriosis" later in this chapter for more info). In reality, endometriosis can take on many varied disguises, and surgeons must be trained and experienced to recognize them.

Lesions: Up close and personal

When bits of endometrial tissue turn into endometriosis, the resulting lesions don't look like your regular menstrual flow. So, what *does* endometriosis look like to the naked eye? Well, it depends. The tissue can appear very different from one woman to another when a surgeon views it through the laparoscope or with his own eyes. Endometriosis from different areas in the same woman can even look totally different from each other.

Endometriosis can be any one of a number of colors — black, blue, red, white, brown, or clear — depending on where it is, how old the lesions are, and what kinds of cells they contain. The tissue can be flat, raised, regular, or irregular; it can be thin, thick, deep, or shallow. The endometriosis can consist of many adhesions or none. In short, endometriosis is variable in appearance; it has no definitive descriptions.

The classic description of endometriosis, which many textbooks still use, is the *powder burn* and *stellate* lesion. Early surgeons saw these structures as obviously abnormal tissue because the abdominal cavity and pelvis have a pink color and the ovaries are white. ***Note:*** Your pelvic cavity has other shades of red, blue, and gray hanging around, but nothing is dark gray to black (powder burn) with whitish, thin bands of firm tissue that spread out from the structure (the starlike, *stellate,* lesions).

The colors of a rainbow: Significant differences

Endometriosis can have many different appearances depending on the stage (See the section "Staging Endometriosis" later in this chapter) and age of the disease. In fact, a patient can have all the different lesions at the same time! The lesions can appear as clear vesicles, or they can be yellow-brown, red, dark red, dark brown, or black areas on the effected surfaces. Your doctor may encounter the following features of these colored lesions:

✔ **Clear:** Although *clear* isn't exactly a color, the clear blebs (little bubble-like areas) are the earliest signs of endometriosis. They may be hard to see, but, as instruments have improved, the blebs have become clearer to the surgeon. Still, many doctors ignore them or misdiagnose them as bubbles (from the procedure's fluid and gas) or as artifact. A surgeon must have experience and training to find and confidently diagnose these structures as endometriosis.

✔ **White, yellowish to light brown:** This next stage of lesions is more visible, but a surgeon may misinterpret the lesions as remnants of the *corpus luteum* (the leftover shell of the egg follicle) or other fairly normal conditions (such as bruising from instruments to blood vessels under the peritoneum). These lesions are often flat but may be raised slightly. They're soft, so a surgeon can usually rub them off the surface of a structure. This stage of lesions can occur anywhere, and it's *metabolically* (chemically) very active.

✔ **Red:** These lesions vary from bright red (like fresh blood) to dark red, almost brown. They can occur anywhere and take on various shapes — round, elongated, long and thin, and so on. These lesions may be more invasive because they're older than the white to light brown variety. Red lesions may be deep and nodular, which leads to scarring. When a surgical instrument enters one of these lesions, a dark fluid (old blood) often emerges. These structures are very obvious and common examples of endometriosis.

✔ **Dark gray to black:** The classic lesions have a gun-powder burn color and represent the disease's end stage. The immune system has attacked the disease, and the endometriosis is now scarred and mostly nonresponsive to the menstrual cycle hormones. However, the damage is done. Lesions have destroyed or distorted nearby tissues, and scarring has stuck organs together (called a *frozen pelvis*) or caused pain and dysfunction.

All these lesions can occur in the same patient at the same time. Because the earlier blebs and yellow lesions are the most metabolically active, women who have them also have the most symptoms. Researchers note that the women with the least apparent disease can have the most symptoms. The reason for this apparent paradox is that these women have plenty of endometriosis — it just hasn't been correctly recognized.

Looking at endometriosis under the scope

You would think that endometriosis always looks the same under the microscope, right? Well, no. Even after a biopsy and under the microscope, this disease doesn't always look the same, even in the same woman.

To diagnose this disease, the endometrial tissue, glands, and stroma must be present in the wrong place. But, in 30 to 50 percent of cases, the biopsy fails these criteria. How can this be? Several reasons may be possible.

✔ **The surgeon doing the biopsy may just miss the real lesion.** An area of endometriosis has many tissue variations. The inflammatory process can cause a change in color and distortion of the anatomy. And an area at the edge that looks good to biopsy may just be a reaction to the disease process and not the actual endometrial implant. The actual lesion may be much deeper and not visible. The surgeon doesn't want to cause harm while diagnosing the problem, so he may not biopsy deeply enough to reach the actual active endometriosis.

✔ **The surgeon may not recognize the active areas.** The textbooks describe classic endometriosis as black, stellate (star-shaped) lesions. But this definition is only for the end stage of the disease, so the biopsy may only contain scar tissue and old inflammatory cells and debris, *not* endometriosis. The surgeon may not even recognize the active areas because they may be too small, hidden, or unusual in appearance. Sometimes the earliest lesions are clear and hard to see. Or the surgeon may biopsy red areas that are actually bruises from the instruments.

✔ **The pathologist doesn't see any glands or stroma.** Endometriosis implants can become so distorted that the pathologist can't see any glands or stroma. The only evident glands are scattered and distorted, separate from any recognizable stroma. Pressure from the retained menstrual blood can squeeze the cells, making an area look different from endometrium. Imagine a shag carpet squashed so flat that its pile looks like part of the backing; this view is similar to what the pathologist may see.

Staging Endometriosis

If your doctor diagnoses you with endometriosis, she may use a staging system developed by the American Society for Reproductive Medicine (ASRM) that categorizes endometriosis into four stages based on

- ✔ The amount of endometriosis present
- ✔ The location of the endometriosis
- ✔ The severity of the disease

Surgeons further classify endometriosis as *superficial* or *deep:*

- ✔ **Superficial endometriosis** lies more on the surface of a structure.
- ✔ **Infiltrative** or **deep endometriosis implants** are deeper than 5 to 6 millimeters.

Your doctor can only make this classification in your diagnosis during surgery. With endometriosis staging, lower numbers are better. The following classifications determine the points and stages of endometriosis:

- ✔ Superficial endometriosis of the peritoneum (1 to 3 centimeters) = 2 points
- ✔ Deep endometriosis of the peritoneum (greater than 3 centimeters) = 6 points
- ✔ Deep endometriosis of the ovary (less than 1 centimeter) = 4 points
- ✔ Deep endometriosis of the ovary (1 to 3 centimeters) = 16 points

The four stages of endometriosis have the following range of points and general descriptions:

- ✔ **Stage I:** Minimal; 1 to 5 points
- ✔ **Stage II:** Mild; 6 to 15 points
- ✔ **Stage III:** Moderate; 16 to 40 points
- ✔ **Stage IV:** Severe; More than 40 points

Some staging classifications also categorize the color of the endometrial implants:

- ✔ The red lesion category includes red, red-pink, and clear lesions.
- ✔ The white lesion category includes white, *peritoneal defects* (these are distorted areas of the pelvic surface sometimes called *windows*), and yellow-brown lesions.
- ✔ The black lesion category includes both black and blue lesions.

Part III
Treating Endometriosis

The 5th Wave — By Rich Tennant

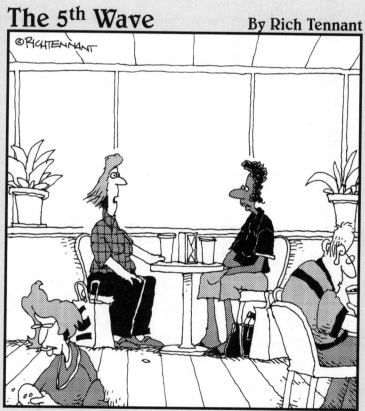

"There are some side effects to my course of treatment, like headaches, nausea, and weight gain, not unlike Thanksgiving weekend at my in-laws'."

In this part . . .

Your doctor has diagnosed that you have endometriosis. Now the question becomes, "How do you treat it?" In this part, we discuss all the current treatments for endometriosis — from pills to major surgery — and talk about which ones work best. We also consider alternative medical therapy and describe the ways a teen's endometriosis may be treated differently from an adult's. Finally, we share ways to keep the pain of endometriosis from taking over your life.

Chapter 10

Relying on (Prescription) Drugs to Treat Endometriosis

In This Chapter

▶ Figuring out how drug therapy fights endometriosis

▶ Looking at your medication options

▶ Giving nonhormonal options a try

▶ Staying optimistic about the future

*U*nfortunately, no medications are available to cure your endometriosis. However, certain drugs may shrink the endometrial implants for a time and reduce pain. Other drugs treat the pain and inflammation and keep them at bay for a while. However, none of the available medications is perfect; most of them have side effects ranging from annoying to serious. What works for your neighbor may not work for you.

With so many drawbacks, why do doctors prescribe medications for endometriosis? Because the meds do help with symptoms — even though the relief may be temporary — and the meds can help avoid surgery. Oftentimes the medications can get you through the tough times until you get pregnant or the disease runs its course. In this chapter, we discuss the most commonly prescribed medications and their pluses and minuses. We also tell you what you can do to alleviate side effects.

Understanding Medical Treatment: How Drugs Fight Endometriosis

Medication therapy isn't a permanent cure for endometriosis. Although it may help with symptoms for a period of time — maybe up to a year or two after treatment stops in the case of the hormonal therapies, dietary changes, and natural substances — medication eventually becomes ineffective and the symptoms come back. The goal of drug therapy is to reduce, not cure, the inflammation and pain, and minimize the destructive complications, such as adhesions and abnormal bleeding.

Different classes of medical therapy work in different ways. Some medications relieve pain and decrease inflammation although they don't directly affect the endometriosis. Other therapies suppress the growth of the endometrial tissue and cause the endometrial implants to shrink down and become inactive.

None of the medications currently available totally eliminates endometriosis, nor do any of them affect adhesions and anatomic distortions already present. Even after hormonal treatment, endometriosis is still there and gradually reactivates after your ovaries start working again. Active endometriosis returns gradually 12 to 24 months after you stop treatment.

When you start considering medication for endometriosis, the goal may hardly seem worth the effort. Some medications take two to four months to become effective, and you can only take them for six months or so. You wonder whether it's worthwhile to suffer through the side effects and then continue the drug for such a short time after you're pain-free. Don't feel discouraged though. These meds can still help. This section gives an overview of how medications work to fight endometriosis in your body.

Mimicking pregnancy

Some of the most common hormonal treatments for endometriosis are designed to trick your body into thinking you're pregnant. The symptoms of endometriosis usually improve during pregnancy because

- The high levels of pregnancy hormones and progesterone effectively suppress the ovaries. Under this suppression the hormone fluctuations of the normal menstrual cycle don't exist.
- The high levels of progesterone stop the endometrium from growing, and you don't have periods.

Medications accomplish this trick by occupying (and blocking) certain receptors in different parts of the brain. This blockade of the receptors stops the ovaries from going through their natural menstrual cycle with all the associated hormonal changes. As a result, your body can experience relief from decreased endometrial growth and decreased periods.

In pregnancy, the high level of hormones has a *negative feedback* on receptors in the *hypothalamus* (a gland in the middle of the brain just above the pituitary gland; see Chapter 5), and this feedback shuts down ovulation. The hormones cause the gland to suppress the release of follicle-stimulating hormone (FSH)

and luteinizing hormone (LH) from the pituitary gland (see Chapter 5 for more details on the menstrual cycle). Birth control pills, progesterone- and estrogen-like compounds, and certain male-like hormones work the same way. They all occupy the receptors in the hypothalamus and fool the gland into thinking you don't need to make an egg. As a result, the endometrial implants aren't being stimulated to grow and bleed, and this decreases the symptoms of endometriosis.

Mimicking menopause

Other hormone treatments work in a way similar to negative feedback (they work on receptors), but these treatments work on the pituitary gland (the gland just below the hypothalamus), tricking the body into thinking that it's in menopause. In natural menopause, the symptoms of endometriosis also decrease for several reasons:

- ✔ Ovaries can't make estrogen.
- ✔ The hypothalamus and pituitary gland go into overtime trying to make you ovulate.
- ✔ Levels of the hormones FSH and LH soar very high, attempting to stimulate the ovary to mature an egg. Because there are no eggs though, nothing happens.

GnRH agonists or antagonists (two classes of drugs) simulate menopause except for one difference: Instead of increasing FSH and LH (which leads to more eggs and more hormones!), these medications remove the stimulus to your ovaries by lowering LH and FSH. The result is, ideally, no menstrual cycles, no hormones, and the number-one goal — decreased amounts of endometrial tissue and endometriosis.

Looking at Hormonal Medication Options

Doctors use a number of hormonal medications to treat endometriosis; some treatments work better for some people, and others work better for other people. Which medication works better for you often depends on your tolerance to the side effects that each medication causes.

Why do hormones decrease the symptoms of endometriosis? Because they induce a state similar to either pregnancy or menopause. (See the section "Understanding Medical Treatment: How Drugs Fight Endometriosis" earlier in this chapter for further explanation.) Endometriosis symptoms generally disappear at those two times and may stay away for long periods of time (probably forever in menopause!).

Hormonal treatments and their effectiveness: Just the numbers, please

Hormonal medications are the most commonly used treatment for endometriosis. Just how effective are hormonal treatments? Check out the following statistics:

✔ Up to 20 percent of all women who receive treatment have pain that returns after hormone treatment.

✔ Around 37 percent of women who use hormone therapy for mild endometriosis have pain five years later.

✔ Generally, 66 percent of women who have conservative surgical treatment have a recurrence of endometriosis within two years after the surgery.

✔ Around 74 percent of women who use hormone therapy for severe endometriosis have pain five years later.

All medications to treat endometriosis don't work the same way, but they all strive to achieve the same goals:

✔ To decrease pain

✔ To control other symptoms

✔ To lessen the damage endometriosis can cause

However, hormonal treatments aren't for everyone. Don't use any of these hormonal medical therapies in this section if you're trying to become pregnant.

Do these hormonal treatments cure endometriosis? That's debatable. Like most other treatments for endometriosis, hormone medications aren't a permanent cure. However, they may be able to help you out. This section delves into the many hormonal treatment options you have and considers their advantages and disadvantages.

Popping the Pill: Oral contraceptives

You're probably familiar with oral contraceptives (OCs), more commonly called birth control pills (BCPs) or just the *Pill*. But you may not know how versatile they are. Preventing pregnancy is just one of their uses (although that use has certainly changed society!).

Breaking down the Pill: Biochemistry 101

The estrogen compound in most oral contraceptives in the United States is a form of *estradiol,* the hormone your ovaries make. However, the progestin element offers some variety (five related to testosterone and one unique compound). As a result, more than 40 types of BCPs are on the market, all with varying combinations of estradiol and one of the progestins. They're available in many different doses and schedules. In general, the monophasic pills (all pills contain the exact same ingredients) are better than the *biphasic* or *triphasic* variations (different ingredients depending on the day of your cycle) for endometriosis.

Tweaking contraceptives to treat endometriosis

BCPs contain combinations of an estrogen and a *progestin* (the synthetic form of progesterone, also called *progestogen*). BCPs are often effective in treating the pain and bleeding problems associated with endometriosis. Birth control pills work because they fool your body into thinking it's already pregnant. They suppress the actions of the reproductive hormones LH and FSH and prevent ovulation. Because BCPs contain a progestin every day (unlike your ovaries, which make progesterone only after ovulation), they also inhibit the growth of endometrial tissue. Some women have light or no periods while on them.

Variations in doses are mostly inconsequential but you may do better on one BCP than another because of the different amounts of *estradiol* (the estrogen compound in most BCPs in the United States) or progestin in each pill. Different doses of estradiol and progestin may cause different side effects. Don't despair if one doesn't work; your doctor may just suggest a different combination. You have plenty to choose from! (Check out the sidebar "Breaking down the Pill: Biochemistry 101" in this chapter for more info.)

Most BCPs for endometriosis are *monophasic,* meaning that you take the same exact combination of drugs every day. Your doctor may recommend that you take an *active* pill daily for three to four months without a break to better simulate pregnancy and suppress endometriosis. Historically, the normal schedule for BCPs is three weeks of hormones (active pills) and one week of blanks (nonactive pills).

Moving (and improving) contraceptives in the 21st century

Most contraceptives are taken by mouth — because they're *oral* contraceptives! But today, contraceptive skin patches and even vaginal rings (a diaphragm without the innards) can dispense estrogen and progesterone in slow-release doses. These patches and rings last for a week at a time, and then you change them. Ortho Evra is an estrogen/progestin patch and NuvoRing is a vaginal insert. ***Note:*** Patches may increase menstrual cramping.

Most of the BCPs for endometriosis now contain lower estrogen doses than they had 20 years ago; they're the so-called *low-dose* pills. Most BCPs use the same synthetic estrogen, ethinyl estradiol, but the amounts can vary from 20 to 50 micrograms.

Your doctor may prescribe BCPs with a more potent progestin to further suppress endometriosis (progestins tend to decrease the growth of the endometrium). Another possible combination is estrogen with an *androgen* (male hormone) to further suppress the ovaries.

Different types of progestin have different potency, milligram per milligram, so a 1.0 mg dose of one progestin may cause more side effects than 3.0 mg of another type of progestin. Just because the dose of progestin is higher, don't assume your doctor is giving you a stronger pill. Check out Table 10-1 to see some of the most common BCPs.

Table 10-1	Common Birth Control Pills for Endometriosis		
Name	**Ingredients**	**Side Effects**	**Type of Pill**
Alesse-28	Ethinyl Estradiol 20 mcg; Levonorgestrel 0.10 mg	Headache, nausea, vomiting, breakthrough bleeding, acne	Higher androgenic, higher progestin, lower estrogen, monophasic
Demulen 1/35, Zovia 1/35 E	Ethinyl Estradiol 30 mcg; Ethynodiol diacetate 1.0 mg	Nausea, vomiting, weight gain	More progestogenic, low androgen, monophasic
Desogen	Ethinyl Estradiol 30 mcg; Desogetrel 0.15 mg	Headache, dizziness, nausea, breakthrough bleeding	Very low androgenic, monophasic
Levlen, Nodora, Nordette	Ethinyl Estradiol 30 mcg; Levonorgestrel 0.15 mg	Nausea, vomiting, spotting, weight gain, acne	Higher androgenic, higher progestin, lower estrogen, monophasic
Loestrin 1.5/30	Ethinyl Estradiol 30 mcg; Norethindrone acetate 1.5 mg	Acne, excess hair growth	Higher androgenic, higher progestin, lower estrogen; monophasic

Name	Ingredients	Side Effects	Type of Pill
Loestrin 1/20 Fe	Ethinyl Estradiol 20 mcg; Norethindrone acetate 1.00 mg	Acne, excess hair growth	More androgenic, monophasic
Lo/Ovral	Ethinyl Estradiol 30 mcg; Norgestrel 0.3 mg	Nausea, vomiting	More progestogenic, monophasic
Ortho Cyclen	Ethinyl estradiol 35 mcg; Norgestimate 0.25 mg	Breast tenderness, mood changes, nausea	Lower progestin, monophasic
OrthoNovum 1/35	Ethinyl Estradiol 35 mcg; Noresthindrone acetate 1.00 mg	Headaches, nausea, mood changes	Higher estrogen, lower progestin, monophasic
Yasmin	Ethinyl estradiol 30 mcg; Drospirenone 3.0 mg	May increase potassium levels; spotting, fluid retention, nausea	Anti-androgenic, higher progestogenic, monophasic

Living with the side effects

Estrogen and progestin each cause different side effects, some very serious and some more minor. In addition to the pill-specific effects listed in the previous table, the minor side effects of estrogen and progestin in oral contraceptives include the following:

- Abdominal swelling
- Ankle swelling
- Bleeding between periods
- Breast tenderness
- Increased appetite
- Nausea
- In rare cases, *deep vein thrombosis* (blood clots)

Breast cancer and the Pill: Is there a connection?

Ever since birth control pills (BCPs) first came on the market, their relationship to breast cancer has been a concern. Unfortunately, studies don't have a clear consensus on this issue. The studies also cannot determine which women, if any, are at risk. A 2002 study showed no increase in breast cancer in women who take BCPs, even in women who have taken them for 15 years or more or who had taken them at young ages. Undoubtedly, more studies will focus on this connection in the future.

If you suspect the prescription is causing high blood pressure or deep-vein blood clots (which can, in rare cases, lead to heart attacks or stroke), you need to immediately call your doctor.

On the reassuring side, a long-term study of 46,000 British women showed no difference in mortality rates between women who took BCPs and those who didn't. In fact, because of the beneficial effects of BCPs, the mortality rate is lower for reproductive-age women who use BCPs than for women in the same age group who don't use them.

Women who smoke have a higher risk of stroke or heart attack when taking BCPs than nonsmokers do. If you smoke, discuss this risk thoroughly with your doctor before taking BCPs — or, better yet, consider not smoking! If you have a family history of clotting or if you've had similar clotting problems, your doctor may want to test your *hypercoaguability* state (the tendency to form clots too easily).

Benefiting (potentially) from the Pill

Some research has shown that BCPs may reduce the risk of ovarian cancer by 30 to 50 percent and the risk of endometrial cancer by 50 percent. These are very important potential benefits for women with endometriosis, who may have an increased risk of ovarian cancer (see Chapter 4). Finally, some *good* news, right?

Other benefits of BCPs are less dramatic (Preventing cancer is about as good as it gets!), but they can make life better. The following are a few other benefits you may notice from taking BCPs:

- They can reduce the severity of acne.
- They can reduce the amount of blood loss during the menstrual cycle and lessen menstrual cramps (see Chapter 5).
- They may add to bone mineral density and reduce your risk of osteoporosis.

Considering progestins alone

Pregnancy often significantly reduces the symptoms of endometriosis because progesterone levels are high. Therefore, medication that raises these hormone levels and tricks the body into thinking that it's pregnant can also reduce the symptoms of endometriosis. One of the progestins, norethindrone acetate, is also used in BCPs and other hormonal contraceptive combinations, and the other, medroxyprogesterone acetate, isn't.

Understanding how progestins treat endometriosis

Pseudopregnancy with progestins for endometriosis started in the 1950s and continues to be of great benefit in some patients. Today, synthetic progesterone (injections or pills) usually prevents ovulation and causes the endometrial tissue to *atrophy* (shrink) over time. So the treatment can reduce the pain of the endometrial implants and possibly control other symptoms of endometriosis.

Up to 80 percent of women with endometriosis have decreased pain while taking progestins. Long-term progestins *decidualize* the endometrium. In other words, they make the endometrium tissue thin and spongelike compared to the thick and complex tissue that estrogen builds. The usual treatment time is at least six months. During the first few months, you may have spotting or irregular bleeding as your periods decrease and then stop altogether.

Knowing your treatment options

The most common progestin for endometriosis is medroxyprogesterone acetate (MPA) with a structure very similar to natural progesterone. MPA may have a slow onset of therapeutic effect, but *adipose* (fat) cells can store it for long periods of time. If it works, you can continue MPA orally or by injection for long periods. MPA acts like BCPs to prevent ovulation. MPA directly inhibits endometrial growth like all progestins. And, because MPA reduces estradiol levels, it may also have an added suppressive effect on the endometrial tissue.

The other common progestins, norethindrone and norethindrone acetate, are in pill form and have similar effects. These drugs have a more estrogenic effect than MPA (so bone loss and other symptoms related to low estrogen may not be as bad), but the effect isn't enough to cause endometrial growth. Although megestrol acetate is seldom a treatment for endometriosis (it's more common in cancer treatment), it can also be an option for some women.

If you've been taking oral progestin and then stop, your periods may take a few months to begin again. If you've been on injections, your periods can take a long time, up to a year, to start back up again and become regular. Because of these delays, you may want to consider another method if you plan on trying to get pregnant soon after stopping treatment. (Table 10-2 lists the different progestin treatment options that you have.)

Table 10-2	Common Progestins and Their Dosages			
Drug	*Brand Name*	*Administration*	*Dose*	*Drawbacks*
Medroxyprogesterone Acetate (MPA)	Depot Sub-Q Provera 104	Subcutaneously	104 mg	Injection, can take up to a year to leave your system
MPA	Depo-Provera	Intramuscular	100 to 150 mg every 2–3 months; can be more frequent in lesser dosages	Injection; long lasting — can take up to a year to leave your system
MPA	Provera	Oral	10 to 60 mg daily	
Megestrol acetate	Megace	Oral	50 mg daily	
Norethindrone	Micronor	Oral	0.35 mg daily	
Norethindrone acetate	Aygestin, Norlutate	Oral	5 to 15 mg daily	

Considering the side effects

Like BCPs, progestins can have side effects. Talk with your doctor if you notice any of these problems. These side effects include

- ✔ **Weight gain:** Sometimes difficult to lose (especially when taking MPA).

- ✔ **Depression, mood changes:** Can be potentially serious.

- ✔ **Irregular bleeding:** May subside after the first month or two.

- ✔ **Bone loss:** If you're on MPA (better known as Provera in its different forms), your doctor may test you periodically for a decrease in bone mineral density.

- ✔ **Decreased *libido* (sex drive):** May not be good for your sex life.

If you don't have severe side effects and you respond well, you can stay on the progestins almost indefinitely.

Debating danazol (Danocrine)

Danazol (brand-name Danocrine) is an oral drug that was extensively used in the past to treat endometriosis. Although it was proven to be effective, its numerous side effects (see "Facing the side effects of danazol" later in this chapter) have resulted in its replacement by more modern medical treatments. However, for some women with endometriosis, it remains an optional medical treatment.

Danazol acts like two kinds of sex hormones, estrogen and testosterone. Its structure is very similar to testosterone, an *androgen* (male sex hormone). Although women normally have androgens, the quantities are smaller than in men. (All's fair with Mother Nature: Men have estrogen but in a lower level than women.) Danazol comes in capsules; the most common dose for endometriosis is 100 to 400 mg twice a day for three to nine months.

Contemplating danazol: How does it treat endometriosis?

Like all hormone therapies and surgery for endometriosis, danazol doesn't cure the disease. However, danazol can help with endometriosis in the following ways:

- **Shuts down your monthly cycle:** Danazol raises androgen levels in your blood stream and lowers your estrogen levels by suppressing production in the ovaries. This change puts the body in a menopause-like state but doesn't affect the pituitary gland.

- **Shrinks endometrial implants:** Like progesterone, danazol may have a direct effect on the endometrial tissue. That is, it may suppress the growth of the endometrium directly, not as a result of just lowering estrogen. Biopsies of the endometrium have shown this suppressive effect.

- **Decreases pain from implants by depriving them of estrogen stimulation:** Without estrogen, endometriosis can't grow.

Some research shows that danazol may also inhibit the immune system and thereby decrease the inflammatory response to endometriosis. Up to 90 percent of women who use danazol report improvement in symptoms of endometriosis. Relief can come within a few months after starting treatment and typically lasts 6 to 12 months after stopping treatment. Symptoms return within a year for one-third of patients.

Facing the side effects of danazol

For years, danazol was the first-line hormonal therapy for endometriosis. But doctors rarely prescribe it now as an initial treatment and limit its use to six to nine months at a time because of its side effects when it is used. Danazol's side effects are common, affecting 80 percent of women who take the drug. Most of these side effects go away within several months after stopping treatment (but some may be permanent).

Side effects include

- **Acne:** Occurs in around 13 percent of patients.

- **Decreased breast size:** Uncommon but probably annoying!

- **Depression and emotional changes:** May include nervousness, anxiety, and emotional ability.

- **Fluid retention:** Occurs in about 6 percent of patients.

- **Flushing:** Occurs in about 6 percent of patients.

- **Increased cardiovascular risk:** The rise in cholesterol is a real problem because the drug increases LDL (the bad one) by more than 35 percent and, worse, lowers HDL (the good stuff) by more than 50 percent. It also adversely affects *apolipoprotein* levels, another indicator of increased cardiovascular risk.

- **Increased risk of ovarian cancer:** Be sure to discuss this effect with your doctor.

- **Increase in male characteristics, such as deepening of the voice and increased facial hair and body hair (*hirsutism*):** A change in voice can be permanent. Many women find these side effects unbearable and stop the medication prematurely. In our experience, more than 50 percent of women couldn't, or wouldn't, tolerate these side effects and stopped taking danazol before they had a clinical response.

- **Muscle cramps:** May include muscles spasms or tremors, joint lock up, or swelling.

- **Oily skin and hair:** Occurs in around 2 percent of patients.

- **Sugar level changes:** This medicine may affect blood *glucose* (sugar) levels. If you notice a change in the results of your blood or urine glucose test, or if you have any questions about this effect, check with your doctor.

- **Skin rash:** Danazol may cause your skin to be more sensitive to sunlight. Even short exposure to the sun can cause a skin rash, itching, redness, or severe sunburn. When you begin taking this medicine, take precautions: avoid intense sunlight; wear sunglasses, a hat, and long sleeves when you do go out; apply a good sun block; and avoid tanning salons and tanning beds.

- **Weight gain:** Occurs in around 4 percent of patients.

Danazol shouldn't be taken in pregnancy because it can harm a developing fetus. You must use a barrier method of contraception (condoms or diaphragm) while taking danazol.

While you're taking danazol, your menstrual period may not be regular or you may not have a menstrual period at all. This change is normal. If regular menstruation doesn't begin within 60 to 90 days after you stop taking this medicine, check with your doctor. Danazol's effects on hormone regulation are usually reversible. But stopping danazol can cause FSH and LH secretion to rebound, resulting in increased fertility.

Danazol doesn't cause bone loss, as some other hormone treatments do, but it does cause other complications that you should be aware of. You shouldn't use danazol if you fall into any of the following categories:

- Breast-feeding
- Chronic liver, kidney, or heart disease, which can become worse with danazol therapy
- High cholesterol
- Inherited disorder of skin pigment *(porphyria)*
- Pregnancy or possibility of pregnancy during treatment (danazol can harm a fetus)
- Abnormal vaginal bleeding without a known cause

Trying GnRH agonists

GnRH agonists are injected or implanted medications that have found wide use as a treatment for endometriosis. They work by causing a *medical menopause* with extremely low levels of estrogen (much like natural menopause). Although they're an effective treatment for endometriosis, they aren't without significant side effects.

To understand how *GnRH agonists* work, you first need to understand *gonadotropin-releasing hormones* (GnRH). GnRH is a vital part of the menstrual cycle. The hypothalamus delivers GnRH to the pituitary in a *pulsatile* fashion (that is, in short bursts) about every 90 minutes. GnRH lasts a very short time because it breaks down very rapidly while working on receptors in the pituitary gland to release FSH and LH. (Checkout Chapter 5 for more information on these two hormones.)

Understanding how GnRH agonists treat endometriosis

GnRH agonists deliver a constant stream of a molecule very similar to GnRH to the pituitary gland. Two to three *amino acids* (the building blocks of proteins) in the agonist are different from those in natural GnRH, and this small difference makes them stick around much longer than the natural GnRH. The agonist fits on the pituitary gland's receptors in place of the real GnRH and stays there.

The pituitary gland isn't used to this constant stimulation (the pituitary usually sees GnRH briefly every 90 minutes). This adjustment results in a phenomenon called *down regulation* (the pituitary gland becomes exhausted and can no longer make FSH and LH), which eventually suppresses the hormones LH and FSH to very low levels.

Suppressing LH and FSH means the ovaries aren't stimulated and no ovulation occurs. As a result, estrogen levels drop very low (a *hypoestrogenic state*). Because estrogen levels normally stimulate growth of endometrial implants, suppressing the estrogen levels decreases the implants and decreases the pain of endometriosis. With no menstrual cycle (due to no ovulation), the endometrium doesn't grow and shed periodically, and you experience less inflammation from endometriosis and bleeding problems get better.

All the GnRH agonists seem to have a similarly positive effect on pain relief. Clinical studies have compared these compounds to placebos (inert substitutes) and danazol (which used to be the standard medical therapy). In these trials, patients noted significant reduction in pain of all kinds (*dyspareunia* — pain with sex; *dysmenorrhea* — painful menstruation; generalized pelvic pain). For instance, GnRH reduced dyspareunia in one year in 75 percent of women who used the medication.

Unfortunately, as with all other treatments, symptoms recurred in most women after some period of time. One study with Lupron found that 57 percent of the patients had recurrence of painful periods within one year of stopping Lupron.

Decreases in pain are presumably due to the low estrogen levels and lack of ovulation. However, the low estrogen levels are also responsible for most of the side effects with these medications. For this reason, many doctors do an *add-back* therapy, that is, a medication or combination of medications that is low enough to maintain the positive effects of the GnRH agonist and high enough to keep symptoms of low estrogen levels to a minimum. The following medications are possible add-back therapies:

- Low doses of estrogen
- Estrogen and progestin
- Progestin alone
- Bisphosphonate (such as Actonel or Fosamax — drugs that prevent bone loss but don't increase your estrogen levels)
- Progestin and bisphosphonate

You can discuss with your doctor which therapy may be best for you.

Looking at the different GnRH agonist options

When you begin taking GnRH agonists, a *flare* effect occurs. (Before the hormone levels start to decrease, they actually increase — flare — for the first four to ten days, causing a possible initial increase in symptoms in the first week or two of treatment.) To help prevent, or at least blunt, this effect, you can start the GnRH agonist about a week after you ovulate. This mid-luteal-phase (middle of your cycle) dosing helps your own hormones block the initial flare and subsequent ovulation. Ask you doctor about the best time to start the agonist.

You can take GnRH agonists a number of ways: injections into the muscle, a nasal spray, or implants under the skin. However, two major drawbacks to using GnRH agonists are that they're expensive and unavailable in tablet form. Table 10-3 lists the common brand names and doses of GnRH agonists.

Table 10-3	GnRH Agonist Medications for Endometriosis			
Drug	**Brand Name**	**Administration**	**Dose**	**Drawbacks**
Goserelin	Zoladex	Subcutaneous implant	3.6 mg once a month	
Leuprolide acetate	Lupron	Subcutaneously	0.2 mg daily	Daily injection
	Lupron Depot	Intramuscularly	3.75 mg once a month or 11.75 mg every 3 months	Injection
Nafarelin	Synarel	Nasal spray	1 spray twice a day	Daily dose

Many women may find nafarelin (Synarel) easier to take because it doesn't involve needles or implants. You take it twice daily in a nasal spray. In one study, nafarelin shrank endometrial implants and significantly relieved symptoms in 85 percent of patients and delayed recurrence of endometriosis after surgery. Compared to leuprolide, nafarelin was less expensive, had fewer side effects, provided a better quality of life — and didn't use needles! Unfortunately, the nasal spray can be hard to standardize and use, so these benefits may not actually be as good in normal use.

Facing the side effects

Although GnRH agonists can make some women's lives easier by treating their endometriosis, this drug isn't for everyone. The following people shouldn't take GnRH agonists:

- ✔ **Women who haven't gone through puberty yet.** If you're a young woman, GnRH agonists prevent you from developing peak *bone mineral density* (BMD, a way to measure bone mineral content) and may increase your risk for osteoporosis later in your life. (Check out *Osteoporosis For Dummies* by Dr. Carolyn Riester O'Connor and Sharon Perkins [Wiley] for more on osteoporosis and peak BMD.) GnRH agonists may also delay puberty.

✔ **Women who are pregnant.** Researchers aren't sure, but GnRH agonists may be harmful to a developing fetus. They also will decrease estrogen and progesterone and may cause miscarriage. Although you're unlikely to become pregnant while using a GnRH agonist, to be completely safe, you should use a barrier method of contraception while you're on these drugs. If you think you're pregnant, tell your doctor immediately.

✔ **Women who have pernicious anemia.** This anemia results from a lack of *intrinsic factor,* a protein that helps you absorb vitamin B12 from the stomach. Decreased estrogen levels with GnRH agonists can worsen symptoms.

You may experience a number of unpleasant side effects while on these medications. Not surprisingly, these are the same symptoms you may experience in menopause. Some common side effects are

✔ **Menopausal symptoms, including hot flashes, night sweats, and mood swings:** Just like menopause, these symptoms are annoying and life altering. Several treatments are available. Ask your doctor.

✔ **Headaches:** May be severe and can be treated by over-the-counter meds, such as ibuprofen.

✔ **Insomnia:** Sleeplessness or awaking in the middle of the night without being able to get back to sleep can cause irritability and emotional changes.

✔ **Bone loss:** Because GnRH agonists decrease your estrogen to menopausal levels, long-term use can result in irreversible bone loss. You can experience 4 to 6 percent bone loss in a six-month treatment period; most of the lost bone regenerates within six months of stopping treatment. Add-back therapy (giving estrogen in addition to Lupron) may allow you to have more extended time (more than six months) or repeat treatment.

✔ **Vaginal dryness:** This may cause painful sex and can be treated with lubricants or local hormone cream.

Handling hot flashes

Hot flashes are one of the most annoying side effects of GnRH agonists, just like they're one of the most annoying side effects of menopause! You can minimize those effects however. To decrease hot flashes, try eliminating the following triggers:

✔ Alcohol (which can make you flushed and hot all on its own!)

✔ Caffeine

✔ Diet pills

✔ Hot (spicy) foods

✔ Hot tubs

- Saunas

- Smoking

- Stress

    For example, if being late stresses you out, make sure you get to your destination early! Reducing stress may not be easy, but it's certainly worth the trouble, not only for reducing hot flashes but also for making your life easier and more fun overall! (We discuss ways to decrease both pain and stress more in Chapter 12.)

You can also decrease the effect of hot flashes. For example:

- Wear layered clothing, so it's easier to undress (one layer at a time, please!) when you start to overheat.

- Use only cotton sheets on your bed; no synthetics.

- Dress in cotton or cotton derivatives; skip synthetic materials that don't let your skin breathe.

- Keep a glass of ice water nearby and sip frequently to keep your insides cool.

- Have a fan in your bedroom — and at your desk, if possible.

I'm burning up: Hot flash facts

The body's drop in estrogen (which certain hormone medications can artificially induce) causes hot flashes. The decreased estrogen affects the hypothalamus, which controls body temperature. Because estrogen receptors are in other parts of the brain and in the skin, the lack of estrogen may directly affect these areas also.

The decreased estrogen causes the hypothalamus to think your body temperature is too hot and sends signals to your blood vessels, heart, and nervous system to start processes to cool you down. Suddenly your heart starts to pound and blood vessels dilate to bring more blood to the skin surface to be cooled (which makes your face look red and your sweat glands release more sweat).

Do you feel like you're about ready to pass out because you're so hot? Do your friends and family think you're a bit strange when you're wearing shorts and a sleeveless shirt on a chilly November day? Don't let those folks bother you. Grab a cold drink, a fan, and arm yourself with these interesting hot flash facts:

- An *aura*, (a feeling that a hot flash is about to begin) often precedes a hot flash.

- Hot flashes usually last just a few minutes, but they can last up to an hour and recur several times during the day (more than 50 times a day in some studies!).

- Hot flashes usually affect your upper body the most, especially your face and chest.

- Hot flashes can cause nausea, dizziness, headache, or heart palpitations.

- Your skin temperature can rise as much as 6 degrees during a hot flash (that's skin, not internal body temperature).

Low-dose antidepressants can help with hot flashes because they disrupt *epinephrine* and *serotonin,* the signals that transmit the go-ahead for hot flashes. Up to 60 percent of women notice a decrease in hot flashes with this treatment, according to one study.

Dealing with the other side effects

The side effects of GnRH agonists can usually be dealt with by taking over-the-counter medications for headaches and pain, sleep aids, or vaginal lubrication aids. If you notice side effects from these drugs, you may want to consider one of the newer types of treatments, such as GnRH antagonists (see "Looking at GnRH antagonists" later in this chapter.)

Inserting an IUD for pain relief

If you had an intrauterine device (IUD) in the past, the thought of using it for pain relief may seem a little foreign to you. After all, most IUDs are pretty uncomfortable at first, so how can one decrease pain?

IUDs are primarily a birth control device, so if you're planning on getting pregnant, an IUD isn't the method to use to decrease endometriosis! However, unlike Depo-Provera (whose effects can last for months after your last injection), an IUD has no effects after you remove it, so you can try to get pregnant soon after.

Understanding how an IUD can relieve endometriosis pain

Studies indicate that the LNG-IUS IUD (Mirena) may effectively relieve pain in endometriosis. This IUD is impregnated with levonorgestrel, a progestin. This IUD reduces endometrial cell-proliferation and increases cell self-destruction. Progestin from the IUD mainly affects the uterus and cervix, causing fewer systemic side effects than other forms of progestins.

The LNG-IUS has several advantages:

- ✔ It can decrease dysfunctional uterine bleeding up to 90 percent.
- ✔ It may lessen or stop menstrual bleeding altogether after the first two to three months.
- ✔ It's less likely to have side effects than oral progestins.
- ✔ It's more effective in preventing pregnancy than copper IUDs.
- ✔ It may decrease your chance of developing pelvic inflammatory disease.
- ✔ It can remain in place up to five years.

Determining if an IUD is right for you

IUDs can be inserted any time, as long as you're not pregnant. The easiest and safest time to insert one is during your menstrual cycle. Insertion takes place in a doctor's office in just a few minutes. Insertion can cause cramping and light bleeding, but you may notice less discomfort if you've had a vaginal delivery.

An IUD may not be a good choice for you if

- You have pelvic inflammatory disease.
- You have a sexually transmitted disease.
- You have an active cervical or vaginal infection.
- You have uterine abnormalities.
- You had a serious pelvic infection in the three months following pregnancy.
- You have more than one sexual partner or a sexual partner who has more than one sexual partner.
- You get infections easily (including immune-system problems), have leukemia or AIDS, or abuse intravenous drugs.
- You possibly have uterine or cervical cancer.
- You have unexplained bleeding from the uterus.
- You have liver disease or a liver tumor.
- You have or have had breast cancer.
- You have had, or are at risk of having, an *ectopic pregnancy* (pregnancy occurring in the fallopian tubes).
- You are allergic to levonorgestrel, silicone, or polyethylene.

Make sure you discuss all the pros and cons with your doctor before deciding on an IUD.

Considering serious side effects

Because IUDs are a foreign body in your uterus, they can cause serious complications; call your doctor immediately if

- You don't feel well or have a fever over 100.4 degrees Fahrenheit.
- You can't feel the strings attached to your IUD or they seem to be misplaced (longer or shorter than usual).
- You have symptoms of a vaginal infection, such as pain, odor, and discharge.
- You have abnormal spotting or sudden bleeding.

Living with normal side effects

An IUD can cause side effects, especially in the first few months after insertion. The following are normal, but if they're especially severe, ask your doctor if you can take anything to combat them. Normal side effects of a progestin-coated IUD include the following:

- Acne
- Back pain
- Breast tenderness
- Cramping
- Headache
- Menstrual changes, such as heavier flow or less flow than normal
- Mood changes
- Nausea

About 12 percent of women with the Mirena IUD have ovarian cysts. In most cases, these cysts disappear spontaneously over two to three months.

Checking Out Nonhormonal Options

Nonhormonal options are usually the first-line drugs for endometriosis pain. Most of these medications are available over the counter, but some do require a prescription. Doctors also may suggest or prescribe these nonhormonal treatments if you can't handle the side effects of hormones or you're trying to get pregnant. You can read more about nonhormonal treatments and other painkilling methods in Chapter 13, where we discuss managing chronic pain.

Using NSAIDs

Nonsteroidal anti-inflammatory drugs (NSAIDs), such as ibuprofen and Naprosyn, are the mainstay and usually the first choice of treatment for endometriosis symptoms. NSAIDs help reduce pain and the inflammation in many diseases. You can buy them over the counter or in higher doses with a prescription. (Check out Chapter 13 for more helpful info about NSAIDs.)

These medications are safe to use (as directed), and they can reduce the pain of endometriosis (such as mid-cycle pain and painful periods) and help decrease the inflammation. This anti-inflammatory benefit can potentially decrease inflammation that leads to adhesions and scarring. Of course, these medications can't help with adhesions and scar tissue that are already present.

For many women, NSAIDs work well enough to make their discomfort tolerable. They're most effective when you take them as soon as, or even before, the symptoms start. As with all pain management, you're most successful when you get ahead of the pain and stay there.

Trying other painkillers

If NSAIDs don't give you enough relief to continue with everyday functioning, then your doctor may prescribe more potent pain relievers. These drugs belong to the class of narcotics and similar medications. Refer to Chapter 13 where we discuss these painkillers in depth.

Looking at What the Future Holds

A number of drugs may be available in the near future for the treatment of endometriosis. Some of these drugs are older and are already effective for other diseases, and they may prove helpful in endometriosis. Other drugs are brand new. Do they all hold promise for the future? Undoubtedly, some of them do; others may fall by the wayside. A few of these treatments are already in use in Europe. In this section, we look at some possible drugs of the future.

Looking at GnRH antagonists

Although these drugs aren't specifically approved to treat endometriosis, some doctors do prescribe them to treat the disease. GnRH *antagonists* are the new kids on the block in hormonal medications to treat endometriosis. They seem to have several real benefits, especially with side effects. Two common GnRH antagonists are Cetrorelix acetate (Cetrotide) and Ganirelix acetate (Antagon). They aren't approved yet for endometriosis, and they're very expensive, much more so than agonists (8 to 20 times more expensive!).

Gauging how GnRH antagonists treat endometriosis

GnRH antagonists are very similar to GnRH agonists, but they work much more quickly than agonists. GnRH antagonists are a synthetic peptide that competes with GnRH for its receptor site, just like agonists. Unlike the agonists that initially stimulate the pituitary gland to release its store of FSH and LH, antagonists block the action of the receptor. This blockage of GnRH action results in the pituitary gland decreasing its output of FSH and LH immediately.

GnRH antagonists aren't long-lasting drugs, so they're usually given subcutaneously, like insulin, through daily injections. One GnRH antagonist, Cetrotide, comes in a higher dose (3 mg) for a once- or twice-a-week dose over eight weeks.

Identifying the side effects to GnRH antagonists

Serum estradiol remains higher with this therapy (around 50 pg/ml), so side effects related to low estrogen are less prevalent. In one study, endometriosis patients undergoing this treatment reported a symptom-free period, with no mood changes, hot flushes, libido loss, vaginal dryness, or other symptoms.

Antagonist side effects aren't as severe as those from agonists. Antagonist effects include

✔ Headache

✔ Nausea

✔ Itching and redness at the injection site

Pursuing antiprogestins

Antiprogestins are promising new drugs for endometriosis because they reduce both estrogen and progesterone receptors. Currently scientists are testing two antiprogestins:

✔ **Gestrinone:** As the most studied antiprogestin, gestrinone (Dimetriose) seems comparable to GnRH agonists in reducing pain but with fewer menopausal symptoms. Gestrinone also seems to have a less negative effect on bone density. In one study, bone density even increased slightly. The side effects are similar to androgens like danazol (see "Debating danazol [Danocrine]" earlier in this chapter). Gestrinone isn't currently available in the United States.

Treatment with gestrinone includes 2.5 mg doses, two or three times per week. Some of the negative effects of gestrinone include

• Abnormal uterine bleeding

• Acne

• Excess hair growth

• Headache

• Weight gain

✔ **Mifepristone (Mifeprex):** In one six-month study, mifepristone improved symptoms and reduced endometrial implants without causing menopausal side effects. Long-term use, however, may cause changes in the uterine tissue and cell proliferation. Experience with this drug for endometriosis is limited.

Selecting SERMS

Selective Estrogen Receptor Modulators (SERMs) are drugs that behave like estrogen in some tissues and like estrogen blockers in others. One well-known SERM, tamoxifen (Istubal, Nolvadex, Valodex), seems to worsen endometriosis, but others, such as raloxifene (Evista), may decrease endometrial implants and decrease pain.

Fulvetrant (Faslodex) is an estrogen blocker, and studies have looked at its effectiveness for uterine fibroids and endometriosis. More testing is needed in this area.

Examining aromatase inhibitors

Aromatase is an enzyme that makes estrogen from other hormones, and it's essential for most estrogen production. Researchers are studying drugs called *aromatase inhibitors* for effects against endometriosis because they block the production of estrogen. Research also shows that women with endometriosis may have abnormal levels of aromatase in these tissues.

Aromatase inhibitors for breast cancer and other disease states include anastrozole, letrozole, exemestane, and vorozole. A 2004 study showed that a combination of letrozole and progestin reduced endometriosis and decreased pelvic pain. More studies are underway.

Testing SPRMs

A new class of drugs, Selective Progesterone Receptor Modulators (SPRMs — make sure you don't add an E after the P!), have both agonist and antagonist properties and may prove beneficial in suppressing endometrial implants. SPRMS, also known as *mesoprogestins,* react differently in different tissues, and may be used in place of GnRH agonist and antagonist drugs that have negative side effects.

One drug in this class that is being tested and is effective in reducing non-menstrual pain and dysmenorrhea in patients with endometriosis is asoprisnil. Asoprisnil is undergoing clinical trials and may be available in the next few years.

Worrying about the effect of medication on future pregnancy

If you're hoping to get pregnant in the near future, taking a medication that fools your body into thinking that it's in menopause may not seem like a very good idea. Decreasing your pain is certainly a concern, but decreasing your chances of getting pregnant is a serious compromise.

Your chances of pregnancy right after stopping medications depends on which medication you choose. For example:

✔ Contraceptive effects of birth control pills usually stop a few weeks to months after you stop the Pill, making it a good choice if you want to get pregnant soon after treatment.

✔ After you have an IUD removed, you can start trying to get pregnant right away.

Fortunately, most of today's drugs are short acting and leave the body pretty quickly (except for medroxyprogesterone acetate — MPA). As long as you don't get pregnant within the first few weeks after stopping the medications, you have no chance of the medications affecting the egg, sperm, embryo, or fetus. In fact, discontinuation of the drugs may even enhance your fertility initially.

Finding new treatments (and wrinkles) all the time

Researchers are considering a number of drugs for investigational testing for use in endometriosis. Just a few examples include

✔ **Various immune modulators:** In many ways, immune therapy is still in its infancy. Because immune issues may play a large part in endometriosis, treatment with immunosuppressive drugs may stop the disease before it becomes a problem in those women susceptible to it. (See Chapter 4 for more on immune therapy.)

✔ **New anti-estrogen medications:** These may also prove useful in shrinking endometriosis without the side effects of older medications.

✔ **Botox (botulinum toxin):** Yes, the wrinkle cure has been used with some success in a small number of patients. It doesn't work in any hormonal way but may help relax muscle spasms in the pelvis, reducing pain.

Chapter 11

Contemplating Surgery to Improve Your Endometriosis

Doctors often suggest medical therapy as the first treatment for endometriosis symptoms. However, if you don't already have a definite diagnosis or the medication doesn't work for you, your doctor may suggest surgery. Surgery, then, can determine whether you actually have endometriosis or another disease, and in most cases, your surgeon can treat the disease during the surgery.

Don't take surgery lightly. Risks are always present, even though small, with anesthesia and surgery. But in many cases, surgery is the best option for decreasing the pain and destruction of endometriosis.

Deciding to have surgery is a major decision, but we hope to make that decision a little easier for you. In this chapter, we discuss all the current options, the potential complications, and the benefits of surgically treating endometriosis.

Eyeing the Two Main Surgical Methods

Choosing to have surgery to treat endometriosis isn't simple. The first questions that come up are, "What kind of surgery? Minor or major? Laparoscopy or laparotomy?" Which type of surgery you and your doctor decide upon will depend on whether your surgery will be conservative (leaving as much in place as possible) or radical (removing organs such as the uterus). Throughout this chapter we discuss the surgical methods and options and give you the information you need to make an informed decision.

Before you can make a decision about which surgery method is right for you, you first need to understand the two types of treatment:

- **Conservative surgery:** The surgeon tries to do as little surgery as possible in order to preserve function of your reproductive organs. She may remove cysts, adhesions, fibroids, abnormal tissue, and even a whole ovary if the other ovary is functional. The goal is to help your symptoms but keep the uterus, tubes, and ovaries (at least one good one) so that your menstrual cycle can continue. (See the section "Starting Surgical Treatment Conservatively" in this chapter.)

- **Radical surgery:** Don't let the term concern you. With endometriosis, radical surgery simply means that the surgeon removes your uterus, tubes, and ovaries. (We discuss radical surgery in depth in the section "Opting for Radical Surgery" later in this chapter.)

If you've unsuccessfully tried conservative surgery and every medical option possible to relieve your symptoms *and* you don't want to get pregnant in the future, radical surgery may be your best option. Sometimes the surgeon leaves one or both ovaries in, but this decision may undermine the success of the radical surgery.

In the vast majority of cases, surgery for endometriosis means choosing an approach for the surgeon to see inside the pelvis and abdominal cavity. Because every surgery requires an incision of some size somewhere, the location and size of that incision dictate the type of surgery. Your surgeon has two choices:

- **Laparoscopy:** This method is less invasive and uses a small incision, much less than an inch, to allow access to the abdominal cavity. This choice probably sounds good to you — why have a big incision when you can have a small one?

- **Laparotomy:** This method uses an incision ranging from a couple of inches to 12 inches or more in length. For example, cesarean section scars are laparotomy incisions. These incisions can be horizontal across the lower abdomen or vertical from the pubic bone to the umbilicus and above. This method is an *open* procedure, allowing your surgeon to see and feel more.

DOCTOR'S NOTES

When endometriosis isn't the problem: Finding the real culprit

If endometriosis is *not* your main problem, then surgery may expose the real culprit. Your surgeon may be able to remove that new problem right then, or you may need another treatment altogether.

Various surgical scenarios allow the surgeon to identify the source of pain. For instance, an appendix stuck to other areas by adhesions from chronic inflammation can cause right lower-abdomen pain. During surgery, the doctor can remove the appendix and, as a result, reduce the symptoms.

However, no two situations are ever the same, and no two patients are identical. Just because someone you know had one type of procedure and swears by it doesn't mean that procedure is the right choice for you. You may end up swearing *at* it! This section looks more closely at laparoscopy and laparotomy and helps you see the advantages of each surgical method.

One option: Having a laparoscopy

Laparoscopy has become the most common way to diagnose and surgically treat endometriosis. The procedure has come a long way since the 1970s when surgeons used it exclusively for tubal ligations and simple diagnoses. In its early days, the telescope optics and the brightness of the light sources were barely adequate to see fuzzy shapes, and surgeons had only a few crude instruments. These limitations minimized the usefulness of laparoscopy.

However, with the explosion of technology in surgical instruments (refer to "Naming the Surgical Tools" later in this chapter for more specifics) and training in this procedure over the past three decades, laparoscopy has become very popular. For example, many training programs include extensive labs with computer-aided simulations and animal labs that offer doctors invaluable experience and training. Numerous post-graduate courses are available for doctors who didn't get this training in their residency program — probably because it hadn't been invented yet!

However, even with all this progress, not every gynecologic surgeon can do advanced laparoscopic surgery. Be sure you ask your surgeon about his qualifications because he needs to feel comfortable about his skills — and so do you! *Note:* Just because a doctor doesn't want to work through the laparoscope doesn't mean he's a poor surgeon. Actually, the opposite is true; doing a procedure through the scope may not be in your best interest. Discuss the pros and cons of each approach with your doctor.

Proceeding through a laparoscopy

Laparoscopy is practical for almost any type of surgery imaginable, including hysterectomy, removal of ectopic pregnancies, appendectomy, gall bladder removal, bowel resection, stomach stapling for obesity, removal of lungs, and even radical surgery for cancer. The list gets longer every day.

In gynecologic surgery, a laparoscopy has the nickname of *belly button surgery* because it almost always uses a small incision in, or just below, the umbilicus. (Obviously you need to shelve any navel embellishments or jewelry for this surgery!) Rarely, the entrance incision is somewhere else on the abdominal wall.

A laparoscopy (check out Figure 11-1) usually follows these steps:

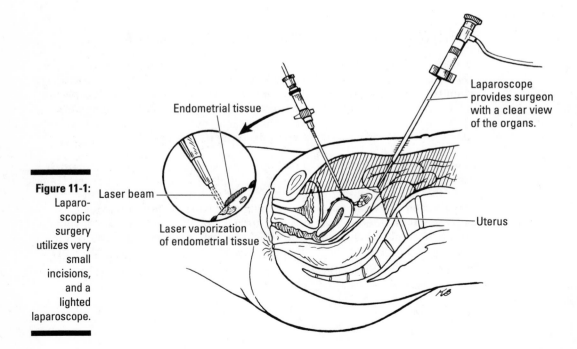

Figure 11-1: Laparoscopic surgery utilizes very small incisions, and a lighted laparoscope.

Endometrial tissue

Laser beam

Laser vaporization of endometrial tissue

Laparoscope provides surgeon with a clear view of the organs.

Uterus

1. **An anesthesiologist or an anesthetist puts you to sleep.**

   (Check out the next section for more anesthesia information.)

2. **The surgeon performs a vaginal exam before the surgery while you're asleep or relaxed.**

   This exam can be more accurate than one in the office because you're more relaxed (you can't get much more relaxed than asleep!), and your bladder is empty and doesn't get in the way (see Chapter 3 to see the close proximity of the uterus and bladder). You have a catheter during the surgery, and it may remain until you're fully awake.

3. **The surgeon makes a small incision into your abdominal cavity.**

4. **Using a small, blunt needle or a similar device, the surgeon inserts gas (usually carbon dioxide) into the abdominal cavity.**

5. **The surgeon slides a *trocar* (a tube with a valve to prevent loss of the gas) into the cavity, allowing him to place the scope and see inside.**

   Because the surgeon can't see or avoid possible abnormal anatomy, he must place the needle and trocar (most have fairly sharp ends!) *blindly* into the area. This step is the most risky part of the procedure.

6. **The surgeon makes at least one additional incision (and usually two or three) as an *accessory* port below the umbilical incision.**

   These incisions are usually about a half-inch long and provide access to the site for other instruments, such as scissors, lasers, or graspers during the procedure. Sometimes a larger accessory port is necessary for removal of big pieces of tissue or organs.

7. **A camera at the end of the scope (some have the camera at the tip that goes inside you but most are on the end that is outside you) feeds the image to a monitor (large TV) so the surgeon and assistants can see their work.**

   Because the image is limited to two dimensions, the surgeon must rely on his experience and use great care to prevent complications. Picture printers, VCRs, or CD recorders can record your surgery for future reference (and may be available for your records).

8. **Because the surgeon can now see inside the cavity with the laparoscope and avoid vulnerable structures, he can insert the accessory ports safely.**

9. **Using a gentle probe or a grasper to move organs, the surgeon looks around the entire abdominal cavity, checking out your liver, gall bladder, intestines, bladder, and pelvic organs.**

   He can deal with any problems at this point or document them for future care.

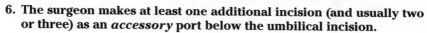

10. **Your surgeon may do a *dilation and curettage* (D&C) or hysteroscopy (a technique to examine the inside of the uterus with a smaller telescope).**

    These techniques allow him to be sure the inside of the uterus has no abnormalities, and he may run dye through the fallopian tubes to check for blockage.

11. **At the end of the procedure, the surgeon closes all incisions under the skin with dissolving sutures or with tissue glue closure that requires no sutures.**

    You may have a small bandage over the incisions to keep them clean (thus another nickname — *band-aid surgery*). Sometimes a harmless string emerges at the incision site and either dissolves or can be removed.

If you've had a previous laparotomy or have a known infection in the abdominal cavity, the chance of running into adhesions and intestinal or bladder injury on insertion of the needle or trocar can be high. In this case, your surgeon may make a slightly larger opening into the abdominal cavity first and then place a blunt trocar to avoid the risky blind insertion with a sharp instrument. However, because studies don't show that this approach greatly reduces injury and is larger and more time consuming, it's fairly uncommon.

Considering anesthesia during laparoscopy

Almost all laparoscopies require general anesthesia, especially if your doctor expects to remove or rearrange tissues. General anesthesia allows for better and more predictable relaxation of the abdominal muscles, which makes the surgery safer and easier.

The newer anesthetic medications

- ✔ Are very safe and gentle on your system
- ✔ Put you to sleep quickly, easily, and safely and allow you to awaken just as quickly
- ✔ Have an amnesiac effect so you don't remember any discomfort
- ✔ Often include an analgesic so you have pain relief before you perceive any pain (a definite plus!)

Usually a person from the anesthesia department interviews you about your medical and surgical history before the surgery and tells you about the drugs and what to expect. A representative from your doctor's office, the hospital, or the anesthesia department will also contact you with specific instructions for you to follow before your arrival.

On the day of surgery, the following steps occur:

1. **A nurse places an *intravenous line* (the IV) in your arm to provide your future medications quickly and easily — and without more needles.**

2. **You may receive a sedative to help you relax while you wait.**

   (If you have any anxiety or fears, this medication can be a godsend — a strange place with many new faces can be scary!)

In the operating room, the following take place:

1. **You're moved onto the operating table, and the anesthetist or anesthesiologist gives you several medications.**

2. **A mask is placed over your mouth with oxygen to ensure that you have enough oxygen during the surgery.**

3. **As soon as you're deeply asleep and your muscles are relaxed, a tube or similar device is placed through your mouth or nose into the trachea (wind pipe) to**

   - Be sure you receive enough oxygen.

   - Prevent stomach contents or excess saliva from getting into your lungs.

Anesthesia has greatly improved over the years. Still, don't plan on driving or making important decisions for 24 hours!

Using MAC during surgery: Advantages and disadvantages

Some surgeons and anesthesiologists perform uncomplicated and quick procedures (usually tubal ligations or purely diagnostic procedures) with local anesthesia and intravenous sedation known as *Monitored Anesthesia Care* (MAC). The plus side: You aren't as deeply asleep with MAC, and you don't have a breathing tube.

MAC has some disadvantages for abdominal surgery, however, so be sure you know the facts before you opt for this approach. Some disadvantages are

✔ Your abdominal organs may not be as relaxed as they are with general anesthesia.

✔ Although the surgeon can numb the incision areas with a local anesthetic (such as Novocain), he can't adequately anesthetize the internal covering of the cavity or the organs that he moves and pokes. As a result, you may have some very uncomfortable moments, and you can't just stop in the middle of the procedure!

✔ The pressure of the gas that separates the organs can make you feel like you can't breathe — not a pleasant feeling and highly anxiety-provoking.

Treating endometriosis during laparoscopy

While your surgeon is looking inside you, what can he do if he finds endometriosis (or any other problem for that matter)? The answer depends on what you discussed when you signed the informed consent.

For example, if this is purely a diagnostic procedure, the surgeon looks around, possibly puts dye through the tubes, and may break up minor adhesions. If you hope to get pregnant and signed a consent for the surgeon to take any necessary steps, he can also try to make the anatomy as normal as possible. If you've had multiple surgeries and this surgery is an attempt to end the problem forever, he can do a hysterectomy and remove the tubes and ovaries (check out "Having a hysterectomy" later in this chapter for more information).

In short, your doctor's actions during the laparoscopy depend on your previous discussions about possible complications and risks, the severity of your symptoms, your previous history, your expectations, your desire for pregnancy now or in the future, your age, and the comfort level of the surgeon (that is, his skill level, his assessment of the risks and benefits for you, and his understanding of your expectations).

Passing through the recovery phase

People have different pain tolerances, so predicting when you'll be back to normal after laparoscopy isn't easy. Some patients return to work the next day, and other people take weeks. Your recovery also depends on the actual procedures during surgery. Cutting a few adhesions and removing implants and cysts can be fairly pain-free because these structures have no pain nerves. But if your doctor has removed a lot of peritoneum or vaporized or cauterized endometriosis, you may have more pain because the peritoneum has pain fibers that respond to any disturbance.

Your doctor can let you know about returning to normal activities, but again, a lot depends on the surgery and how your body responds to it. Be sure to ask about sexual activity. Each surgeon has suggestions on timing, but some of the decision depends on the extent and type of surgery (such as vaginal work, D&C, or a hysteroscopy).

Taking care of your incision

The wounds on the skin of the abdomen can hurt just like any other cut. Many surgeons use a local anesthetic, such as marcaine, in these sites to help relieve pain. The size of the incision can also, of course, add to the discomfort. And types of closure also affect your recovery. Sutures through the skin are more painful than sutures underneath, and a tissue glue closure normally causes the least pain.

No matter what kind of closure or incisions you have, you can decrease the recovery discomfort in several ways:

✔ Keep the wounds clean and covered until your doctor tells you to remove the bandage.

✔ Don't let clothing (especially elastic bands or belts) or jewelry rub against the wounds.

✔ Use a mild soap to gently lather the area, then rinse it well and replace the bandage.

✔ Apply an ice pack for 30 minutes and then remove it for 30 minutes as often as feasible the day of surgery. (For the first 24 hours, an ice pack can help decrease the swelling and inflammation.)

✔ After this first 24 hours, heat can help healing in the area. Three or four times a day, use heat just above body temperature for 20 to 30 minutes.

Your doctor prescribes pain medication based on the extent of the surgery, including ibuprofen to opioids. If you're not getting adequate pain relief from your medication, let your doctor know.

Ouch! Why your throat may hurt

Perhaps the worst part of the immediate recovery is the sore throat from the breathing tube. Though the anesthesiologist may give you medication to prevent it, most people still feel the effects. The discomfort usually doesn't last long, and you shouldn't see any blood. The treatment is the same as for any sore throat: lozenges, warm saltwater gargles, or analgesics.

Before you leave the recovery area, ask the anesthesiologist about any special difficulties you may have had during surgery so she can help you deal with them. If your sore throat persists or gets severe or if you see blood in your sputum or have trouble breathing, let your doctor know immediately.

The breathing tube is necessary because your abdominal muscles need to relax for surgery. The anesthesiologist administers a paralyzing medication to relax these muscles, but the drug also reduces your ability to breathe on your own. So, the anesthesiologist inserts an endotracheal tube into your bronchus to provide additional oxygen and to prevent you from *aspirating* (getting something into your lungs — not good). Although the endotracheal tube is the safest and most common instrument, other devices are also available, such as the laryngeal mask airway (LMA) or the nasotracheal tube, but they all accomplish the same goal.

Another option: Choosing laparotomy

Laparotomy means to enter the abdominal cavity via a large, or relatively large, incision. With the advent of mini-laparotomy techniques, the incision may be as small as 4 centimeters (about an inch and three-fourths), which is still bigger than the 1-centimeter incision for laparoscopy but far smaller (and easier to heal) than the common 12-inch wounds a few years ago. Before the boom of laparoscopic technology and training, a laparotomy was the only way to really treat endometriosis. Even today, most training programs teach procedures using laparotomy.

Sizing up a laparotomy

During a laparotomy, your surgeon makes a vertical or horizontal incision. The cut can go from the top of the pubic bone to the navel (and beyond, if necessary), or it can be across the lower abdomen, from the top of one hip-bone to the other. The size of the incision depends on the procedure and the need for exposure of structures.

Most gynecologic cases (such as cesarean sections) use a *transverse* (horizontal) incision that extends from a couple of inches to more than 12 inches, depending on the procedure. Most general surgeries use a vertical incision, and some gynecologic cases may also require this approach. Ask your surgeon which incision he plans to use and why.

Noting the treatment advantages of laparotomy to laparoscopy

Sometimes a laparotomy is necessary or more beneficial than a laparoscopy. Although laparotomies do result in a larger incision and slower healing time, they have the following advantages over laparoscopy:

- **Laparotomy gives the surgeon as much room as he needs to perform a procedure.** The incision can be big enough to get instruments, hands, and assistants' hands into the area. Because *exposure* (accessibility) is the mantra of surgery, the laparotomy was the only approach for many years. This need for exposure is still true of many procedures, especially those that require extensive tissue removal or reconstruction.

  Furthermore, a laparotomy allows the surgeon more room to readily repair damage to the ureter, major blood vessels, intestines, bladder, uterus, and other organs.

- **Most surgeons are trained to do laparotomies.** Most training programs still teach doctors to do major procedures, such as hysterectomy, *myomectomy* (removing fibroids), *oophorectomy* (removing ovaries), and *salpingectomy* (removing ovaries and tubes), via laparotomy. However, this preference may change as more gynecologists receive training in laparoscopy and as the equipment becomes more available.

- **Laparotomy makes viewing and removing extensive adhesions and distorted anatomy easier.** With the exposure of a laparotomy, the surgeon and his assistants can actually place their hands into the pelvis to feel for problems and expose areas better. This accessibility is very important when dealing with dense scar tissue, anatomic distortions and malformations, and large growths (such as fibroids and cysts).

- **Laparotomy allows easier removal of potentially dangerous lesions from the pelvis.** The surgeon may not want anything to spill from the pathology he is removing, particularly if cancer is a concern. But spillage from endometriomas, dermoid cysts, and even fragments of fibroids can also cause problems. Laparotomy gives the surgeon a better chance to remove all the pathology easily and cleanly.

✔ **Laparotomy lets the surgeon do more extensive removal of lesions while avoiding vital structures.** Most surgeons are better trained to do extensive surgery via laparotomy and can do it quicker and with less risk of injury to other organs and structures.

Granted, the few surgeons who perform advanced laparoscopic surgery will say that all these advantages are also possible through the scope. And that's true, but very few surgeons are capable of performing all these procedures as well via laparoscopic surgery. Your doctor may feel more confident with laparotomy, and the doctor's level of confidence is important!

Recovering from laparotomy

For a laparotomy, you can follow all the same guidelines as for a laparoscopy (see the section, "Passing through the recovery phase" earlier in this chapter). These guidelines include ice the first 24 to 48 hours (to decrease swelling and pain) and then regular heat on the incision to help healing.

However, the recovery process for a laparotomy is a bit more complicated than a laparoscopy because the incision is larger and surgery is more complex. Most patients stay overnight after laparotomy for the following reasons:

✔ **The wound is usually too painful and your movement too restricted for the first 24 to 48 hours for you to be comfortable at home.** Regular pain medication is important and may not be available at home. The hospital staff can monitor the powerful pain medications after a laparotomy to be sure that you don't have a problem with blood pressure or breathing.

✔ **The digestive system sometimes doesn't work well after laparotomy.** A problem called *ileus* (the intestines just stop functioning) can occur and lead to major problems. The problem can be hard to monitor at home, and the resulting complications can be very serious.

✔ **The wound runs the risk of bleeding.** The hospital staff can watch your incision for the first 24 hours or so.

The incision can disrupt the abdominal muscles and their attachments, and it opens up the *fascia* (the tough white tissue that supports the abdominal wall and attaches muscles to bones). Remember these facts about the fascia:

✔ The fascia must heal before full strength and function of the abdominal muscles returns.

✔ During this healing process, movement of any kind can be painful.

✔ The fascia takes about two weeks to regain most of its strength, but tenderness can remain for a while longer.

The laparotomy wound is more likely to get infected than a smaller laparoscopic incision. Contact your doctor if you have redness, firmness, or increasing pain and discharge from the wound because any of these symptoms can signify infection.

Most surgeons close laparotomy wounds with metal staples or sutures of other material that must be removed. These closures can come out in three to five days, but occasionally they need more time. (Your doctor can make that call.) Be sure to keep the sutures clean and free from irritation. Sometimes the sutures are under the skin and dissolve away on their own. Although most of these sutures don't need removal, you should take the same precautions as for the above-ground variety.

Due to all these recovery factors, your return to work and other normal activities can't be as quick as with a laparoscopy. Ask your surgeon about returning to normal activities, but resign yourself to at least two weeks (and probably four to six weeks) of minimal activities.

Naming the Surgical Tools

Wouldn't it be great if your physician could wave Dr. McCoy's diagnostic *tricorder* in *Star Trek* over your body to make a diagnosis? Despite all the technological advances in the past three decades, surgeons still have to rely on today's surgical tools to help them treat endometriosis.

Various companies have developed ingenious devices for many more procedures via laparoscopy. These devices can

- ✔ Make entrance and exit easier and safer
- ✔ Grasp tissue gently and minimize trauma
- ✔ Remove tissue neatly
- ✔ Cut with less bleeding and collateral damage
- ✔ Prevent spillage of irritants and pieces of tissue

Nevertheless, the surgeon must still make an incision to see and work inside your pelvis and abdominal cavity with a laparoscope. The usual size of scopes today is 5 or 10 millimeters (⅕ to ⅖ of an inch) in diameter. This requires an incision of less than an inch, but it still requires an incision. Newer scopes (as small as 2.8 mm) aren't common yet, but they're on the way.

This section looks at some of the surgical tools for a laparoscopy or laparotomy, the technology behind these tools, and your doctor's decisions about tools for your surgery.

Cutting with knives and scissors

Many surgeons still use the tried-and-true scalpel (knife) and scissors. Surgeons use the scalpel — almost exclusively — for the initial incision in laparotomies and laparoscopies. The scalpel is useless after the initial incision in laparoscopy, but some surgeons use scalpels in laparotomy to remove adhesions, organs, and other pathology.

Scissors are very common in laparotomy because surgeons have room to get their hands in the incision. Scissors have several advantages as tools:

- They're cheap.
- They can be sterilized to use over again.
- They do a fine job of cutting.
- They allow a surgeon to feel what he's doing with his hands.
- They have a variety of uses.
- They're very safe because they don't use any other energy source. They don't cause collateral damage like other methods (such as cautery) can.

Scissors are available for use in laparoscopy as well, with long handles that fit through the tiny incisions. They have the same safety profile as laparotomy scissors, and surgeons are comfortable with them. However, the cost is higher than for laparotomy because most laparoscopic scissors are disposable and have a one-time use.

Vaporizing tissues: Electrosurgery

Almost as old as the scalpel and scissors is electrosurgery, which converts energy into heat. Electrons are generated at a frequency in the range of AM radio stations, hence the term *radio frequency* for this energy. The varying types of electron waves produce different effects in tissue. Two types of currents are

- **A *cutting* current:** A continuous, high-frequency flow of electrons without going to zero so electrons constantly flow to the tissue. This method causes instant vaporization of the water in the cells so they explode! This instantaneous vaporization of the cells prevents spread of harmful heat to surrounding tissues, so it minimizes collateral damage to nearby structures and helps to lower the chance of adhesions and other complications.

> ✔ **A *coagulating* current:** The current goes to zero between the peaks. This interrupted current causes dehydration, not vaporization, of the tissues and denatures the proteins. (Think of cooking eggs where the clear proteins turn white and firm.) Although this effect stops bleeding, it allows heat to build up in the tissues and is more likely to cause collateral damage.

Some surgeons use electrocautery to burn away the endometriosis. This method is very effective in getting rid of the disease, but the destructive energy of this device can spread over 1 centimeter (there are approximately 2.5 cm per inch). Using electrocautery is like using a nuclear bomb; you destroy the target but you also do extensive collateral damage. Newer devices have been developed to minimize this problem but all have some drawbacks.

Both laparotomy and laparoscopy use electrosurgery. Some newer devices combine paddles for coagulation with a knife blade for speed, and other devices add this energy to scissors for coagulation while cutting. Each method has advantages and disadvantages.

Beaming away the tissues: Lasers

Laser is an acronym for *light amplification by stimulated emission of radiation*. Laser is a finely focused beam of electromagnetic radiation of a certain wavelength. These wavelengths are in or around the visible light spectrum.

Through the magic of television and movies, many people have formed ideas about lasers and their uses. And because of this introduction, laser is the most misunderstood term in surgery. People may think laser surgery means no cutting and no incision, as if surgeons just aim the laser through the skin and the problem evaporates. In fact, many doctors advertise that they do laser surgery, perhaps implying that it is magic and special. But laser surgery is simply one of many means to an end — the cutting and removal of various tissues and pathology.

The radiation in laser isn't the same type as in X-rays or bombs that can cause cancer. Laser radiation's energy is in the form of *photons* (pockets of light that electrons create when they go to lower energy levels in atoms). Simply put, laser is concentrated light that's similar to the intense, focused light of a magnifying glass when it burns paper or wood, except laser contains only one color of light. The biggest problems with lasers are the cost (literally tens of thousands of dollars), their bulkiness in tight surgical areas, and the need for specially trained personnel.

Several kinds of lasers are available for use in all parts of the body. But the main lasers in gynecologic surgery are

- **Carbon dioxide:** Best for cutting and vaporizing tissue
- **Potassium-titanyl-phosphate (KTP):** Causes coagulation rather than vaporization; used to treat deep endometriosis and bleeding
- **Neodymium-yttrium-aluminum-garnet (Nd: YAG):** Penetrates deeply into tissue
- **Argon:** An inert gas; used similarly to KTP

Surgeons can apply lasers to tissue in various ways, such as glass fibers, crystal tips, and mirror-focused beams, to name a few. As with electrosurgery, the tissue reactions vary due to different power densities and wavelengths. All lasers can be used in open (laparotomy) or closed (laparoscopy) cases. (Sorry, Dr. McCoy, none of these work without an incision for gynecologic surgery — not yet anyway!)

Using the harmonic scalpel

The relatively new kid on the block is an ultrasonic device called the *harmonic scalpel*. This device uses rapid vibration (55,000 per second!) to disrupt the proteins in tissue. You may know this from the device your dentist uses to clean your teeth. The vibration or movement of the tips or blade causes *cavitation* (collapse) of the tissue and disruption of the proteins with implosion of the cells. Besides the rapid movement of the device over very small distances, no other energy source is used, so the risk of damage to surrounding structures is minimal, just like the tartar on your teeth is removed without damage to your teeth or gums.

The ultrasonic device comes with different tips to do a variety of tasks. Your surgeon can use them in both open and closed surgeries for removing adhesions, fibroids, cysts, ovaries and tubes, the appendix, the whole uterus, and many other tissues. Besides excision, they can also destroy or ablate tissue, including endometriosis. The biggest drawback of this device is the questionable ability to prevent some types of bleeding so a second instrument, like the electrosurgery machine, may be needed.

Putting everything back together

Any time your doctor makes an incision, he needs to seal it in some way. But if the thought of stitches or metal clips bothers you, welcome to the world of *Star Trek* closings!

The following are just a few of the ways your doctor can close your incision without staples or exposed sutures:

- ✔ Sutures that dissolve under the skin so you won't ever see them
- ✔ Tissue glue for small incisions — no sutures at all

Ask your surgeon how he plans to close your wounds so you're prepared for it when you wake up.

Knowing which tool is better

So futuristic, science-fiction tools are still a few years away, but how does a surgeon decide which tools to use today, and does that choice make a difference in your treatment? Current studies don't show that one tool is superior to all others in every circumstance, but surgeons tend to strongly advocate one device as the best and only one they use.

However, having a surgeon who's proficient in all (or most) of today's technologies is a good idea. (Just ask what he prefers.) Each patient is different and each instrument has its own strengths and weaknesses. Also, what happens if the only tool your doctor uses is unavailable? He's out of luck — and so are you! Fortunately, surgeons have many tool choices, and he should be able to use most of them.

Starting Surgical Treatment Conservatively

You may assume a surgery is conservative or radical depending on the method. In other words, you may think laparoscopic surgery is conservative and laparotomies are radical. However, the terms *conservative* and *radical* have nothing to do with the *method* of incision. Instead, they refer to the surgical *procedure* your doctor performs. Both radical and conservative procedures can be done via laparotomy or laparoscopy.

This section looks at some of the more conservative procedures your doctor may perform during your surgery. Some of these techniques directly tackle the endometriosis, and others help reduce pain. Conservative surgery for endometriosis is possible via laparoscopy or laparotomy.

Cutting away adhesions

The simplest conservative treatment for endometriosis is the removal of *adhesions* (scar tissue) around the ovaries, tubes, and uterus. The risks of this treatment are minimal (unless the scar tissue is very dense and around vital structures), but the results can be dramatic. Surgery is via a laparoscopy or a laparotomy, using scissors, electrosurgery, laser, harmonic scalpel, or a blunt instrument to simply break down thin, filmy adhesions.

If adhesions are causing your pain, you should feel better almost immediately after they're removed. If your problem is infertility, cutting adhesions around the tubes and ovaries and squirting dye through the tubes may significantly improve your chances of getting pregnant.

Trying ablation of endometriosis

No matter which approach you choose (laparotomy or laparoscopy), dealing with endometriosis lesions through *ablation* (surgical destruction) or *excision* (removal) remains controversial. Some surgeons prefer to remove only lesions involving important structures. Other surgeons remove every last bit of disease they can see. Who's right? Both — and neither. You should discuss these issues and the pros and cons with your doctor.

Your doctor may use any or all of the instruments in the section, "Naming the Surgical Tools" earlier in this chapter. Some instruments are better than others for certain procedures, and some surgeons use more than one device during a procedure.

Using the different tools, your doctor can ablate implants in several ways (check out Figure 11-2):

- **She can scrape or pick off superficial, loose implants from the structure.** This method has the following benefits:
    - Causes minimal disruption of the surface
    - Involves little, if any, bleeding
    - Provides a biopsy specimen for pathology
- **Your doctor can excise the lesions.** If the lesions are deeper or don't come off the surface easily, she may have to cut out them. This method
    - May damage the structures below or around the implants when the implant is removed, so the surgeon must be careful.
    - Requires the surgeon to take a margin of normal-looking tissue with the implant because microscopic endometriosis reaches some distance around the main, easily visible lesion.

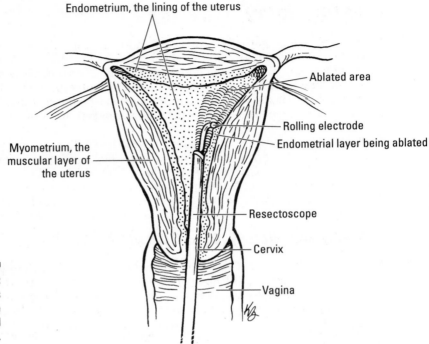

Endometrium, the lining of the uterus

Ablated area

Rolling electrode

Endometrial layer being ablated

Myometrium, the muscular layer of the uterus

Resectoscope

Cervix

Vagina

Figure 11-2:
Surgeons can ablate endometrial lesions.

✔ **Your doctor can destroy the lesions.** If she doesn't remove the implants, your surgeon can rely on electrosurgery, laser, or ultrasonic energy to destroy them. Each method has advantages and disadvantages, but the goal is to totally destroy the implant with the least amount of damage to surrounding tissues.

Any instrument that can cut the surface with the disease can also remove the implant entirely. Scissors are fine but may cause bleeding; electrosurgery can cut and coagulate the bleeding, but the energy may cause collateral damage. Lasers and ultrasonic devices can cut and remove tissue with the same caveats as the electrosurgery. Likewise, any of these tools can be used to ablate the tissue. Which method is best?

- Electrosurgery with a needle-point probe and cutting current can be very accurate and effective. It also works well on lesions with blood or liquefied tissue.

- The carbon dioxide laser causes minimal peripheral damage, and its tiny spot size can be very precise. However, this laser isn't as good as other lasers or electrosurgery for lesions with blood of liquefied tissue and lacks the ability to stop bleeding.

- Because the KTP and nd-YAG lasers are effective through fluid and are absorbed by the pigment in endometriosis, they can be good in larger lesions. They're particularly good in the treatment of endometriomas. But because they coagulate and don't vaporize, they have a greater chance of damaging surrounding tissues.

- Ultrasonic devices can be used to destroy the lesions, but they may cause collateral damage and don't coagulate well.

No matter which method the surgeon uses to excise or destroy the lesions, *denuded* (bare) tissue remains, leaving the underlying tissue without its slick covering. Because the denuded tissue is vulnerable to new adhesions, surgeons have devised various methods to prevent these raw areas from forming adhesions. These methods include

- Taking *omentum* (the sheet of fat that's covered by peritoneum) from the perineum to cover the denuded tissue

- Adding various commercial adhesion-preventing fluids or patches made from animal tissue or synthetic material

The larger the area of disease that the surgeon excises, the greater the chances of bleeding, adhesion formation, and injury to a blood vessel of another organ.

Removing ovarian cysts — How much?

The ovary is a special case when treating endometriosis. Surgeons have no standard for treating these lesions, but your surgeon must be careful not to decrease ovarian reserve (see Chapter 7) if you plan to become pregnant in the future.

If surgery removes parts of the ovary with the endometriosis or inadvertently destroys parts by collateral thermal damage from a device, then primary follicles are also lost. Because every woman has a finite number of eggs, anything that decreases this number can lead to premature ovarian failure, premature menopause, and infertility.

The Catch-22 is that not treating the underlying endometriosis can lead to the same fate! This problem is especially true of *chocolate cysts (endometriomas)*. The surgeon must try to remove or destroy all the disease while saving the ovarian tissue.

Should a surgeon remove endometriomas? Most specialists think they should take the endometriomas to save ovarian tissue from destruction. Medical therapy with GnRH agonist doesn't appear to be effective for endometriomas (see Chapter 10 for more on treating endometriosis with medication). In cases where pregnancy is the goal, in vitro fertilization (IVF) without removal of small endometriomas may work well. Because science has no one right answer at this time, surgeons must deal with each case individually.

If a surgeon plans to remove an endometrioma or any other cyst, he has two basic concerns:

- He needs to take out the whole cyst, wall, and all its contents, if possible. Any spilled contents of the cyst must be removed.

- He doesn't want to harm the normal ovary, but he does want to leave as much healthy ovarian tissue as possible. The patient's desires for future pregnancy and her age are important factors. If she doesn't hope to become pregnant and has no concerns about early menopause, then the surgeon can be more aggressive in dealing with a cyst.

In some cases the cyst may have totally destroyed the ovarian tissue, so the surgeon must remove the whole ovary to prevent future problems. Still, these are rare cases; generally the surgeon should try to save as much of the ovary as possible. Although surgeons can remove cysts laparoscopically, some cases may be safer via laparotomy to be more precise and to save more ovarian tissue.

Looking at LUNA

Laparoscopic Uterine Nerve Ablation (LUNA) is a conservative surgical procedure used to help *dysmenorrhea,* or painful periods, which can be caused by endometriosis. During the procedure, the surgeon can cut, burn, or otherwise destroy bundles of para-sympathetic and sympathetic nerves. These nerves carry pain sensation from the uterus, and scientists believe the nerves are involved in painful menses. (See Figure 11-3 for an illustration of nerves in the pelvis.) Because the nerves don't seem to have any other important function, such as sexual response, destroying them doesn't appear to have any other significant risks.

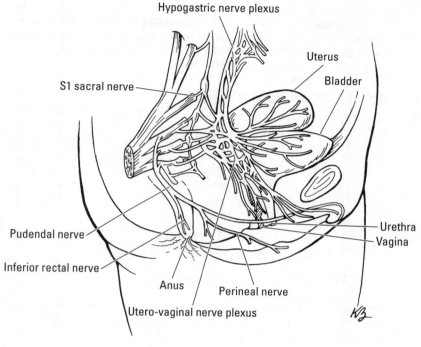

Hypogastric nerve plexus

Uterus

Bladder

S1 sacral nerve

Urethra

Vagina

Figure 11-3:
Surgeons
may cut
nerves in
the pelvis to
give relief
from pelvic
pain.

Pudendal nerve

Inferior rectal nerve

Anus

Perineal nerve

Utero-vaginal nerve plexus

What's involved with LUNA?

A surgeon can perform LUNA via laparotomy or laparoscopy in the following way:

1. **After the surgeon opens the pelvis, the cul-de-sac is exposed.**

   (See Chapter 3 for a biology recap.)

2. **He pushes the intestines out of the way and identifies the uterosacral ligaments.**

   The nerves run in the ligament. The ligaments meet and form the *ganglion* (group of nerve cells) that attaches to the uterus at the junction of the cervix.

3. **The surgeon uses one of two methods to interrupt these nerves:**

   - He cuts the uterosacral ligaments where the ligament meets the uterus.

   - He ties off or cauterizes the tissue with electrosurgery or laser to prevent bleeding (because a blood vessel is there also). He then cuts the ligament to interrupt the nerve.

Because the ureter runs very close to this area, the surgeon must be careful that the energy source doesn't damage it. Bleeding is the other major complication. The uterine artery and its major branches are nearby. Damage to them can lead to dangerous bleeding. Surgeons must also be careful not to injure deeper blood vessels and nerves.

Does LUNA really decrease pain?

Many women wonder if LUNA really works. Good question! As with many procedures, some surgeons swear by it and some swear at it. Studies suggest that LUNA may decrease dysmenorrhea in 80 percent of women with the problem. Although few women get total relief, most women notice some improvement in their symptoms. Because LUNA is fairly easy and safe and because it requires no special equipment or skill, many doctors suggest LUNA for women with painful periods who haven't responded to traditional methods.

Decreasing endometrial pain: Presacral neurectomy

Another way of decreasing pain from the pelvis caused by endometriosis is to interrupt the nerve fibers that carry pain messages from the pelvic organs and covering. These fibers are part of the sympathetic nerve system; the tiny nerves come from both sides of the pelvis and form visible nerve fibers on the surface of the sacrum, hence the term *presacral*. These nerves don't have any other known function, so cutting them only affects pain sensation. For instance, these nerves don't affect labor or pushing during childbirth, nor do they affect sexual response.

What's involved with presacral neurectomy?

This procedure was only done via laparotomy until recently. Now, skilled endoscopic surgeons can do it safely and effectively as an outpatient procedure. Still, the surgeon must be careful not to injure the *aorta* and *vena cave* (the biggest blood vessels that take blood away from and to the heart, respectively) and the plexus of veins on the surface of the sacrum. These injuries may cause catastrophic bleeding. Injury to the intestines is also a common complication.

In a presacral neurectomy (PSN), the surgeon

1. **Moves the intestines out of the way to expose the covering of the sacrum at the base of the spine.**

   This peritoneal covering is part of the peritoneum all over the abdominal cavity.

2. **Cuts and peels away the peritoneum to see the nerve fibers.**

   These fibers may be in one bundle or in many separate nerves.

3. **Isolates and cuts all of the nerve fibers.**

4. **Repairs the peritoneum and replaces the intestines.**

Does PSN really help decrease pain?

That answer depends on which authorities you believe. Advocates say that 70 to 80 percent of women have relief with the procedure. Detractors say that the results aren't nearly that good and the benefit doesn't justify the risk. Some reasons PSN isn't routine are

- ✔ The surgery is very difficult and dangerous.
- ✔ The anatomy of the nerves is so variable that complete dissection often isn't successful.

Incomplete cutting of all the nerves appears to cause the failed surgeries. Because of the controversy, difficulty of the surgery, and variable results, surgeons usually save PSN as a last option.

Opting for Radical Surgery

Unfortunately, some women don't get enough relief from their endometriosis with medications or conservative surgery. These women have two choices:

- ✔ They can live with the problems and adjust their lifestyle to suit the disease.
- ✔ They can have radical surgery, removing the uterus, ovaries, and fallopian tubes in the hopes of ending the problem for good.

But even radical surgery isn't 100 percent effective for ending all the symptoms of endometriosis.

"How can this be?" you ask. If a woman has no more ovaries to feed the implants, no uterus to supply the endometrium, no tubes to transport the disease, and nothing to stick together, why does she still have problems? Doctors and researchers don't really know the reason. A couple of theories include

- ✔ The effect of microscopic endometriosis lesions on the peritoneal surface in the pelvis, on the intestines, or on the bladder
- ✔ The metaplasia theory (see Chapter 4), where the cells of the pelvic lining can change and become endometrial tissue
- ✔ The abnormal inflammatory response of immune cells and other mediators to the presence of even microscopic disease

Whatever the reason for incomplete relief from radical surgery, you must be aware of the possibility and accept this risk. Discuss the expectations, risks, and benefits with your surgeon before radical surgery (or any treatment for that matter).

This section looks at the two most common radical surgeries: an *oophorectomy* (the removal of the ovaries) and a complete hysterectomy. In this section we tell you what happens during these procedures and give you the lowdown on the pros and cons.

Removing your ovaries

In some cases, you and your doctor may elect to remove one or both ovaries (an *oophorectomy*) and not the uterus. This decision is unusual but has some good reasons. Sometimes one ovary keeps forming chocolate cysts and adhesions that cause pain and hormonal changes. When more conservative treatment has failed or the disease has recurred quickly, removing the "bad" ovary may be beneficial.

Usually this radical surgery isn't for young women who may want to become pregnant. However, if one of the ovaries seems more involved (the pain isn't in the middle of the pelvis but more on one side or the other), removing that one ovary (and possibly its fallopian tube) may relieve symptoms. In this case, at least one ovary remains, so pregnancy is still possible.

Some women don't want to risk losing all their natural hormones. One ovary can provide plenty of natural hormones to prevent menopausal symptoms with the potential problems of osteoporosis and other menopausal problems.

Freezing eggs for a possible pregnancy

With the advent of assisted reproductive technologies (ART) and in vitro fertilization (IVF), surgeons may remove both ovaries but leave the uterus in place. This choice works for women who need to relieve symptoms from the ovaries but still want the possibility of carrying a pregnancy.

Before the surgeon removes the ovaries, a fertility specialist removes the eggs and fertilizes them and then freezes the embryos. At a later date, the embryos can be thawed and placed into her uterus. Recent technical breakthroughs show that the eggs themselves may be frozen and fertilized later (see *Fertility For Dummies* by Jackie Meyers-Thompson and Sharon Perkins for more on advances in egg freezing).

Performing an oophorectomy

Surgeons remove one or both ovaries via a laparotomy or laparoscopy. The route depends on the anatomy, possible distortion of the normal structures, presence of adhesions, and the judgment of the surgeon. You should discuss the approach with your doctor before surgery.

To remove an ovary, the surgeon

1. **Blocks off its blood supply and cuts some ligaments that suspend the ovary between the sidewall of the pelvis and the uterus.**

2. **Cuts other small blood vessels and attachments between the ovary and tube to free the ovary.**

   This area has few pain nerves, so the procedure itself isn't painful; only the access hurts.

If the surgeon removes the fallopian tube, he uses the same procedure. But the blood supply is much smaller and easier to coagulate, and the tubes have no real ligaments (just fairly filmy attachments) to cut.

Although this procedure sounds fairly straightforward, the surgeon must avoid major arteries in the area and the ureter. Direct damage to these elements or indirect damage from *thermal spread* (damage done to adjacent structures by the energy used) or kinking of the tissue can lead to major complications.

Recovering from oophorectomy

This surgery adds little, if any, discomfort to the incision for access to the pelvis, so recovery centers on the route, laparotomy or laparoscopy. The same caveats for recovery that we mention in "Passing through the recovery phase" earlier in this chapter apply here.

The only major difference with an oophorectomy is the removal of the ovarian hormones and the short- and long-term effects of no estrogen. If both ovaries are gone, essentially all the estrogen and progesterone producers are gone too. This absence of estrogen can cause menopausal symptoms within a few days of the surgery and may last for a variable amount of time, from months to years. Symptoms usually abate eventually. If they don't, your doctor may prescribe hormone replacement, depending on your overall health history, such as history of heart disease or cancer.

If surgery removes only one ovary, the other ovary may shut down for some time. As a result, a woman may have the same menopausal symptoms for the short term. In almost all cases, the remaining ovary begins to make estrogen quickly. Short-term hormonal replacement can help with these symptoms if needed.

Having a hysterectomy

If you're reading your doctor's notes as he writes, you may be stymied by the initials *TAH-BSO*. This is shorthand for *removal of uterus, fallopian tubes, and ovaries.* (*TAH-BSO* stands for *total abdominal hysterectomy and bilateral salpingo-oophorectomy.*)

Most of the time surgery removes the whole uterus, the cervix, and fundus. Some physicians advocate leaving the cervix to enhance pelvic support and improve sexual response after surgery. This is called a *partial* (or *supracervical*) hysterectomy. Sometimes, especially in cases of severe adhesions and a frozen pelvis, the surgeon may leave the cervix for reasons of safety because it may be dangerous to risk injury to the major blood vessels, intestines, bladder, or ureter. Occasionally, your doctor decides to leave an ovary in place (see the previous section for reasons).

Choosing how to approach a hysterectomy

Most surgical procedures, including a hysterectomy, have more than one approach. Until the advent of laparoscopy, two approaches were common: the abdominal incision (laparotomy) or a vaginal removal. All three methods have their advocates. Because no one right choice exists for everyone or every situation, you and your doctor should discuss the route for your surgery.

Making an incision: The abdominal method

In most cases where the surgery involves removing ovaries, the abdominal incision allows easier and less risky access for oophorectomy. Even when a cul-de-sac and other scarring aren't likely or present, adhesions are likely around the ovary in cases of endometriosis. In this situation, a vaginal removal of ovaries is more difficult and dangerous.

A frozen pelvis from severe adhesions makes the abdominal approach a necessity. The laparotomy has all the same advantages we discuss in "Noting the treatment advantages of laparotomy to laparoscopy" earlier in this chapter, and it's often the method of choice for radical surgery. A supracervical hysterectomy via laparotomy is easier via laparotomy, and all gynecologists are trained in this approach. The mini-laparotomy (smaller incision) is another option but offers slightly less access.

Going through the canal: The vaginal method

As the name implies, the surgeon performs a vaginal hysterectomy through the vagina. Obviously, access is much more limited than with a laparotomy, and hands and instruments greatly reduce visibility during the procedure. Because the surgeon can't really get his hands in to feel for structures, he has to rely on that limited sight. With many pelvic surgeries, limited access isn't a major problem for the experienced surgeon, but when dealing with endometriosis, the limitations can become a real disadvantage. As a result, vaginal hysterectomies are less common for endometriosis because they offer little access to probable adhesions and distorted anatomy.

Nonetheless, vaginal hysterectomy has advantages. It's an ideal method for removal of the fairly normal-sized uterus for benign conditions like fibroids, *adenomyosis* (growths in the uterine wall), refractory dysfunctional bleeding, abnormal Pap smears, and *prolapse* (collapse of the uterus into the vagina through the cervix). And because this surgery involves no large abdominal incisions, recovery is usually quicker than with a laparotomy. Unfortunately, many younger surgeons aren't getting enough exposure to this procedure in training programs, and it's an underused procedure in gynecology today.

Using new technology: The laparoscopic method

With the development of laparoscopy for hysterectomy, surgery is minimally invasive and provides better tolerance and recovery for the patient. However, for patients with endometriosis and severe adhesions — where structures are stuck together — a laparoscopic approach may not be safe. If the patient has a possible frozen pelvis, severe adhesions, or a much-distorted anatomy, the surgeon may initially use laparoscopy to assess the viability of that approach. But, if he determines that the route isn't appropriate, he can then convert the approach to a laparotomy.

The scope offers two ways to perform a hysterectomy. Each method has its proponents, but your surgeon makes the final decision.

✔ **Laparoscopic assisted vaginal hysterectomy (LAVH):** This method was the original laparoscopy. A wise surgeon decided that he could accomplish vaginal hysterectomies more easily and safely if he used the laparoscope. The most difficult part of the vaginal hysterectomy was getting the upper attachments and blood vessels under control. These structures (the round ligaments and ovarian arteries) are fairly easy to tie off, coagulate, and cut via the laparoscope. After this upper work is complete, the rest of the procedure can proceed vaginally.

This method also allows surgeons to check for adhesions or anatomical abnormalities and deal with the problems via the scope, under direct visualization. Likewise, a surgeon can evaluate ovaries and tubes and then detach them much more effectively through the scope. So, with only a few tiny incisions on the abdominal wall, LAVH makes vaginal hysterectomies a better possibility.

✔ **Laparoscopic hysterectomy (LH):** This option uses laparoscopy exclusively. As the name implies, the surgeon detaches and removes the uterus (and tubes and ovaries if necessary) from the pelvis via the laparoscope. You may wonder how he gets that large uterus (at least the size of a small pear) out through that tiny incision. Good question! In the LAVH, the surgeon takes the uterus out through the vagina. If a baby can fit, then a uterus is a piece of cake! With LH, as soon as the surgeon has secured the blood vessels and cut the support structures, he can extricate the uterus, tubes, and ovaries through the laparoscopic incision.

Your surgeon has two ways to remove the organs:

- He can enlarge one of the incisions to afford removal of the organs. This may seem somewhat self-defeating because the advantage of an LH is the small incisions. Why not just take the uterus out through the vagina? Two reasons: The uterus may be too big (not usual with endometriosis), or the surgeon performed a supracervical hysterectomy, which offers no opening to the vagina because the cervix is left in place.

- He can *morcelate* (shred) the uterus, tubes, and ovaries into pieces less than a centimeter with an instrument (powered or manual) and then remove the tissue through the normal-size incisions. Because these instruments can cause inadvertent damage, the surgeon must be careful to avoid injury to other organs, such as the intestines or major blood vessels. The other potential problem is that the organs are in pieces, which can make microscopic diagnosis more difficult and can leave other diseases undiagnosed (such as cancer, in the worst-case scenario).

Whichever route your surgeon takes, the two of you must be on the same page. Discuss these options, and be sure that you're comfortable with your doctor's suggestion.

Recovering from hysterectomy

Recovery from a hysterectomy depends on the method. With LH, your recovery is about the same as any other laparoscopy. However, when the surgeon has cut ligaments and other attachments to the uterus, the surgery injures a larger area of tissue. As a result, patients usually have a bit more pain and discomfort with LH than with other laparoscopic procedures.

On the other end of the spectrum is the recovery from a laparotomy (see the earlier section "Recovering from laparotomy"); the removal of the uterus adds some to the discomfort, but most of the pain is incision-related.

The pain level after a vaginal hysterectomy falls between the pain levels of the other two approaches. In this case, the surgeon has removed the same organs, but you have less pain and can return to activity more quickly because you have no abdominal incision. However, this procedure causes more vaginal discomfort because the retractors and other instruments in the vagina and pelvis can cause swelling and inflammation. These conditions add to the pain and discomfort, but not as much as a laparotomy does.

If your surgeon removed your ovaries, the loss of hormones can bring on menopausal symptoms. Check out "Recovering from oophorectomy" earlier in this chapter for more info.

Complications may prolong recovery from hysterectomy. Some of these are common and not severe, including

- ✔ Urinary tract infection (due to the catheter in the bladder)
- ✔ Bowel dysfunction
- ✔ Wound infection from skin bacteria
- ✔ *Atelectasis* (collapse of some air pockets in the lung)
- ✔ Pneumonia
- ✔ Deep vein thrombosis (blood clots in the legs or pelvis)
- ✔ Bleeding

The chance of any one of these complications increases with the length and route of surgery. Laparotomy is most likely to cause complications; laparoscopy is least likely.

Follow all post-operative instructions to minimize the risk of these problems. If you have frequent, difficult, or painful urination, try to drink fluids, and let your doctor know whether the problem persists. Deep breathing may be painful, but it is essential to prevent lung problems. And getting out of bed and moving around can help your bowels work, your lungs fill, and your veins stay free of clots. All of these preventive measures can make your recovery smoother.

Inform your surgeon immediately if you have

- ✔ A cough (especially if you cough up blood) or breathing problems
- ✔ Shortness of breath
- ✔ Constipation or diarrhea
- ✔ Pain in the legs (especially the calves)
- ✔ Chest pain
- ✔ Increasing (rather than decreasing) abdominal pain or redness and pain in the incision
- ✔ Fever after surgery (more than 100.4 degrees Fahrenheit)

Making the Right Surgical Choice

Depending on your symptoms, your doctor may start with conservative surgery, such as a hysteroscopy or a dilation and curettage (D&C). Or your initial surgery for endometriosis may be a diagnostic laparoscope so your doctor can take a look around your pelvis and possibly remove endometrial implants. But if you've already had diagnostic surgery, you may decide to have a more radical treatment that's based on previous results.

After you and your doctor decide to have surgery, you need to choose the proper approach. Your doctor will undoubtedly have preferences based on his findings and will guide you on the pros and cons of all the alternatives.

Unfortunately, surgery isn't always a miracle cure. In some circumstances, surgery may be too risky because it's unsafe for you or because it can do more harm than good. For example, to preserve your chances of getting pregnant, your doctor doesn't want to interfere with your ovaries. But some times the surgeon does everything possible, and the patient still has symptoms or still can't get pregnant. No surgeon is perfect, and no procedure is guaranteed to work.

In the end, you and your doctor have to make the decisions about surgery; if he seems to be proposing one type of surgery over another, ask him why. Many offices today have videos you can watch about different types of surgery and their risks and benefits; offices that don't offer this usually have written information you can take home and mull over at your leisure. Rarely is surgery for endometriosis a life-or-death decision, so take the time to really understand what's involved before making a surgical decision.

Chapter 12

Considering Alternative Therapies and Remedies to Relieve the Pain

*N*ever before have so many people looked for alternatives to traditional Western medicine — herbs, acupuncture, Eastern medicine, and other alternatives are all getting a close look. But you may be asking: Why the popularity of alternative treatments? After all, traditional medicine today is as advanced as it's ever been and improving all the time. So why are so many people looking for alternative treatments?

Part of the reason is that traditional Western medicine focuses on illness, devoting far more time to curing disease than to preventing it. Alternative treatments tend to focus on integrating the mind, body, and spirit in treatment and prevention. More people today are aware of the mind's influence on health and want to incorporate an integral approach into their treatment. Sometimes traditional medicine doesn't have the answers you're looking for. When your doctor says, "There's not much more we can do for you," you may decide to look to nontraditional methods to decrease pain or treat endometriosis.

This chapter looks more closely at alternative treatments and remedies, including those that rely more on the mind-body connection and those that utilize hands-on treatment, like massage and chiropractic.

Being Aware of Alternative Medicine Pitfalls

Because alternative medicine isn't as stringently regulated as traditional medicine, you need to be on your guard against undertrained and improperly trained practitioners, as well as outright snake oil salesmen. Although many alternative treatments have become almost mainstream in their acceptance by the general public and medical personnel and have strict guidelines for practice, others have little in the way of regulation to make sure that practitioners are consistent and effective.

For this reason, you must remember one caveat above all others when choosing alternative medical treatment: Consumer, beware! Pursuing alternative medicine treatments can have potentially serious drawbacks. This section looks at those drawbacks.

Finding a competent practitioner

Be sure the practitioner you choose is licensed if the treatment has a licensing procedure. Many alternative treatments, such as acupuncture and chiropractic, have strict criteria for licensure. Finding a practitioner that uses techniques outside mainstream medicine can be more challenging than finding a traditional medical doctor. One of the drawbacks to alternative therapies is that licensing of practitioners isn't as stringent as the licensing of medical doctors, so you may not know whether your practitioner has had adequate training. A well-intentioned but untrained practitioner can do a lot more harm than good!

In order to find a competent practitioner, we recommend you start with the governing boards or licensing bodies of the professions that have them, such as Traditional Chinese Medicine (TCM), naturopathy, or acupuncture, to name a few. (We list the governing bodies of many alternative treatments in the sections describing them.) If you want to find out or you're unsure whether a profession is regulated, a number of sources can help.

- ✔ The **National Center for Complementary and Alternative Medicine (NCCAM),** which is associated with the National Institute of Health (NIH), is a good place to start. The NCCAM provides an amazing amount of information on alternative treatments, including licensure information, clinical trial updates, and articles on finding an alternative practitioner. They don't make physician referrals, however. The NCCAM even has an online chat with a health information specialist Monday through Friday 8:30 a.m. to 5 p.m. EST. You can reach the NCCAM at

> NCCAM Clearinghouse
> P.O. Box 7923
> Gaithersburg, MD 20898
> Phone 888-644-6226
> TTY 866-464-3615
> 301-519-3153 (international)
> Web site http://nccam.nih.gov/

- ✔ For information on dietary supplements, try the **NIH Office of Dietary Supplements (ODS).** Its Web site is www.ods.od.nih.gov.

- ✔ The **Food and Drug Association (FDA)** can also provide valuable information on supplements and their safety at www.cfsan.fda.gov. You can reach the FDA by phone at 888-723-3366.

After you find a regulated profession and need to find a practitioner, you can use the same criteria for finding a practitioner that we suggest in Chapter 8 for finding a doctor.

If the treatment you're considering isn't regulated, finding a practitioner is more difficult. You may have to rely on two methods: asking friends and acquaintances for references and listening to your gut. It's important not to sign up for anything until you've met with your potential practitioner in person and asked some of the following questions. The answers you get may give you a feeling for whether or not this practitioner is knowledgeable in his or her field.

Meet with your potential practitioner before you start working with her for a "get to know you" appointment. Doing so is especially important if there's no licensing board to check with. Make sure you ask her the following questions:

- ✔ What are your qualifications? What kind of training have you had and for how long? Where was your training done?

- ✔ How many years have you been in practice?

- ✔ Are you associated with a recognized professional organization, and are you listed as a member in good standing?

- ✔ Is treatment covered by health insurance?

- ✔ How much will treatment cost?

- ✔ How long will treatment take?

- ✔ What kind of results can I expect?

- ✔ Do you have any patients who would be willing to talk to me about their successful treatment?

Asking these questions can help you make an informed decision about the qualifications of the practitioner you're considering.

Protecting yourself from dangerous (or useless) pills

Many people think that herbs and food supplements in health food stores can't possibly be harmful. This assumption isn't true — deaths from herbal preparations have occurred and are documented. Many herbs are powerful, especially if you *mix and match* without guidance from a professional. Most employees at your local health store are undertrained (if trained at all) in the products and possible interactions and are no more a professional than you are, although you may find exceptions.

One problem with alternative therapies that use food supplements, herbs, vitamins, and other natural medicines is that no governing body has scientifically studied or compared most of them to more traditional treatments or *placebos* (compounds that don't contain any active ingredients). You can't verify what's in that bottle of natural medicines, herbs, supplements, or vitamins that you buy. The amount of medication in each dose may vary from bottle to bottle or even dose to dose. Furthermore, many of these herbs and food supplements contain added ingredients that have effects such as anti-inflammatory drugs and amphetamines. These added ingredients — not the herb — may actually be the source of your relief. Many herbs also stimulate the immune system; some herbs can make other diseases worse. Evening primrose oil, for example, can increase the risk of seizure activity. These important facts are almost never on the label.

In contrast, pharmaceutical companies that sell traditional medicines must complete very thorough studies, governed by the FDA, that establish the dose and quantify the benefits and risks. The FDA also makes sure that each dose is uniform and that the substance is *pure,* with no contaminants.

We're not just two people from the traditional medical world bad-mouthing the alternatives. Far from it. We've used alternative treatments with patients and ourselves. But independent agencies have tested many over-the-counter (OTC) vitamins and supplements and have shown wide variations in doses and potencies — even in compounds manufactured according to United States Pharmacopeia (USP) standards. Strict scientific studies on some forms of *natural therapy,* notably those for menopause, have found that these therapies are no more effective than placebos.

If you're seriously considering alternative treatments, first check with your primary care physician. You also need to keep the following pointers in mind:

> ✔ **Be sure that you only use products from reputable companies or stores, and get your information on supplements from people who know their product well.** Small stores that have been in business for years often have knowledgeable owners who are passionate about supplements. The local big box vitamin store, on the other hand, is more

likely to hire people who need a job, not people who know — or care — about supplements. This rule isn't hard and fast; you may find an extremely knowledgeable salesperson at a large chain store. Ask the person you're taking advice from how long she's worked in the store, and what her training is before you load hundreds of dollars worth of supplements into your cart.

✔ **If you find a product that works for you, use it under supervision of a trained professional.** He can ensure that you're taking the product correctly.

✔ **Ask questions of any practitioner that suggests a treatment.** Ask questions about the efficacy, safety, quality, and potency of the therapy.

✔ **Search reference sources about studies on these products.** Try to find legitimate studies that test many women (at least a hundred in each group, not just a few) and that compare the therapy to a placebo or other documented therapy. NCCAM has information on many clinical trials that have been done with alternative therapies.

If you can't get answers from the professionals or references about these therapies, then be wary. The products may do more harm than good and cost you dearly in the long run.

Accessing Acupuncture

You may be familiar with *acupuncture,* the art of inserting fine, sterile needles into different areas of the body for treatment of any number of disorders. Acupuncture, which is part of Traditional Chinese Medicine (TCM), came into use in the United States in the 1970s and is often used for pain relief. Some traditional medical doctors now train in the use of acupuncture. TCM acupuncturists often combine treatments with the use of herbs.

This section looks more closely at how acupuncture can help ease your endometriosis pain and how you can find a licensed acupuncturist.

Easing the pain with just a little prick

Are you looking for a little extra pain relief from your endometriosis? Acupuncture may be an option. Acupuncture and herbal medicines are frequent treatments for endometriosis and other pelvic disorders. These herbal medicines include plant elements, such as roots, barks, flowers, and fruits, and the formulas prescribed vary from person to person. Common acupuncture points in the treatment of endometriosis are the ears, abdomen, wrists, feet, legs, and back. Needles remain in place for 20 to 45 minutes.

So how does acupuncture really work? An acupuncturist inserts needles into certain points on your body to stimulate nerve endings and release *endorphins* (neurotransmitters) that have pain-relieving qualities. You may need up to six treatments before you feel significant pain relief.

Some of the goals of acupuncture and herbal medicines are to break up stagnation of blood by moving blood from one place to another, thus stopping the pain. Each point of needle placement and herb has its own therapeutic importance in the treatment of endometriosis depending on the TCM diagnosis of the individual.

If you're needle-phobic, don't rule out acupuncture altogether. The needles are about the width of a human hair; insertion is far less uncomfortable than your average blood test.

Finding a licensed acupuncturist

Acupuncture became an officially recognized treatment for pain by the National Institutes of Health (NIH) in 1997, so you can find a physician trained in acupuncture more easily now than even ten years ago. Physicians can be certified in acupuncture after taking a 200- to 300-hour training course. They're then members of the American Academy of Medical Acupuncture (AAMA).

The FDA regulates acupuncture needles and tools, so standards are high but the FDA doesn't regulate the practitioner, so be careful. You can get a listing of medical doctors in your area who perform acupuncture by contacting the AAMA at its toll-free number at 800-521-2262 or by searching its Web site at www.medicalacupuncture.org.

Acupuncture-trained physicians are licensed or certified through the National Certification Commission for Acupuncture and Oriental Medicine. To confirm your practitioner's certifications, check out the NCCAOM's Web site at www.nccaom.org.

Considering a Chiropractor

Millions of people visit a chiropractor each year, and many make regular visits. According to the *Annals of Internal Medicine,* chiropractic is the largest, most regulated, and best recognized of the complementary and alternative medicine professions. Doctors of Chiropractic have at least four years of post college education at accredited chiropractic schools and must pass boards to be licensed to practice.

Understanding what a chiropractor does

Chiropractic physicians use hands-on manipulation, called *chiropractic adjustment,* of muscles and joints (particularly in and around the spinal column) to treat a number of diseases and to decrease pain by restoring mobility to tissues that have become restricted in their movement, causing inflammation and pain. Because pain from endometriosis can involve the back and the nerves that run from the spinal column to the pelvis, chiropractic manipulation may decrease its pain.

Chiropractors use more than 20 different techniques to manipulate tissues. You can go to two different chiropractors and have two completely different experiences depending on their individual approach to manipulation. You can find a good explanation of commonly used chiropractic techniques online at www.becomehealthynow.com/category/chirotechniques/.

Finding a chiropractor

You may think finding a chiropractor is fairly easy because most strip malls and office complexes seem to have a chiropractor's office. As easy as these offices may be to find, we still suggest you follow the Chapter 8 guidelines for finding a good doctor when you're looking for a chiropractor. Take the time to meet with your prospective chiropractor and ask him about his training and methods. (For example, chiropractors use different manipulation methods, some of which may be more painful for you.) Ask if he's treated other patients with endometriosis, and what results you can realistically expect.

Many chiropractors will want to see you on a regular basis, such as once or twice a week. Some insurance companies will pay for chiropractic visits. You can verify a chiropractor's certification by visiting the National Board of Chiropractic Examiners' Web site at http://www.nbce.org/.

Using Heat and Massage for Pain Relief

Sometimes simple methods work well for relieving pain. Heat can be a great muscle relaxer. Sometimes just soaking in a warm tub or resting with a heating pad or hot water bottle can relieve pain. Some heating pads supply moist heat, which can be even more effective than dry heat.

You can also make your own packs by warming slightly dampened towels in the microwave. Remember that microwaves don't apply heat evenly, and make sure the towel doesn't get too hot in one spot; you could end up with a painful burn in addition to your other aches and pains. One advantage of using warm towels is that you can mold them to your aching areas, which is difficult to do with commercial heating pads.

Massage can be a great way to lessen your endometriosis pain, even if the relief's only temporary. You can also use massage therapy to decrease pain, relax muscles, and relieve tension. The following types of massage may help you:

- ✔ **Acupressure** applies pressure to specific trigger points to release tension in muscle fibers.

- ✔ **Deep-tissue massage** applies pressure to connective tissue and muscles to release tension.

- ✔ **Shiatsu** is a form of acupressure that combines pressure on trigger points with long strokes, stretching, and manipulation.

- ✔ **Swedish massage** uses long firm strokes on heavily muscled areas and softer strokes on more delicate tissues to release stress and relax tense muscles.

Some massage therapists may incorporate aromatherapy (see the section "Breathing Your Way to Feeling Better: Aromatherapy" later in this chapter for more info) into the massage because the body absorbs these essential oils through massage. As a result, you get two benefits for the price of one.

If you're choosing a massage therapist, look for someone who has graduated from an accredited school (accredited by the Commission for Massage Training Accreditation [COMTA]) and is a member of the American Massage Therapy Association or the Associated Bodywork and Massage Professionals. You can find Web sites listing members at www.amtmassage.org or www.abmp.org.

Some malls and airports have massage therapists set up so you can shop and then drop onto the table for some relaxation, but make sure the person doing your massage is a trained therapist. Furthermore, some nationwide clinics claim to offer a unique, deep, external and internal massage technique that can break down scar tissue. This therapy is expensive, unproven, and can be harmful. Always discuss this sort of therapy with your regular doctor and follow his recommendation; he knows your scar tissue better than anybody!

Relying on Relaxation Techniques

Your mind is a powerful tool. In fact, several mind-body therapies rely on *mind over matter* — the idea that you can overcome or control physical sensations, such as pain, with mental effort to actually reduce pain. This type of therapy can be a valuable part of treatment for pain because it's nonaddictive, has no unpleasant side effects, and gives you the sense of controlling your own body. The following different techniques use your mind to overcome pain:

✔ **Biofeedback** teaches you how to use your body's response to decrease pain and stress through a technique called *positive reinforcement*. Often the technique begins with the use of a machine that records your heart rate and other vital signs as they change in response to stimuli. Eventually you understand how to respond positively to pain by relaxing muscles, breathing deeply and slowly, and using visual imagery or positive thoughts to distract you from the pain.

✔ **Guided imagery** helps you relax tense muscles by using visual images of places that you find peaceful and relaxing. You can also use this technique in conjunction with music therapy.

✔ **Hypnosis** puts you into a *trance state* of extreme suggestibility and relaxation. A therapist can show you how to use a type of self-hypnosis that is similar to relaxation training.

✔ **Meditation** can calm and focus the mind. This therapy promotes relaxation by using two principles:

  • **Focusing repetitively** on a word, sound, phrase, sensation, prayer, or even muscular activity.

  • **Developing a passive attitude** toward any intrusions and then returning to the focus.

✔ **Mindfulness training** is a meditation technique aimed at reducing stress and decreasing pain by increasing awareness of the present moment.

✔ **Music therapy** can combine relaxing music with relaxation therapy to decrease anxiety and reduce tension.

✔ **Relaxation training** enables you to relax tense muscles and reduce anxiety that can intensify pain.

✔ **Religion** and prayer, along with any spiritual beliefs, may work for some people. Though controversial and hard to prove, a study by Johns Hopkins showed that people who are more spiritual are also more able to cope with chronic diseases. The study didn't show any improvement in the disease, but the more spiritual patients were happier and felt better about themselves and their health.

✔ **Spas and balneotherapy** have treated chronic pain syndromes for centuries. *Balneotherapy* (bathing in hot mineral water) has a reputation as a healing technique. Although no scientific research exists, both practices can relax and soothe pain.

Stretching with Yoga and T'ai Chi

People have practiced yoga and T'ai Chi for centuries. Although their original purpose was to improve the mind-body-spirit connection, yoga and T'ai Chi are most popular in the United States for their combination of gentle and controlled movements that provide a no- or low-impact workout for people in almost any physical condition. These exercises can ease tense muscles, reduce pain, improve flexibility, and enhance a person's strength, balance, and endurance.

This section uncovers where you can find out more about yoga and T'ai Chi and explains how these two arts can benefit you and ease your endometriosis pain.

Finding out more about yoga and T'ai Chi

Yoga and T'ai Chi are gentle enough for almost everyone, and they're adaptable to your physical level. Nearly every college, gym, hospital, YMCA, and neighborhood recreation center offers some type of yoga or T'ai Chi instruction. Most classes are relatively inexpensive and may be covered under your health plan if your doctor prescribes them.

If you want to find a program, check out www.yogafinder.com or www.taichinetwork.org. You can take group classes or have individual instruction (definitely more pricey). Books and DVDs can also guide you through the movements of yoga and T'ai Chi at home, which is helpful if you don't feel like reaching for all those positions in front of a dozen strangers. Keep in mind, though, that the home schooling approach is harder without a few lessons from a pro first. *Yoga For Dummies* by Georg Feuerstein and Larry Payne (Wiley) and *T'ai Chi For Dummies* by Therese Iknoian (Wiley) are good starts if you want more information before signing up for a class.

Finding a qualified instructor isn't always easy because just about anyone with a correspondence course under her belt can call herself a yoga instructor. Yoga Alliance, a teacher-organized group, recommends at least 200 hours of expert training to qualify as a yoga instructor. At the last count, 8,000 instructors in the United States have met that standard. So finding a qualified instructor near you should be easy.

Looking closer at the benefits of yoga and T'ai Chi

The pain of endometriosis often causes tense muscles, which makes overall pain even worse. Gentle stretching and controlled movements like those performed in yoga and T'ai Chi can help relax muscles, decreasing pain.

Yoga's and T'ai Chi's benefits include

- Stress reduction
- Relaxation

✔ Improved circulation

✔ Improved muscle tone

✔ Enhanced cardiovascular health

One school of thought proposes that progesterone receptors stop functioning in the presence of adrenaline, the stress hormone. When that happens, you may have an imbalance of estrogen and progesterone effects that can increase symptoms of endometriosis. Calming exercises can relieve stress and facilitate more balanced hormones. Relaxing with yoga, for example, can calm and relax you. When you're more relaxed, you may not notice your endometriosis symptoms as much as if you were stressed.

Using a TENS Unit

A Transcutaneous Electrical Nerve Stimulation (TENS) unit uses electrical impulses to block pain signals. Electrodes — on your skin near the pain — transmit a mild electrical current through the skin, blocking the sensation of pain for several hours. TENS units cost around $100, and the electrodes run around $30 for a pack of four. Electrodes are good for 15 to 30 uses. TENS units run on batteries, and most are small enough to hook to your belt, so you can keep moving while you're wearing one. Patients control the unit by turning it on and off; some units can be programmed for a pre-set amount of time, such as 30 minutes.

Use a TENS only under the supervision of your doctor or physical therapist; your insurance company may reimburse the cost as long as you have a prescription. You can also rent a TENS unit before buying one to make sure it helps you with your pain. Many medical companies let you rent one for a month and apply the rental fee to the purchase price if you decide to buy the unit.

If you have a pacemaker, a TENS unit may interfere with your pacemaker. Talk to your doctor before considering a TENS unit.

Trying Traditional Chinese Medicine

Traditional Chinese Medicine (TCM) categorizes endometriosis as a *blood stasis* disease with formation of lumps. The Chinese name for endometriosis is actually *neiyi,* meaning *internal lump.* TCM relates blood stasis in the lower abdomen to back and pelvic pain. In addition, *qi stagnation* (restricted blood flow due to emotional distress) and *coldness* (decreased metabolism and circulation — sometimes called *kidney yang deficiency*) cause the blood stasis.

Since 1979, Chinese researchers have studied endometriosis extensively, especially in Shanghai. This research has centered on basic herbal preparations used to treat qi (the basic problem in endometriosis). The Chinese believe the mixture revitalizes blood flow and, as a result, minimizes the symptoms.

In the 1800s, TCM physician Wang Quingren, forerunner of endometriosis treatment in China, developed two blood-vitalizing formulas for the lower body that are still widely used in TCM today. One formula is *Shaofu Zhuyu Tang* (*shaofu* means *lower palace*) and the other formula is *Gexia Zhuyu Tang* (*ge* means *diaphragm,* while *xia* means *below*). The two formulas are similar and contain many of the herbs listed in Table 12-1.

Table 12-1	Common TCM Herbs and Their Uses	
Herb	*Purpose*	*How Taken*
Cinnamon twig or bark (guizhi or rougui)	Improves circulation, warms the body, decreases pain	Usually paired with tang-kuei, peony, or red peony to improve circulation and relieve pain
Cnidium (chuanxiong)	Promotes circulation, decreases pain	Usually paired with tang-kuei to treat pain and regulate menstruation
Corydalis, yanhuuo	Promotes blood circulation, alleviates pain	Added to formulas for treatment of painful syndromes, especially of the abdomen
Oyster shell (muli)	Softens masses	Used for abdominal masses
Persica (taoren)	Breaks up static blood to relieve pain	Usually paired with either moutan, rhubarb, or carthamus to vitalize blood circulation
Red peony, chihshao	Improves blood circulation	Usually paired with either salvia or moutan or both to improve blood circulation
Rhubarb, dahuang	Promotes blood circulation, relieves swellings, laxative when carbonized, inhibits bleeding	Usually combined with persica for abdominal masses and constipation
Tang-kuei, danggui	Nourishes blood, circulates blood, improves qi circulation	Nourishes blood, circulates blood, improves qi circulation

Herb	Purpose	How Taken
Trogopterus (also know as pteropus), wulingzhi	Vitalizes blood, decreases pain	Almost always paired with typha, based on Shixiao San (an ancient formula)
Typha (also known as bulrush), puhuang	Vitalizes blood, reduces pain; when fried or carbonized, inhibits excessive menstrual bleeding	Almost always paired with trogopterus, based on Shixiao San (an ancient formula)

If you're combining the methods of a TCM practitioner with traditional Western medicine, make sure all your caretakers know what you're doing! Trying to mix and match treatments is a good way to end up in trouble; herbs and supplements from health food stores or TCM practitioners can be every bit as potent as medicine from your local pharmacy — mixing the two can cause serious side effects.

So how do these herbs work? Researchers believe they may increase blood flow and give a boost to the immune system.

Considering Herbal Medicines

Herbalists, homeopaths, and naturopaths also use herbs to treat diseases, including endometriosis. *Herbalists* use herbs to strengthen the immune system and restore health, *homeopaths* use minute amounts of minerals to cure disease, and *naturopaths* use a natural, balanced approach of herbs and dietary changes to allow the body to heal itself. This section looks at these more in-depth and identifies how each one treats endometriosis.

Trying an herbalist

Herbalists use herbs to rebalance the hormone levels in the body and strengthen the immune system. Herbalists tend to associate endometriosis with a variety of causes, such as emotional stress, anxiety, constitutional weakness, surgical history, exposure to cold temperatures during menstruation, diet, chronic illness or weakness, or a history of genital infections, so they prescribe specific herbs depending on each person's unique history. If you're looking for a qualified herbalist, check out the Web site www.yinyang house.com/directory/ for a list of practitioners.

Although modern medicine may criticize the use of herbs, plants and herbs historically are at the root (pun intended) of today's most-accepted medicines. So, even though modern medicine uses plant and herb extractions, herbalists advocate the use of the whole plant rather than laboratory-purified products.

Some of these herbs and their purposes include the following:

- **Chamomile flower** reduces inflammation.
- **Ginger root** relaxes muscles.
- **Goldenseal** relaxes uterine muscles and decreases abnormal bleeding.
- **Motherwort** reduces pelvic congestion.
- **Red raspberry** reduces pelvic congestion.
- **Red root** reduces pelvic congestion.
- **Shepherd's purse** helps decrease abnormal menstrual bleeding.
- **Squaw vine** reduces pelvic congestion.
- **Turska's formula** decreases pain.
- **Vitex,** also called *chaste tree berry,* helps balance estrogen and progesterone.

Working with a homeopath

Homeopaths administer diluted plant, animal, and mineral derivatives to help an individual's body to correct the illness. Homeopathic medicine's premise is *like cures like,* which means that the medicine must cause symptoms similar to the disease in order to cure it.

Homeopathic treatment of endometriosis is individualized. At one time, it was quite mainstream; in 1900, one out of five doctors in the United States practiced homeopathy. However, it lost popularity as medical science and education advanced. Some medical doctors today can also be licensed homeopathic physicians. If you're looking for a homeopathic practitioner, or just want to know more about homeopathy, check out www.homeopathic.org/find.htm for a list of practitioners and tons of other info.

The FDA regulates the homeopathic medications manufactured by established pharmaceutical companies under strict guidelines. The dosages involved in homeopathic drugs are minute, so minute that detractors say they can't possibly be of any benefit. Homeopaths, however, believe that only a tiny amount of a substance is necessary to cure illnesses with symptoms similar to those the drug produces.

The following medications are common recommendations by homeopaths for endometriosis:

- **Belladonna** for menstruation with sensation of heaviness and heat
- **Calcarea phosphoricum** for excessive periods with backache
- **Chamomilla** for heavy menses with dark, clotted blood and pains
- **Cimicifuga racemosa** for unbearable pain radiating from hip to hip

Seeing a naturopath

Naturopathic medicine uses herbal remedies, diet, hydrotherapy, and lifestyle changes; it emphasizes the body's "God-given" ability to heal itself in the proper environment. Naturopathy is also about maintaining wellness and relieving stress (from mental, nutritional, environmental, or physical factors) without pharmacologic medications. Approximately 1,500 naturopathic physicians practice in the United States.

Naturopathy emphasizes the body's power to heal itself. Developed in the late 19th century, naturopathy regards the body's natural state as one of equilibrium, which an unhealthy lifestyle can disturb. Naturopathic doctors (NDs) look for underlying causes of a problem instead of treating symptoms alone.

Endometriosis treatment in naturopathic medicine involves a holistic approach to all areas of a patient's lifestyle, including diet, cleansing, and hormone-balancing herbs. Treatment may also include herbs for pain relief and external preparations to clear toxicity in the abdominal area.

Several accredited naturopathic schools are located in North America; programs consist of four years post-graduate education. In some states, a State Board of Examiners licenses and regulates naturopaths, requiring applicants to pass a national or state board examination. Several naturopathic professional organizations also require the candidate to pass a proficiency test in naturopathy in order to join their organization. You can find an accredited ND at www.findnd.com or www.naturopath.org.

Breathing Your Way to Feeling Better: Aromatherapy

Aromatherapy may sound like it belongs on the perfume counter, but this approach isn't just about sniffing different odors. Aromatherapy utilizes the essential oils of plants both for their scent and for their medicinal properties. These aromatic oils can be extracted from the seeds, bark, leaves, flowers, wood, roots, or resin of a plant.

Experts don't see aromatherapy as a cure for endometriosis but as an aid to strengthening the body's immune system to heal itself. Some of the oils for endometriosis, touted to decrease adhesions and help heal the body, include the following:

- ✔ **Chamomile** soothes, relaxes, acts as an analgesic, and reduces spasms.

- ✔ **Jasmine** soothes, relaxes, acts as an antidepressant, and reduces spasms.

- ✔ **Lavender** calms, acts as an anti-inflammatory, and reduces spasms.

- ✔ **Oils of rose** relaxes, acts as an antidepressant, and reduces spasms.

You may want to consult with an aromatherapy expert in your area; ask your local health food store for the names of knowledgeable people. Just remember that aromatherapy isn't a state-licensed or regulated practice.

Considering Immunotherapy

Many doctors already use immune therapy in cancer patients as well as patients with autoimmune disease, a category it seems endometriosis may fall into. (See Chapter 4 for more on the immune system and endometriosis.)

The link between the immune system and endometriosis

Can immune therapy help decrease endometriosis? The following three areas of research may support the idea of immune treatment for endometriosis:

- ✔ Implants of endometriosis cause increased peritoneal fluid, which contains increased numbers of immune cells (leukocytes and others). These cells release chemical substances *(cytokines)* that may help endometrial implants grow, cause adhesion formation, reduce fertility, and increase frequency of miscarriages.

- ✔ New research shows women with endometriosis often have increased autoantibody levels, suggesting that endometriosis is an autoimmune disease. Common systemic symptoms like cyclic headaches, ovulation dysfunction, recurrent flu-like syndromes, joint pain, chronic fatigue, irritable bowel symptoms, and possible increased rate of miscarriage may be caused by the increase in autoantibody levels.

- ✔ Research may link the female sex hormones (estrogen and progesterone), testosterone, follicle-stimulating hormone, and luteinizing hormone to the immune system. Hormonal and menstrual cycle irregularities are common with endometriosis.

A normal immune system checks the growth of endometrial tissue outside the endometrial cavity, just like it would check the growth of any *neoplastic* (new or tumor) cells found where they don't belong. However, most women with endometriosis may have malfunctioning immune systems that don't destroy stray endometrial cells before they have a chance to take up residence. Most immune therapy involves intravenous infusions or injections of medications that stimulate the immune system to reject and destroy tumors and growths. This section briefly looks at a few treatment options.

Naming the two main treatment options

Immune therapy is successful with other types of autoimmune disease, and because of the link of endometriosis to autoimmune diseases, researchers suggest that immune therapy may work against endometriosis. Because the FDA hasn't approved any of these more aggressive treatments for endometriosis, we include them in this chapter. The two main treatments include

- **Intravenous immunoglobulin (IVIG):** IVIG is a sterile protein preparation derived from human blood, given intravenously. IVIG is being used in other autoimmune disorders with some success, but some studies have found no real benefit to IVIG. The biggest problem with this treatment is the cost, $2,500 to $4,000 per treatment, which most insurance companies don't cover because IVIG isn't approved for use in endometriosis.

   IVIG comes from the same blood pool used for transfusions, so it's quite safe, because these products are specially treated to filter out and kill viruses. The IVIG products available in the United States and the United Kingdom have, according to manufacturers, not resulted in a single HIV transmission in more than 2 million administrations.

- **Pentoxifylline (Trental):** Trental is an oral medication that normalizes the activity of a wide range of immune cells that may contribute to endometriosis. One study done by Dr. Michael Vernon in Kentucky found that Trental treatment caused endometriosis to shrink in animals, and a study in Spain showed the pregnancy rate for women treated with Trental was 31 percent compared to 18 percent for women treated with *placebo* (sugar pills).

   Trental has an advantage over IVIG because it's fairly inexpensive, is taken by mouth, and less than 1 percent of patients report noticeable side effects. Tell your doctor you're taking this medication before any type of surgery, including dental surgery, because increased bleeding is a possible side effect.

Considering biologic response modifiers

Medications called *biologic response modifiers,* such as adalimumab (Humira), infliximab (Remicade), and etanercept (Enbrel), have been used for many autoimmune diseases, but are still under investigation for endometriosis. Biologic response modifiers inhibit cytokines, which decrease pain and inflammation.

These drugs are expensive and must be given intravenously or by injection. They may also increase the risk of infections. Some can have a bad effect on the neurological system, making them unacceptable for use in some patients.

Chapter 13

Managing the Chronic Physical Pain

Chronic pain can drive you to despair. When you suffer from acute pain, say from a bad infection, you know it will eventually end and you'll feel better. But chronic pain gives you no such assurances. You can only hope the pain lessens after treatment or that some medication can keep it at bay.

Even with the treatments your doctor gives you, permanently defeating the pain of endometriosis may take a long time. But defeating pain one day at a time may be possible, although you need patience to figure out what combination of drugs, exercise, or therapy works for you. Pain from endometriosis can occur at different times in your cycle and in different places in your body. You can look at your progress by keeping a detailed diary of your pain, your symptoms, and your treatments. (See Chapters 2 and 10 for more on keeping a diary.)

Keep track of the medications you've tried and what works best for you. Some days you may find one medication works better, some days another, depending on your symptoms. You'll never remember what worked best if you don't write it down though!

In this chapter, we tell you how to keep the pain of endometriosis under control as much as is humanly possible. We cover the different types of over-the-counter (OTC) medications and prescription drugs as well as other methods that can help you manage the pain.

Defining Chronic Pain

Chronic pain is difficult to understand. Often the pain continues long after the original injury has healed, leaving other people to wonder why you're not better. For example, "Didn't your surgery fix all that?" is a typical attitude from uneducated family and friends.

So what exactly is chronic pain?

 ✔ Pain that may not have a definable cause

 ✔ Pain that continues for longer than six months

 ✔ Pain that may not respond well to conventional medical therapies

What's the first step to decreasing pain? Know your enemy. (Read Part I to get the lowdown on endometriosis and how it affects your body.)

The next step? Know what works for you. Everyone responds differently to pain medication, and chronic pain can change the way you respond to medications that you may have used effectively in the past. When pain becomes chronic, you may need to increase the dose of medications you take, try new medications, or move up to prescription-strength medications.

Self-Medicating with Over-the-Counter Meds

Drugstores can be deceiving. With so many medications on the shelf, surely some medicine can help, right? The trouble with OTC medications for pain is that many of them have the same ingredients — just different packaging with different names by different companies — so the varieties of medicine aren't as diverse as they first seem.

This section helps you identify the two main types of OTC painkillers and then discusses a few pointers you need to consider when taking an OTC medicine to battle your pain.

Comparing the types of OTC painkillers

When you're walking the aisles of your neighborhood pharmacy, you basically can choose from two types of OTC pain medicines, or *analgesics.* You have acetaminophen, better known as Tylenol, which relieves pain but doesn't decrease inflammation, and *nonsteroidal anti-inflammatories* (NSAIDs), which include aspirin and newer NSAIDS, such as ibuprofen, which relieve both pain and inflammation. We discuss all the options in the next sections.

Acetaminophen

Acetaminophen, sold as Tylenol, is the most common OTC analgesic in the United States. Acetaminophen relieves pain and reduces fever but doesn't decrease inflammation or inhibit platelet function. For this reason, it doesn't cause stomach irritation or increase bleeding tendencies. Although it's very safe when taken in recommended dosages, overdoses can result in fatal liver disease.

Acetaminophen is often sold as a prescription drug in combination with opioid medications, available only by a prescription for stronger pain. You can buy the medicine OTC in 325 milligram and 500 milligram tablets and it can be safely taken in doses up to 1,000 milligrams four times a day.

Because acetaminophen doesn't cause the stomach upset and bleeding problems common to aspirin and NSAIDs (see the next two sections), it may be a safer long-term choice for self-medication for some people. However, because acetaminophen doesn't block the inflammation that is a large part of endometriosis, it may not be effective in the long run.

Aspirin

Aspirin is one of those modern medicines that was first discovered in nature thousands of years ago. As early as 400 B.C., the Greek physician Hippocrates prescribed tea made from the bark of the willow tree to relieve pain and fever. In the 1800s, salicin was extracted in the laboratory from willow bark and the spirea plant and transformed into the more active acetylsalicylic acid, known today as *aspirin.* Aspirin is sold in tablets containing 325 mg or 500 mg.

Today aspirin remains one of the most commonly used pain relievers. Aspirin inhibits *prostaglandins,* the chemicals responsible for uterine cramping. This decreases pain, fever, and inflammation. (See the sidebar in this chapter, "How do NSAIDs work" for more information.) Although aspirin is the grand-daddy of all NSAIDs, it isn't as effective as its newer relatives.

Newer nonsteroidal anti-inflammatories (NSAIDs)

NSAIDs work differently than other analgesics (see the sidebar, "How do NSAIDs work?" in this chapter for more info), and because NSAIDs reduce inflammation, they may be more effective in reducing pain than plain analgesics. NSAIDs inhibit *prostaglandins,* the chemicals responsible for uterine cramping. The most common newer OTC NSAIDs include the following brand and generic names:

- Ibuprofen (Advil, Motrin, Nuprin) sold OTC in doses up to 200 mg, depending on the brand name (400, 600, and 800 mg are available by prescription)
- Naproxen (Naprosyn) 250 mg, 375 mg, 500 mg
- Naproxen Sodium (Aleve, Anaprox) 220 mg, 275 mg, 500 mg

NSAID daily doses shouldn't exceed 2,400 mg unless you're told to take more by your doctor.

NSAIDs' enzyme-inhibitor effect also increases your risk of bleeding and stomach ulcers. If you want to take an OTC NSAID on a regular basis, discuss it with your doctor first. Side effects of increased bleeding and stomach ulcers can make NSAIDs dangerous if you have any of the following issues:

- Congestive heart failure
- Gastroesophageal reflux disease (GERD)
- Liver disease
- Renal (kidney) disease
- Stomach ulcers

NSAIDs have a large list of potential side effects besides the more serious problems of bleeding and stomach ulcers. Allergic reactions are common. In addition, you may experience any of the following:

- Constipation
- Diarrhea
- Drowsiness
- Fluid retention
- Headache
- Nausea
- Rash
- Vomiting

In addition, NSAIDs decrease blood flow to the kidneys and can raise blood pressure in individuals with hypertension. NSAIDs can also interfere with the metabolism of certain medications, such as lithium or methotrexate. Finally, NSAIDs can increase symptoms in asthma sufferers.

How do NSAIDs work?

NSAIDs work by blocking the production of *prostaglandins,* the chemicals produced in the uterus (as well as a number of other places) at the time of your period. They cause the cramping that helps shed the uterine lining if you're not pregnant, and can cause diarrhea, fever, pain, and inflammation. Because prostaglandins are responsible for uterine cramping, medications that reduce their effects can help block menstrual cramping.

Prostaglandins are produced within the body's cells by the enzyme cyclooxygenase (COX). There are two COX enzymes, called, logically, COX-1 and COX-2. COX-1 enzymes support platelets and protect your stomach lining; taking aspirin or NSAIDs frequently decreases the protective effects of COX-1 and can cause bleeding and ulcers in some people. Some NSAIDs are more effective in blocking COX-1 than others and vary in their tendency to cause ulcers and promote bleeding.

Acetaminophen appears to block COX enzymes only in the central nervous system. For this reason, acetaminophen decreases pain and fever but doesn't decrease inflammation or platelet function.

A promising new class of NSAIDs, COX-2 inhibitors, selectively block only the COX-2 enzymes. This approach initially looked good for pain management because these drugs reduce pain and inflammation while protecting the stomach and platelets. A few years ago, however, COX-2 inhibitors reportedly appeared to increase the risk of heart problems, and some COX-2 inhibitors were taken off the market. COX-2 inhibitors that are still available require a doctor's prescription.

Choosing meds wisely

Start with your doctor when you need more information about OTC pain relief medications. However, if you're wandering around the 24-hour drugstore at 4 a.m., calling the doctor may not be a good idea — not if you want him to *stay* your doctor. If a pharmacist is on duty, she can help you out by telling you which drug products have basically the same ingredients. You can also keep the following in mind when you're considering OTC drugs:

- ✔ **Keep an eye out for the same ingredients.** As you can see by reading the previous section, some medications, such as brand-name Motrin and generic ibuprofen, contain the same ingredients. This information is important to know so you don't overdose, thinking you're taking two different drugs.

- ✔ **Take single drugs rather than combination drugs.** Taking single drugs, such as plain aspirin, is better than taking combination drugs, like Excedrin, which contains acetaminophen, aspirin, and a hefty dose of caffeine. Combination drugs may give you ingredients you don't need and may increase the chance of drug interactions.

▶ **Ask your doctor for a prescription — and if he gives you one, have it filled!** Many times doctors hand out prescriptions at your appointment and you never have them filled because you've seen the names of the drugs on the pharmacy shelves. But doctors can prescribe drugs like ibuprofen in higher dosages than you can buy them OTC. Although you can certainly take four 200 mg pills rather than one 800 mg pill, why would you want to? And it costs more to take several pills instead of one.

Trying Prescription Medications

OTC medications often aren't enough to treat chronic pain. You may also need to take prescription pain medication, at least at certain times of the month. However, you may find that taking pain medication on a schedule is more effective than waiting until the pain builds up.

This section looks at the different types of prescription medications that can help you manage your pain. In this section, we cover prescriptions NSAIDs, Ultram, opioids, antidepressants, and antiseizure drugs.

Taking prescription NSAIDs

Some prescription pain medications are the same medications you can buy OTC but in higher dosages. One example of an NSAID available both OTC and by prescription is ibuprofen, which comes in doses up to 200 milligrams OTC. You need a doctor's prescription to buy ibuprofen in doses of 400 to 800 milligrams.

Some common prescription NSAIDs (and their brand names) that require a doctor's prescription are

- ▶ Diclofenac (Cataflam, Voltaren)
- ▶ Etodolac (Lodine)
- ▶ Fenoprofen (Nalfon)
- ▶ Flurbiprofen (Ansaid)
- ▶ Ibuprofen (Advil, Motrin)
- ▶ Indomethacin (Indocin)
- ▶ Ketoprofen (Orudis, Oruvail)
- ▶ Meclofenamate (Meclomen)
- ▶ Meloxicam (Mobic)
- ▶ Nabumetone (Relafen)

✔ Naproxen (Anaprox, Naprelan, Naprosyn)

✔ Oxaprozin (Daypro)

✔ Piroxicam (Feldene)

✔ Sulindac (Clinoril)

✔ Tolmetin (Tolectin)

COX-2 inhibitors are drugs that block certain prostaglandin-producing enzymes. (See the sidebar "How do NSAIDS work?" for more info.) The only COX-2 inhibitor still available by prescription is Celecoxib (Celebrex). In 2004, the FDA removed other COX-2 inhibitors from the market because studies showed an increased risk of heart disease in patients taking them.

Considering opioids

Opioids are a powerful prescription-only class of pain relievers related to the granddaddy of all pain relievers, morphine. Also called *narcotics,* opioids include the natural opium alkaloids, the semisynthetic opioids derived from them, and the fully synthetic opioids. They all bind to opioid receptors found principally in the brain and gastrointestinal tract.

The following includes some common prescription opioids, with their brand name in parentheses:

✔ Codeine (Tylenol 3)

✔ Hydrocodone (Vicodin)

✔ Hydromorphine (Dilaudid)

✔ Meperidine (Demerol)

✔ Morphine

✔ Oxycodone (OxyContin, Percocet, Percodan)

Long-term use of these medications can lead to physical dependence and tolerance; you may need increasingly larger amounts to achieve the same effect. Addiction to opioids can occur if the drugs are misused, taken in larger doses or more often than prescribed, or mixed with other medications.

Table 13-1 lists drugs by classification and schedule, which is the way the Drug Enforcement Administration (DEA) defines the uses of certain drugs. Schedule I drugs have high abuse potential, have no medical use, or haven't been proven to be safe, so we don't list them. Because most opioids fall into Schedules II to IV, we concentrate on them.

Table 13-1	Controlled Substances Classification II–IV	
Schedule	**Characteristics**	**Examples (Brand Names)**
Schedule II	High potential for abuse.	Fentanyl (Sublimaze, Duragesic)
	Has an acceptable medical use.	
	Abuse may lead to severe physical or psychological dependence.	Hydromorphone (Dilaudid)
		Morphine (MS Contin, Duramorph)
		Oxycodone (OxyContin, Percodan, Percocet, Tylox)
Schedule III	Less abuse potential than Schedule I or II drugs.	Butalbital (Fioricet, Fiorinol)
	Has an acceptable medical use.	Codeine (Tylenol #3)
	Low to moderate risk of physical or psychological addiction.	Hydrocodone bitartrate (Lorcet, Lortab, Vicodin)
Schedule IV	Low abuse potential.	Dextropropoxyphene (Darvon, Darvocet)
	Has an accepted medical use.	
	May lead to limited physical or psychological dependence.	

Some doctors are hesitant to prescribe opioids because of the risk of addiction; other doctors are so negative about prescribing opioids that you may leave their office in tears, feeling as if you've been treated like a drug addict for even asking about them. (See the nearby sidebar, "Opioids can lead to dependence and addiction" for more info.)

Finding a doctor who understands pain and is willing to treat it can be an important part of your care. However, doctors who are willing to treat pain are very different from doctors who indiscriminately overprescribe opioids. How can you tell the difference? Your doctor is prescribing responsibly if he

✔ Asks about whether or not the drugs are helping, rather than just handing you another prescription

✔ Prescribes only a small amount of medication at a time rather than a year's supply

✔ Discusses alternative pain-relief methods to try along with the pills

  ✔ Is concerned about overmedicating you and discusses the signs of over-medication with you

  ✔ Listens to your concerns about possible addiction

Many combination pain relievers are opioids mixed with aspirin or aceta-minophen. Table 13-2 lists some of the most common pain relievers and their compositions.

Table 13-2	Common Pain Reliever Combos
Drug	*Description*
Tylenol #3	Acetaminophen 300 mg + Codeine 30 mg
Percocet 7.5	Acetaminophen 325 mg + oxycodone 7.5 mg
Percodan	Aspirin 325 mg + oxycodone 5 mg
Vicodin	Acetaminophen 325 mg + hydrocodone bitartrate 5 mg

Trying Ultram

Tramadol (Ultram) is in a class by itself. Tramadol is an analgesic that has its effects in the brain. Its mode of action resembles that of opioids, but researchers believe that it has much less potential for abuse and addiction than the opioids. It's not derived from natural sources nor is it chemically related to opioids. For these reasons, it hasn't been classified as a controlled substance. Ultram is effective in relieving moderate pain and causes less res-piratory depression than opioids.

REMEMBER

Opioids can lead to dependence and addiction

Anyone who takes opioids for any reason will develop some degree of tolerance and depen-dence over time. There's a difference, however, in tolerance, dependence, and addiction.

  ✔ **Tolerance** is the tendency of the body to adapt to the effect of opioids; over time, the body requires higher and higher doses to produce the same effect.

  ✔ **Dependence** is the tendency of the body to experience unpleasant side effects if a person stops taking the drug abruptly.

  ✔ **Addiction** is a psychological dependence to the side effects of opioids, such as eupho-ria. The craving for the side effects leads to taking medication when not medically nec-essary. Addiction causes continued use even when that use becomes self-destruc-tive. Addiction is most common in people who are taking medication purely for recre-ational use; addiction is less common in people using the drug for legitimate pur-poses, such as pain management.

Even though Ultram isn't classified as a controlled substance, as an *atypical opioid,* it can produce many of the same euphoric effects and has a potential for abuse and addiction.

Some of Ultram's most common side effects are

- Agitation
- Blurred vision
- Constipation
- Diarrhea
- Dizziness
- Drowsiness
- Dry mouth
- Headache
- Mood changes
- Nervousness or anxiety
- Sweating
- Upset stomach

Like any medication, Ultram can also cause allergy symptoms and rare, but serious, side effects. If you experience hives, swelling, fast heartbeat, seizures, or hallucinations, you should, of course, notify your doctor immediately and go to the nearest emergency room.

Taking antidepressants

At first glance, you may think this section is in the wrong chapter. How can taking prescription antidepressants help with pain? Actually, antidepressants can help decrease chronic pain in several ways. The two most obvious ways are

- **Improved sleep** so pain decreases
- **Decreased depression,** which is a common side effect of chronic pain (Check out Chapter 15 for more information about depression and your emotions.)

However, there's much more to this story. Many studies have shown that some classes of antidepressants have analgesic properties and have reduced chronic pain in more than 50 percent of the people studied.

Tricyclic antidepressants

The antidepressants that have been studied the most for pain relief are tricyclic antidepressants. These antidepressants may work on pain by

- ✔ Blocking pain pathways
- ✔ Increasing endorphin release (*Endorphins* help regulate mood and block pain.)

Some of the most common tricyclic antidepressants (and their brand names) are

- ✔ Amitriptyline hydrochloride (Amitril, Elevil, Endep)
- ✔ Desipramine (Norpramin)
- ✔ Doxipin hydrochloride (Sinequan)
- ✔ Imipramine hydrochloride (Janimine, Tofranil)
- ✔ Nortriptyline (Aventyl, Pamelor)

Dosages for pain relief are often lower than dosages for treatment of depression. The drug may take several weeks to be effective, so don't be ready to give up if you don't see any results within the first week or two.

Antidepressants do have side effects. Check out Chapter 15 for more information.

Other antidepressants

What about other antidepressants not in the tricyclic family? A number of newer antidepressant drugs on the market fall into categories that are nearly unpronounceable. Three new categories are

- ✔ Serotonin and Noradrenergic Reuptake Inhibitors (SNaRI), like venlafaxine and duloxetine
- ✔ Noradrenergic and Specific Serotoninergic Antidepressants (NaSSA), like mirtazapine (Remeron)
- ✔ Noradrenaline Reuptake Inhibitors (NaRI), like reboxetine

SNaRI antidepressants are some of the most investigated of the new drugs shown to be effective in the treatment of different kinds of pain, and appear to have fewer side effects than TCAs. Duloxetine (Cymbalta) and venlafaxine (Effexor) have both been found to be effective in treating chronic pain. Mirtazapine (Remeron) is an NaSSA that is more sedating than some of the other antidepressants and may be helpful if you're having trouble sleeping.

Selective Seratonin Reuptake Inhibitors (SSRIs) are useful for relieving neuropathic pain. Citalopram (Celexa), fluvoxamine (Luvox), paroxitene (Paxil), fluoxetine (Prozac), and sertraline (Zoloft) are all SSRIs. See Chapter 15 for more on antidepressants and their effects.

Considering antiseizure medications

Some doctors prescribe antiseizure medications for neuropathic and chronic pain, including pain associated with endometriosis. Two of these proven antiseizure medications are carbamazepine (Tegretol) and gabapentin (Neurontin).

The most common side effects to antiseizure medications are

- Dizziness
- Fatigue
- Headaches
- Sleeplessness

Creaming Away the Pain

You may think a painkiller in the form of a cream or patch may sound too good to be true. However, pain medications, such as fentanyl, work quite effectively as skin patches. Logically, other pain medications may eventually work the same way.

Medications that are absorbed through the skin into the bloodstream avoid the *first pass* effect; in other words, they don't pass through the stomach and liver. The most significant benefits to *transdermal* (through the skin) applications of medications are

- Fewer side effects, such as stomach upset
- Faster onset of pain relief than oral medication
- Possibly more of the drug reaching the pain site
- Possibly longer-lasting relief

A number of drugs are available either in cream form or in a patch; both types are absorbed through the skin. Some examples are as follows:

✔ **Over the counter**

- **Aspercreme:** An aspirin cream.

- **Ibugel:** A gel that contains 5 percent ibuprofen and was as effective as oral ibuprofen 400 mg in one study; approved for sale in Europe but undergoing clinical trials in the United States.

- **Menastil:** A topical anesthetic sold in a lipstick-sized container. The manufacturer claims Menastil is specifically effective against menstrual cramps and the symptoms of endometriosis.

✔ **Only by prescription**

- **Fentanyl:** An opioid pain reliever that is available in transdermal form and must be prescribed

- **Lidocaine:** A well-known anesthetic that is applied via a patch and available by prescription

- **Zonolon:** A tricyclic antidepressant cream that contains doxipin and is available by prescription

Is it worth giving topical medications a try before taking pills? It may be if you have a sensitive stomach or have liver problems. However, remember that these gels and creams do contain active medication; you can't slather yourself in them!

Exercising Away Your Pain

Exercise can really help decrease chronic pain; the key to beneficial exercise is to start slow, do only what's comfortable at first, increase gradually, and most important of all, don't give up too soon! Getting started on an exercise program takes perseverance. The most important step you can take is the first one: just get up and do it!

Gentle stretching exercises may be all you can manage at first, but as you limber up, you may find a yoga or T'ai Chi class helpful in pushing you a bit without injuring anything (check out Chapter 12 for more info).

Kegel exercises can also help with endometriosis pain by strengthening the pelvic muscles and bladder. The best way to practice Kegels initially is to find the pelvic muscles by trying to stop the flow of urine by squeezing the muscles. After you've isolated the muscles, you can "Kegel" frequently during the day. Kegels can help get your pelvic muscles back into shape after childbirth as well!

Walking is one of the most beneficial exercises of all. It requires no equipment other than a good pair of walking shoes. You can add hand weights as you become more fit, and increase your speed and distance.

The best thing about exercise? It releases *endorphins,* chemicals that boost your sense of well-being. (See Chapter 16 for more on exercise when you have endometriosis.) Exercise may also reduce estrogen levels, and estrogen promotes growth of endometrial implants.

Using Heat and Massage for Pain Relief

Sometimes simple methods work well for relieving pain. Heat can be a great muscle relaxer. Sometimes just soaking in a warm tub or resting with a heating pad or hot water bottle can relieve pain. Some heating pads supply moist heat, which can be even more effective than dry heat.

You can also make your own packs by warming slightly dampened towels in the microwave. Remember that microwaves don't apply heat evenly, and make sure the towel doesn't get too hot in one spot; you can end up with a painful burn in addition to your other aches and pains. One advantage of warm towels is that you can mold them to your aching areas, which is difficult to do with commercial heating pads.

You can also use massage therapy to decrease pain, relax muscles, and relieve tension. Check out Chapter 12 for more on massage and other alternative treatments that can alleviate your pain.

Chapter 14

All Things Teens: Diagnosing, Treating, and Coping with Endometriosis

*N*ot too many years ago, doctors thought teenagers couldn't have endometriosis, and many moms taught their daughters that pain, cramps, and abnormal bleeding were just a normal part of becoming a woman. Now that doctors have diagnosed endometriosis in girls as young as 11 years old, they're more aware of endometriosis as a possible cause for a teen's painful periods.

In this chapter, we discuss how doctors can diagnose and treat endometriosis in young patients, and how parents can keep communication open with their teenage daughter (as well as with her doctor), can help teens feel well enough to stay in school, and can preserve fertility in teens.

Making a Diagnosis in Teens (And Preteens)

The symptoms of endometriosis in teens (and even some preteens) are similar to those for women in their 20s or 30s, with the most common symptom being painful periods, or *dysmenorrhea*. (Check out Chapter 2 for a complete rundown of common symptoms.) The difference in teens, though, is that many parents and doctors don't consider endometriosis as a diagnosis for the painful cramps that can keep a teen home from school or in bed a few days each month.

Diagnosing endometriosis in teens starts with suspecting the disease and actively looking for it. Doctors who look do find it. Statistics show that

- ✔ From 4 to 10 percent of teens with severe menstrual cramps will be found to have endometriosis.
- ✔ Teens make up 5 to 6 percent of all endometriosis patients.
- ✔ More than 40 percent of women who have endometriosis say that their symptoms started during their teen years.

Sadly, the average time between the start of endometriosis symptoms and diagnosis is nearly ten years. But early treatment is likely to result in less serious disease down the road and can help preserve normal reproductive function.

The only way to truly diagnose endometriosis is surgery, but you may not want to consider this route right off the bat. When doctors make a *presumptive* diagnosis of endometriosis, they're saying that all the symptoms fit and endometriosis is likely the cause, but they haven't proved 100 percent that endometriosis is present.

This section focuses on you helping your teen by talking with her about severe menstrual pain, helping her with the initial gynecological exam so her doctor can make a presumptive diagnosis, and understanding what other problems your teen's doctor has to rule out before diagnosing endometriosis.

Letting teens know that severe menstrual pain isn't normal

Many teens think that cramps and severe pain with their periods and in the middle of their menstrual cycle is just a normal part of being a woman — because their parents and friends told them. But believing this myth often leads to a delayed diagnosis and treatment that can have long-lasting consequences.

Many teens (just like many adults!) play "Can you top this?" when discussing medical issues. Unfortunately, if a teen's friends exaggerate their painful periods to sound like ptomaine poisoning, she's going to think painful periods aren't only normal but required.

Although some cramping is normal — up to 50 percent of teens experience cramping during their periods — severe cramping and pain that interferes with normal activities isn't.

Understanding why pain doesn't recur every month

Endometriosis can be easy to dismiss as a possible diagnosis in a teen if she doesn't have painful periods every month. After all, if a teen has the disease, why doesn't it show up every month, rather than every other month, or for two or three months in a row and then not for a few more months?

Many teens don't have pain every month because they don't ovulate regularly. Especially in the first year or so of menstrual periods, an egg doesn't develop and estrogen doesn't rise every month. And because estrogen feeds the growing endometriosis, an *anovulatory* cycle (no egg) may escape severe pelvic pain or cramps. This inconsistency can lead to a false sense that endometriosis isn't present when it may be.

Getting through the gyno exam

The first step to diagnosing endometriosis is a gynecologic exam (see Chapter 9 for more about GYN exams), but many teens have never had one — and would rather not have one!

If grown women are often afraid of pelvic exams, imagine the fear that strikes a teen or preteen who has to undergo such an ordeal! If you're the parent of the teen, you need to help your teen through this experience with a minimum of trauma.

As with most frightening procedures, education is the best tool. Teens need to know what to expect during a gynecologic exam. A doctor or nurse who takes time to explain exactly what occurs and what it feels like is worth her weight in gold. A doctor who takes her time and is extra gentle is also a necessity!

Deep breathing techniques can help nervous teens get through the exam and relax at the same time. Tense muscles make a thorough examination nearly impossible. However, gynecologic examinations are possible without using a *speculum* (an instrument used to hold the vagina open so the doctor can see inside the vagina) or *bimanual* exam (using one hand in the vagina and the other on the abdomen). A *blindly-placed* swab in the vagina (to check for infection or abnormal cells) and an abdominal exam with ultrasound may suffice. A teen may tolerate a rectal exam better than a vaginal exam to determine pelvic abnormalities. All these methods are possible for examining a young woman with fear of a full pelvic exam.

Ruling out other problems

To make a presumptive diagnosis of endometriosis, your teen's doctor may need to rule out other potential problems by looking for the following:

- ✔ **Pelvic organ abnormalities:** The most common symptom experienced by teenagers with a uterine abnormality is severe menstrual cramps caused by backward *(retrograde)* flow of menstrual blood through the tubes. Early surgical correction of such an abnormality can avoid the development of severe endometriosis is some patients. Pelvic ultrasound, performed through the vagina or abdominal wall, can verify that the uterus and ovaries are normal. Unfortunately, unless an endometrioma is present in the ovary, ultrasound can't "see" endometriosis.

- ✔ **Sexually transmitted diseases (STDs):** Doctors must differentiate between endometriosis and a sexually transmitted disease because the diseases have some of the same symptoms *but* need very different treatment. Unfortunately, the first diagnosis many doctors consider when teens have severe pelvic pain is an STD rather than endometriosis.

  Many doctors incorrectly assume that a teen with pelvic pain is having sex. This assumption can be embarrassing for a teen who isn't sexually active and can lead to a lack of trust in a doctor who jumps to conclusions. However, if a teen *is* sexually active, she needs to be honest; otherwise, the doctor may overlook an important problem.

  Doctors can diagnose STDs by taking a blood sample (for syphilis) or a cervical swab (for chlamydia and gonorrhea). If a teen has been sexually active, the speculum may be easier to insert into the vagina than with a teen who isn't sexually active. A Pap test is also necessary if a teen has had intercourse because the test can detect changes in the cervix that may lead to cervical cancer, which the doctor can then treat relatively early and easily.

  Having an STD doesn't mean a teen can't also have endometriosis, so she should follow up after STD treatment if symptoms haven't disappeared!

- ✔ **Sexual abuse:** Healthcare providers have finally begun to realize that sexual abuse can cause symptoms similar to endometriosis. During the exam, the doctor can look for signs.

- ✔ **Other organ system problems:** Intestinal or urinary tract disease can also mimic the symptoms of endometriosis and can be affected by the menstrual cycle (see Chapter 2).

Knowing the Risks When Choosing Treatment for Teens

Treating teens with endometriosis may differ from treating adults in a number of ways because a teen's body hasn't completely developed like an adult's. Teens have special issues, from fear of pelvic exams to preserving their ability to have children. Teens and their parents need to carefully consider the risks that accompany different medications as well as the risks of surgery. This section looks at the important considerations and risks.

Being more conservative (or more aggressive?) when treating teens

Because teens generally aren't planning to become pregnant for a few years, their endometriosis requires treatment that won't affect their chances of pregnancy in the future.

Yet some doctors are hesitant to treat teens aggressively for fear of irreparably damaging growing reproductive systems. This fear, however, can lead to undertreatment, which in turn doesn't prevent the reproductive damage that a more aggressive treatment may have prevented.

Make sure all parties — the doctor, the teenager, and the parents — stay involved and aren't afraid of frank discussions about treatment. (Check out "Keeping Communication Open between Parent and Teen" later in this chapter for more about the importance of communication.) Being too conservative or too aggressive in treatment can have long-term consequences. Everyone involved needs the opportunity to talk through and understand all the risks and benefits.

Realizing that teens may still be growing

You may wonder whether a teen's physical immaturity affects the treatments for endometriosis. In fact, many of the drug treatments for endometriosis can damage growing bones. Because of this concern, doctors need to look at the length of treatment, monitor closely for side effects, and provide *add-back therapy* (check out Chapter 10 for more information on this treatment plan) to offset negative effects.

Examples of problematic teen treatments include estrogen and testosterone. Estrogen can cause the fusion of the growth plate (preventing a child from reaching her full height), and testosterone-like compounds can affect the genital system, hair and breast growth, and the voice. All hormonal medications require cautious use.

Eying the medication risks

Medication choices for teens with endometriosis are somewhat more limited than they are for adults (check out Chapter 10, which discusses medication treatments for endometriosis). Because many medications to treat endometriosis can be harmful to a teen's growth and development, selecting the right medication for a teen (or preteen) is vital.

Treating teens with GnRH agonists

GnRH agonists, such as leuprolide acetate (Depot Lupron) or goserelin acetate (Zoladex), work by shutting off hormones made by the ovaries that lower estrogen levels. As a result, these drugs temporarily shut down the menstrual cycle. Teens on GnRH agonists don't usually have regular periods, although they may have spotting at times.

The FDA has approved these drugs for use up to six months at a time. If used for more than six months, studies have found they can cause permanent changes in bone density. Although decreased bone density has no symptoms, young women with low bone density are at increased risk of fracture related to thin bones after menopause. For this reason, many doctors use add-back therapy, which means that estrogen is prescribed along with the GnRH agonists to protect against bone loss.

Putting teens on birth control pills

Hormonal treatments, such as birth control pills (BCPs), work well but may give parents pause. A large number of BCPs are available today that have differing combinations of estrogen and progesterone — two female hormones. (Some teens tolerate one combination better than another; some treatments are helpful for teens with acne, and others may make acne worse.)

Often doctors direct a patient to take BCPs continuously, without a break in the active pills for three months or more. This may allow for better suppression and periods only a few times a year.

Note: Some pills are packaged in this three-month format that may be tolerated by a teen, but patients may also use regular BCPs, skipping the sugar pills (or *inert* pills) and taking only the active pills for three months straight. With this treatment, monthly menstrual periods don't occur. Although some teens may find this change worrisome; others may find it freeing!

Worrying about birth control pills and sex

Putting a teen on birth control pills (BCPs) can be a guilt-producing experience for parents. On one hand, it reduces your teen's pain, which is a big positive. On the other hand, you may worry that you're giving your teen carte blanche to have sex.

Parents can't help but worry about this conflict; it's what makes parents parents! But the fact is, taking BCPs for endometriosis is different from taking pills just so she won't get pregnant. BCPs are simply a medication for endometriosis. As a parent, you shouldn't feel guilty about putting your child on them.

But this is an important time to have a dialogue with your child. Honest discussion about the reasons for using BCPs and the responsibility of sexual relations is a must. In fact, the topic may be a good lead into a frank, general talk about sex or a reinforcement of past discussions.

Taking BCPs, even for long periods of time, doesn't make getting pregnant more difficult in the future. Today's pills are a much lower dose than those of 20 years ago, and normal periods usually resume within a month or two after stopping the pill.

Using progestin-only pills

Another type of daily pill contains only synthetic progestin. Norethindrone acetate (Aygestin) is one type of progestin-only medication. Patients that can't take hormone medication with synthetic estrogen may take this type of medicine.

Progestin-only medications don't supply estrogen. As a result, some, especially methoxyprogesterone acetate (Provera in its different forms), can cause lower bone density, leading to a higher risk of osteoporosis (brittle bones) if teens take them for a long time. The doctor may also prescribe estrogen for patients with endometriosis who are on this medicine for more than six months. Unfortunately, not all teens get pain relief from progestin-only medications.

Injecting progestins

Another way of taking progestins is by injection. This method is a bit more convenient because a patient has the injection only once every three months. Depo-provera has been around for decades and can give good results. The biggest problems with this treatment are possible irregular bleeding, the absence of menstrual cycles, possible bone loss, and weight gain. Two other possible drawbacks to injections are that:

- Some people, especially young people, are afraid of injections.
- After you inject the medication, you can't remove it, so side effects can persist for a while.

Limiting NSAIDs

Though the *nonsteroidal anti-inflammatory drugs* (NSAIDs), such as ibuprofen or acetaminophen, are safe, too much of any medication can be harmful. These medications are available over the counter so your doctor may not really know how much the patient has really taken. These medications do have potentially severe side effects. Be sure that a healthcare provider is monitoring your teen if she is taking more than a few pills a month.

Identifying surgical risks

As a teen or a parent of a teen with endometriosis, the thought of undergoing surgery to treat endometriosis may be frightening. You may worry about damage to reproductive organs, having a big scar, or something going wrong during surgery.

Studies have shown that treating endometriosis surgically is better sooner rather than later, especially if medical treatment isn't working after six months or so. The endometriosis lesions will cause less damage if a surgeon removes them sooner and symptoms should diminish. You may be doing your child a favor by deciding on surgery because it may prevent big problems or more extensive surgery in the future. As with all other treatments, a discussion with the doctor about risks, benefits, and alternatives is essential.

The good news is that surgery has never been safer. A large incision isn't usually necessary because most surgeries are by laparoscopy and require only a few tiny incisions. (See Chapter 11 for more about surgery options.) Some of your daughter's friends may have had arthroscopic surgery for sports injuries, so your child can feel better knowing her surgery may use a scope too.

Anesthesia today is also very safe because hospitals use less of it. Recovery is short, only a few days, so your daughter can get back to school or other activities quickly. (That can be good news or bad, depending on how she looks at it!)

Keeping Communication Open between Parent and Teen

Being able to talk about endometriosis is important, but parents and teens may both have trouble with this! Even in this tell-all era, many teens have trouble talking to their parents about their periods, and many parents — who didn't discuss menstrual issues with their parents — have difficulty asking their daughters about it. Although teens may discuss everything with their friends (and, amazingly, tend to believe their friends' advice as gospel truth), they're often reluctant to listen to you, the parent.

If you're a parent, your part of keeping communication lines open is to

- **Take complaints about cramps and pain seriously.** Severe cramps and pain aren't part of normal menstruation, so follow up on them.

- **Be nonjudgmental about your daughter's complaints.** Telling her that she's just being a baby or trying to get out of going to school isn't going to encourage her to tell you anything further.

- **Ask open-ended questions about how she's feeling.** Don't try to describe what you think she should be feeling; ask her what she *is* feeling.

- **Not be afraid to suggest a visit to the gynecologist.** If your daughter has endometriosis, the earlier treatment starts, the less harm will be done.

- **Talk to your daughter's school administrator if absences are a problem.** You may need to explain that she has a chronic illness and will be absent from time to time. You don't need to go into great detail about your daughter's private health issues; a doctor's note may be helpful without being too descriptive.

If you're a teen, you can help your parents by remembering these tips:

- **Be honest about what you're experiencing.** Don't minimize your symptoms, even if all your friends have assured you that they feel the exact same way and it's normal. Severe cramps and pain aren't a normal part of periods.

- **Be willing to see a gynecologist.** This isn't high on the list of fun activities to do in your spare time, but an appointment with the GYN is the only way to determine the cause of your symptoms.

- **Trust your parents.** They really only want to help, and watching you suffer can make them crazy.

Helping Teens Live with Endometriosis

Teens can be notoriously bad about taking care of themselves when they have a chronic illness. In fact, some studies show that teens with chronic illnesses are more likely to take chances and live dangerously than the average teen. The best way to help teens live with a chronic disease is to involve them in their care.

Being a teen with a chronic disease and feeling like you have no control can be bad enough. But living with a disease that involves reproductive organs is even worse because you may be too embarrassed to talk about it to friends and family (yes, even in this day and age!).

Teens with endometriosis need to learn about it, and they need to learn how to deal with it. As much as possible, these teens should also be in charge of their own medication and treatment.

Chronic illness can affect teens emotionally in a number of ways. For example, chronic illness can

 ✔ Interfere with their ability to be independent

 ✔ Disrupt relationships with peers

 ✔ Limit social activities

 ✔ Affect self-esteem

 ✔ Impose physical limitations

Needless to say, adolescence by itself brings problems to all of these areas; adding a chronic illness to the mix can seriously stress both the teen and her family. The following section provides some helpful tidbits to assist your teen in living with endometriosis.

Handling school absence

More teens miss school for painful menstrual periods than for any other reason, and teens with endometriosis are likely to miss more school days than their friends. These absences can be a source of frustration for teens and parents alike.

If you're a teen with endometriosis and you miss school because of your symptoms, you shouldn't feel guilty. If you're a parent of a teen with endometriosis, don't make your child feel guilty for missing school when her symptoms flare!

On the other hand, if you're a parent, you may suspect that your teen is occasionally using endometriosis as an excuse to avoid gym class, or to skip school once in a while. How can you tell? Most teens in the throes of endometriosis pain are obviously hurting, but the bottom line is, you need to set some rules about missing school. For example, if your teen doesn't go to school, she can't go out later when she miraculously recovers. And too many absences may warrant a visit to the doctor to find out if the disease is worsening or needs different treatment.

Keeping the lines of communication open with the school when absences are unavoidable can help curb discipline problems in the future. Two suggestions for dealing with the school are

✔ Talking to the school administrator to let her know your daughter's situation

✔ Asking your daughter's doctor for a note that can excuse her from physical education when necessary

Watching for signs of depression

Having endometriosis can cause depression in teens, just like it can in adults. Missing out on activities and suffering with pain each month can send teens into an emotional tailspin. Depression is common among people with a chronic illness such as endometriosis and can manifest itself both physically and mentally.

Whether you're a parent of a teen with endometriosis or are a teen with endometriosis, you need to watch for these signs of possibly serious depression:

✔ You're unable to sleep — or sleep too much

✔ Simple activities are exhausting

✔ Nothing seems like fun anymore

✔ Life doesn't seem worth living

✔ Life seems unfair

✔ Being with other people is too much trouble

✔ Normal activities cause anxiety

✔ You have weight loss or gain

✔ You have physical symptoms, such as headaches, chest pain, diarrhea, constipation, or stomachache

✔ You have guilty feelings

✔ You have recurring thoughts of suicide

If you notice these signs, keep a close eye on your teen. Although everyone is entitled to a down day or two, depression that continues more than a few days, that seems to be worsening, or that includes any hint of suicide or wanting to harm herself warrants a visit to the doctor immediately. (Check out Chapter 15 for more on coping with endometriosis.)

Preserving fertility in teens with endometriosis

Although the last thing most teens want is to become pregnant, the day may come when having a baby becomes a priority. For a teen with endometriosis, a medical provider wants to do everything possible to make sure that pregnancy is possible in the future.

Your daughter's doctor needs to be aggressive enough with treatments to prevent long-term damage. Surgery, long-term medication, and other methods of treatment are necessary and shouldn't be delayed. Your daughter's doctor can help decide on the best way to preserve your teenage daughter's fertility while providing the best treatment options for her.

Finding a teen support network

Networking on the Internet is the one exercise most teens are good at. And sources on endometriosis are available just for teens. The Endometriosis Association (www.endometriosisassn.org) publishes a quarterly newsletter just for teens and runs a correspondence network to connect teens that have endometriosis. Teens can choose to e-mail, write, or call each other for conversation and commiseration!

The Endometriosis Association also sponsors a mentor program for teens. A person with a few years of *endo-experience* under her belt answers questions, gives support, and generally provides a helping hand to teens recently diagnosed with endometriosis.

Two other helpful sites include

- ✔ The American College of Obstetrics and Gynecology (ACOG at www.acog.org) has information on endometriosis.

- ✔ Another helpful Web site, sponsored by Children's Hospital Boston, contains articles for parents and teens alike. You can find this information at www.youngwomenshealth.org.

Part IV
Living with Endometriosis

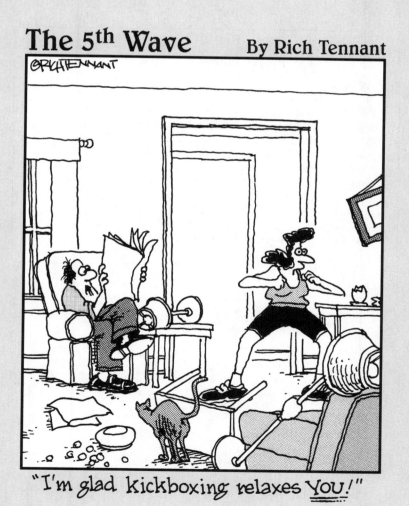

The 5th Wave   By Rich Tennant

"I'm glad kickboxing relaxes YOU!"

In this part . . .

When you have endometriosis, you just gotta live with it, right? Wrong! Although you may think this chronic disease is going to ruin your quality of life, you *can* make daily living easier. In this part, we cover how you can make a real difference for yourself — from eating to exercising (okay, so all these suggestions aren't painless!). We also give you a pep talk on keeping your spirits up when dealing with endometriosis. Last, but not least, we throw in a chapter that's just for family and friends — because they have frustrations with endometriosis too, and they really want to help you.

Chapter 15

Coping with Endometriosis and Your Emotions

....

In This Chapter

▶ Figuring out how endometriosis affects your mental health

▶ Understanding depression

▶ Considering anxiety

▶ Asking yourself if you're depressed or anxious

▶ Treating your depression and anxiety with meds

▶ Sharing your sorrows

....

Does anything make you feel more alone than a disease that others can't see? People with a chronic disease, such as endometriosis, deal with it in different ways. Some never stop talking about the problems, and others never talk about the disease at all. Neither extreme is good for your emotional health.

Trying to find a happy medium is important for your own emotional and psychological well-being. However, no matter how you cope, you may inevitably be depressed or anxious at one time or another. Face it: Endometriosis is very painful, and its symptoms are so overwhelming at times that even the strongest people can experience depression and anxiety.

In this chapter, we help you to emotionally and psychologically handle the frustration of endometriosis in a way that's healthy for you — and the people around you. We look at how endometriosis affects your mental well-being, why women with endometriosis often battle depression and anxiety, how to determine if you're depressed or anxious, and how you can overcome the funk with medications and support.

Understanding How Endometriosis Can Affect Your Mental Health

Initially you may be scratching your head and wondering how we can even suggest that endometriosis may affect your emotional and psychological well being. Endometriosis is a disease typically located in a woman's reproductive organs that causes physical pain, right? How can it affect your mental health?

In addition to causing severe physical pain (check out the symptoms of endometriosis in Chapter 2), endometriosis can severely affect your mental health. When you're in pain, you may feel alone. As often as other people say, "I know how you feel," you can't help but feel that they really don't understand at all. And verbalizing your pain over and over because other people forget about it becomes frustrating. Yet you feel like a hypochondriac when you have to keep turning down invitations and activities you may really want to do. How do you keep the balance between feeling like a martyr when no one understands and being this person whose every waking moment is consumed with endometriosis? It's not easy!

Unfortunately, endometriosis doesn't go away just because you can't see it or decide not to think about it. At times you may feel great and barely give the disease a second thought. Then another period starts, or you have mid-cycle pain, and the problems all come rushing back into your life. (Read more about physical pain relief in Chapter 13.)

Oftentimes people living with physical pain can develop emotional problems, such as depression and anxiety (check out the next two sections). And these emotional problems can even cause the physical pain and symptoms of endometriosis to worsen. Sometimes, though, differentiating between chronic pain and emotional pain isn't easy because many of the symptoms of chronic pain are also symptoms of depression.

When Depression Rears Its Ugly Head: Feeling Down in the Dumps

Depression is common in the general population, never mind people with chronic pain. In fact, depression may affect as many as 50 percent of all chronic pain sufferers because depression can be a normal response to the losses that come with chronic pain. When we also figure in the high percentage of women compared to men — up to three times as many — who suffer from depression (at least in the years before menopause), the potential for a woman with endometriosis to experience depression is very high.

This section looks more closely at depression, identifies the signs of depression, and tells you when you may need to seek professional help.

What exactly is depression?

Depression — feeling sad, losing interest in daily activities, experiencing changes in sleep patterns, and feeling like things will never be the same again — is a normal reaction to loss and drastic changes in life. However, if depression continues for weeks after an event or occurs even without any dramatic life events, you may be clinically depressed. *Clinical depression* is a medical diagnosis indicating that medical intervention is needed. In other words, you're not likely to shake off clinical depression by giving yourself a pep talk or by forcing yourself to get back to your regular routine. About 16 percent of people suffer from clinical depression at one time in their lives.

Clinical depression is more than just having a *down day* or two. Everyone has bad days, and some people have personalities that tend to be more melancholy than others. Clinical depression is defined as sadness lasting more than two weeks that has advanced to the point where it disrupts activities of daily living or social functioning.

Depression can be very complex. Years ago, many people thought the cause for depression was a personality weakness. And today some people believe that depression is strictly a chemical disorder. However, neither explanation is true. Depression is a multifactorial problem; chemical imbalances are certainly a part of depression, but other aspects contribute as well. Some of these contributors are as follows:

- ✔ **Alcohol and drug use:** Daily use of marijuana has been associated with a five-fold increase in depression, according to a study published in the British Medical Journal in 2002.

- ✔ **Family history:** A 2004 statement from the National Institute of Mental Health reports that major depression may be 40 to 70 percent heritable. The statement also notes that development of depression hinges on the interaction of several genes with environmental events.

- ✔ **Life experiences:** Past trauma, abuse, and life-affecting events can all contribute to development of depression.

- ✔ **Medical conditions:** Certain illnesses, including heart disease and hypothyroidism, may contribute to depression; certain prescription medications, such as birth control pills, may also contribute to depression.

- ✔ **Psychological factors:** Low self-esteem and negative thinking can contribute to depression.

The high numbers of depression

According to the World Health Organization, clinical depression is currently the leading cause of disability in the United States as well as other industrialized countries and is expected to become the second leading cause of disability worldwide (after heart disease) by the year 2020. Most depression occurs between the ages of 25 and 44, although it can strike at any age. Most depressive episodes last six to nine months.

What are the signs of depression?

Obviously, a disease with no clearly defined cause, pains that no one can see, and treatments that seem to be of no help can all be upsetting. Some women become withdrawn; others become angry. Some feel guilty over their inability to fulfill responsibilities. Many women feel isolated and alone. You may even begin to doubt your own symptoms, wondering whether this disease really is all in your head.

Medical institutions love to put diseases under neat little codes so the insurance company can pay for them. On paper, then, clinical depression has certain characteristics, and, according to insurance regulations, depressive disorder has at least one of the following characteristics:

✔ Depressed mood

✔ Loss of interest or pleasure

In addition, you have to have four of the following symptoms to be diagnosed with a depressive disorder:

✔ Feelings of overwhelming sadness or fear, or the seeming inability to feel emotion

✔ A decrease in the amount of pleasure derived from what were previously pleasurable activities

✔ Changing appetite and marked weight gain or loss

✔ Disturbed sleep patterns, such as insomnia, loss of REM sleep, or excessive sleep

✔ Changes in activity levels, such as restlessness or a slowing of movement

✔ Fatigue — mental or physical

✔ Feelings of guilt, helplessness, hopelessness, anxiety, or fear

✔ Decrease in self-esteem

✔ Trouble concentrating or making decisions, or a generalized slowing of thought processes

✔ Self-harm or thinking about self-harm

✔ Preoccupation with death or suicide

✔ Reduced memory

If you feel some of these symptoms, you may be clinically depressed, and should see your medical doctor to make sure there's no physical cause first.

How do 1 know when 1 need help?

When you're depressed, you may be the last person to recognize it. Often friends or family may be the first to point out that you may be clinically depressed. Although knowing that you're depressed is the first step to getting help, you may be too depressed to do something about it!

Don't be offended if family members or close friends suggest you need help. Although many people feel psychological help is a sign of weakness, actually the opposite is true. Admitting that you've lost control of your life and need help is much harder than just trying to slog through on your own. Fewer than half of all people with depression seek help, even though depression is very treatable; more than 80 percent of people who seek treatment show improvement.

Determining 1f Anxiety 1s Your Problem

One trouble with chronic pain is that it never seems to end. If you have a broken leg, at least you can look forward to the day your cast comes off and you're good as new. Chronic disease, on the other hand, doesn't give you anything to look forward to — except more pain. You may not be feeling depressed about your condition, but you may have chronic anxiety. This section looks a little closer at anxiety.

Defining anxiety

Anxiety is a state of apprehension and uneasiness where fear and worry affect your moods and behavior. Anxiety is normal in new or stressful situations, but anxiety can become chronic, leading to anxiety disorder. Anxiety can lead to

✔ **Worrying that your condition will never improve.** The one constant you can count on in life is change. And you can hope your symptoms will change for the better. New research is in progress, and new medications are available. Surgery is less invasive and more effective. Don't give up hoping that remedies will improve — chances are they will.

✔ **Worrying that your condition will actually get worse.** Over time, the symptoms from endometriosis often improve — Stages III and IV of the disease tend to *burn out,* so pain decreases (see Chapter 9 for more on staging the disease). As a result, the odds are that your pain will diminish over time, not worsen. And few women have symptoms after menopause. This fact may not be much of a consolation if you're in your 20s, but if you're in that age range, you're bound to see many advances in the treatment of your endometriosis.

Looking for possible signs

Anxiety disorder is a condition characterized by extreme, chronic anxiety that disturbs mood, thought, behavior, and/or physiological activity. If you have anxiety disorder, you're anxious more often than not and find the anxiety difficult to control. You may also

✔ Feel restless, keyed up, or on edge

✔ Be easily fatigued

✔ Have difficulty concentrating

✔ Be irritable

✔ Have muscle tension

✔ Suffer from sleep disturbance (difficulty falling or staying asleep, or restless unsatisfying sleep)

If you have three or more of the preceding symptoms, with symptoms occurring more often than not over a six-month period, you may have an anxiety disorder. See your medical doctor to make sure there's no physical cause; he can refer you to a mental health specialist if necessary.

Treating Emotional Problems with Medication

Experts differ on treatment for depression and anxiety. Although some doctors feel a combination of therapy and medication is most helpful, others believe a trial of antidepressant medication may be adequate.

If you want to try medication without counseling first, your doctor may suggest one of the many antidepressants available. Most of these medications change the balance of the nerve chemicals in your brain. These chemical messengers, called *neurotransmitters,* are released by nerves and then taken up again by the nerves for reuse.

If you find medication alone isn't enough, many therapists, psychologists, and psychiatrists specialize in women's issues. But, if you want a more casual setting, support groups and online bulletin boards and chat rooms may be for you. (Check out "Expressing Your Frustration without Alienating Everyone You Know" later in this chapter.)

If you and your doctor agree that medication is the avenue for you to pursue, this section can help. It looks more closely at the different types of antidepressant medication available that can help you cope with depression and anxiety. (See Chapter 13 for medications that relieve the physical pain of endometriosis.)

Trying tricyclics

Tricyclic antidepressants (TCAs) have been around a long time. They increase the brain's supply of two neurotransmitters, serotonin and norepinephrine, which are abnormally low in people with depression. The following list contains some common TCAs (brand names are in parentheses):

- Amitriptyline hydrochloride (Elavil, Emitrip, Endep, Enovil)
- Amoxapine (Asendin)
- Clomipramine hydrochloride (Anafranil)
- Desipramine hydrochloride (Norpramine, Pertofrane)
- Doxepin hydrochloride (Adapin, Sinequan)
- Imipramine hydrochloride (Janimine, Tipramine, Tofranil)
- Pamelor (Nortiptyline)
- Protriptyline hydrochloride (Triptil, Vivactil)

Doctors usually prescribe TCAs at a low dose initially and slowly increase the dosage until you start to see results. Don't expect overnight results; the difference may not be noticeable for a few weeks.

One problem with TCAs is their effect on other neurotransmitters and brain cell transmitters, which can lead to unpleasant side effects. Some common side effects and the reasons they occur are

- **Blurred vision, constipation, dry mouth, rapid heartbeat, and difficulty emptying the bladder.** Amitriptyline, clomipramine, doxepin, imipramine, and protriptyline are likely to cause these side effects.

- **Dizziness and decreased blood pressure when you're standing.** This side effect is most common if you're taking amitriptyline and is least likely to occur if you're taking amoxapine or nortriptyline.

- **Drowsiness.** Doxepin, amitriptyline, and imipramine are three TCAs that often cause drowsiness.

- **Neuroleptic malignant syndrome.** Some patients taking clomipramine for long periods of time have a small risk of developing this syndrome, which can cause fever, fast or irregular heartbeat, sweating, loss of bladder control, and even seizures.

- **Sexual difficulties.** Many antidepressants cause loss of sexual desire. If this problem is significant for you, bupropion (Wellbutrin) may be an option for you. (See more on Wellbutrin in the section "Looking at the latest antidepressants" later in this chapter.)

- **Sun sensitivity.** TCAs can increase your sun sensitivity. Be sure to use a good sunblock and avoid tanning salons and sunlamps.

- **Weight gain.** Many TCAs cause weight gain. If this is a concern of yours, ask your doctor about switching to one of the newer antidepressants, such as Wellbutrin, Paxil, Prozac, Zoloft, Desyrel, or Effexor, which are less likely to cause weight gain.

If you have any of the following issues, make sure your doctor knows about them before you take TCAs because the drugs may cause complications or interactions in these cases:

- Alcohol abuse (TCAs may increase depressant effects of alcohol)

- Allergies (to TCAs, foods, preservatives, dyes)

- Asthma

- Blood disorders

- Contact lenses (drugs may cause dry eyes)

- Convulsions or seizures

- Glaucoma or increased eye pressure

- Heart disease

- High blood pressure

- Hyperthyroid

- Intestinal problems (TCAs may cause increased risk of serious side effects)

- Kidney disease

- Liver disease (may raise blood levels of TCAs, causing more side effects)

- Manic depression

- Schizophrenia (TCAs may worsen schizophrenia)

✔ Stomach problems (TCAs may cause increased risk of serious side effects)

✔ Urinary problems

If you have a history of heart problems, avoid taking TCAs.

Switching to SSRIs and other new antidepressants

Selective serotonin reuptake inhibitors (SSRIs) are a newer class of antidepressants. They're effective in approximately the same number of people who find relief from TCAs, but, because they react only with one neurotransmitter (serotonin), they have fewer side effects.

Well-known SSRIs that doctors frequently prescribe are escitalopram (Lexapro), citalopram (Celexa), fluoxetine (Prozac), paroxetine (Paxil), and sertraline (Zoloft).

Despite their popularity and fewer side effects, these antidepressants still have some side effects. Some of the more common effects include

✔ Diarrhea (especially with Zoloft)

✔ Dry mouth

✔ Headache

✔ Insomnia

✔ Nausea

✔ Nervousness (especially if you're taking Prozac; you also may not be able to sit still)

✔ Sexual problems

✔ Tiredness (especially if you're taking Paxil)

Looking at the latest antidepressants

The new antidepressants sound like alphabet soup, with names like SNRI (serotonin and noradrenaline reuptake inhibitors) and NRI (selective norepinephrine reuptake inhibitors). Most of these drugs differ from TCAs and SSRIs in side effects rather than in effectiveness.

✔ **Bupropion** (Wellbutrin) is chemically unrelated to TCAs or SSRIs. Bupropion's main side effects are agitation, constipation, dry mouth, headache, insomnia, nausea, and tremors.

- ✔ **Duloxetine hydrochloride** (Cymbalta) is an SNRI. Nausea, dry mouth, constipation, loss of appetite, fatigue, drowsiness, dizziness, increased sweating, blurred vision, rash, and itching are common side effects.

- ✔ **Nefazodone** (Serzone) is chemically unrelated to TCAs or SSRIs. Nefazodone is chemically similar to trazodone (Desyrel), another antidepressant. The most common side effects are agitation, blurred vision, confusion, constipation, dizziness, insomnia, nausea, and tiredness.

- ✔ **Venlafaxine** (Effexor) is a potent SNRI and a weak inhibitor of dopamine reuptake. Venlafaxine can cause similar side effects to other antidepressants. Like most antidepressants, it can cause nausea, headaches, anxiety, insomnia, drowsiness, and loss of appetite. Increased blood pressure can occur, so blood pressure should be monitored. Seizures have occurred.

Avoiding serotonin syndrome

Whenever you switch from one antidepressant to another, you need to allow a washout period so the drugs don't overlap in your system. Failure to do so can cause *serotonin syndrome,* a condition that results from overstimulation of serotonin receptors. Taking antidepressants with certain prescribed medications, over-the-counter herbal meds, and some recreational drugs can also cause this syndrome (check with your doctor or pharmacist for a list of these possible drugs).

Stopping antidepressants

If you've been on antidepressants for some time and you plan to stop taking them, you first need to consult with your doctor. Weaning down your dose gradually is better than going cold turkey. Stopping antidepressants abruptly can cause symptoms such as

- ✔ Agitation
- ✔ Anxiety
- ✔ Blurred vision
- ✔ Dizziness
- ✔ Electric shock sensations
- ✔ Fatigue
- ✔ Hallucinations
- ✔ Insomnia
- ✔ Irritability
- ✔ Myalgia (generalized muscle pain)

- Nausea
- Sweating
- Tingling sensations
- Vivid dreams

Your doctor can slowly decrease your dose while watching for signs that depression is coming back. Your family or friends may notice a change for the worse before you do, so be sure to listen if they voice concerns that you're becoming depressed again, and follow up with your doctor immediately.

Expressing Your Frustration without Alienating Everyone You Know

You probably know when your audience isn't paying attention. They start to twitch, look away, shift from foot to foot, and demonstrate a host of other verbal and physical clues that say, "I'm tired of hearing about this." Of course, their actions may just make you want to shout back, "I'm tired of living this too! Listen to me!" But that approach isn't likely to get you anywhere. Sometimes you need to look elsewhere to express how you feel, especially if the people close to you just can't hear you.

This section looks at who you can turn to for help, including friends and family, support groups, and even a professional therapist.

Finding friends who understand

When all is said and done, the people you want to be around you are your family and friends. They really do want to help, but sometimes they don't know how to go about it. How can you help them help you? Here are some suggestions:

- **Have them read Chapter 17, which is for family and friends.** In fact, you may want to read it too!

- **Don't expect Mr. Macho Man to turn into Mr. Sensitivity overnight.** Your partner cares deeply, but guys generally aren't as good as women at giving sympathy. Or he may show sensitivity once or twice and feel like that's enough. Guys can be educated, but it takes time.

- **Try not to make endometriosis the topic of every conversation.** Ask how other people are feeling sometimes. In fact, don't let endometriosis become the center of your world. Life is short — don't waste it.

✔ **Don't let your feelings get hurt too easily.** Accept that friends have other thoughts on their minds, so they may forget to ask about your most recent surgery, or they may forget that you don't feel like going out right now. The oversights don't mean these folks don't care — they just forget at times.

✔ **Thank your friends and family for what they do for you.** Everyone likes to be appreciated!

However, sometimes your friends and family can't be your support system. Because endometriosis is invisible, some people may have an "out of sight, out of mind" mentality, no matter how hard you try to convey what you're feeling. Sometimes people get tired of hearing about the problem, especially when they can't fix it.

Even if they're your nearest and dearest family and friends, your situation doesn't affect them in the same way it affects you. Yes, they're upset for you. Yes, they feel bad, and they do care what you're feeling. But sometimes they have problems they want to talk about too. Remember, they also have stories to tell. And sometimes you need to listen to them and give them your shoulder to cry on.

Eventually, however, you may have to turn elsewhere — such as to support groups or to a professional therapist — for support (check out the next two sections).

Looking for support from groups

So where do you go when you know your family and friends don't want to hear the word *endometriosis* one more time? You go to people who not only know about endometriosis but also want to talk about it as much as you do!

Two of the most common types of support groups are traditional support groups that usually meet in your local hospital and online support networks, where you can find helpful people wanting to chat at almost all hours of the day and night.

Traditional support groups

Nearly every large city has support groups for women with endometriosis; your weekend paper often lists the meeting times and locations. Or you can call your local hospitals to find out if they sponsor support groups. The drawback to support groups is their limited meeting schedule (usually only once a month), but you can make friends there that you can talk with more frequently. If you're not comfortable talking about your disease face to face in a social setting, check out the next section, which may be just what you're looking for.

Online support networks

Have you ever wondered how on earth people can spend hours with a bunch of strangers in a chat room? Just like people come in all shapes and sizes, so do their reasons for talking online with other women they'll probably never meet. When the common enemy is endometriosis, two important reasons to talk online are

- ✔ **Anonymity:** Online bulletin boards and chat rooms are anonymous. You can talk about your symptoms, feelings, treatments, relationships, successes, and failures without fear of being recognized, patronized, or ostracized.

- ✔ **Empathy:** The people who frequent the boards are, for the most part, women dealing with the same problems and frustrations of endometriosis that you are. You can pour your heart out and someone is sure to understand.

Need some encouragement to jump in? You can find bulletin boards and chat rooms at `www.google.com` or any search engine. When you type *endometriosis bulletin board* or *endometriosis chat room* on the search line, you get more than 100,000 hits! (See Appendix B for a list of some good Web sites that have informative forums.)

Whichever board you finally settle on, here are a few common-sense guidelines:

- ✔ **Maintain some anonymity.** Use made-up names when you chat, including your significant other's name your kids' names. You don't know who's reading, and you want to be able to say your peace without your next-door neighbor reading it — and knowing who you are!

- ✔ **Start slow.** Take time to get the feel of a bulletin board group; by listening to the give and take on a board, you can decide if you really want to *bare all* there.

- ✔ **Never meet a bulletin board friend for the first time at your home.** Some people seem saner online than in person, and you may regret the day you told someone where you lived! Meet in a public place.

- ✔ **Balance questions with support.** Every bulletin board has people who continually ask for advice and support but never share their own wisdom or show their concern for other members.

- ✔ **Remember — Meaning is often lost online.** In conversation, you can hear inflections and see facial expressions that help communicate a speaker's meaning. But these advantages are lost online, so readers need to give writers the benefit of the doubt. If a remark sounds out of place, maybe it was intended as humor, or maybe it was a typo!

  When you're the writer, use the common abbreviations (for example, *LOL* for *laughing out loud*) to make your meaning clearer.

Each online bulletin board is a bit different

As you search through the bulletin board results from your search engine, you notice that each bulletin board is a little different. Keep the following in mind when selecting an online support group. Some basic formats are

✔ **Very tight:** Moderators keep a close watch, deleting problematic postings and banning posters who get out of line with personal remarks.

✔ **Very loose:** Just like the Wild West, anything goes, and it's every woman for herself!

✔ **Very sponsored:** Drug companies and doctors who specialize in infertility or other endometriosis-related issues frequently maintain their own boards.

✔ **Remember — You have a life!** Bulletin boards and chat rooms are addictive. Ask any teenager! But anyone, adults included, can get hooked and spend hours online. Limit your time, or you may end up needing a support group for Internet addictions!

Turning to a therapist

Finding a therapist isn't easy. Therapists can be medical doctors (psychiatrists), psychologists, social workers, or certified counselors. Therapists have different philosophies and methods; a therapy technique that works well for your friend may be a total bust for you.

Your doctor may suggest a certain therapist, and that's a good place to start. But don't feel that you have to stay with someone whose approach isn't helping you. Feel free to try someone else if you don't feel your therapist is right for you. Make sure that you give it a few months first, though; therapy doesn't work immediately. Follow our guidelines in Chapter 8 to find a therapist that you not only can trust, but one that will help you get back to normal.

Chapter 16

Changing Your Lifestyle When You Have Endometriosis

....

In This Chapter

▶ Living well despite endometriosis

▶ Making changes in your work life

▶ Lowering the stress in your life

▶ Taking in the good, leaving out the bad

▶ Getting up and exercising

▶ Detoxing your world

▶ Adding some spice to your sex life

....

*I*n a perfect world, you wouldn't have the inconvenience of endometriosis — but in the real world, you do. However, having endometriosis doesn't have to mean the end of life for you. For the most part, you don't really want to change your life completely. Maybe you're fairly happy with it the way it is. And if you aren't completely happy with your life, you may feel too overwhelmed to make any significant changes.

However, change can be good, even if you're happy with your life the way it is. And if you're too busy or don't know where to start making some lifestyle changes, don't worry. This chapter can help you analyze your lifestyle a bit more closely.

Finding the right job, decreasing your stress, and improving your sex life may not make you forget your endometriosis, but they can add to your life in a way you didn't think was possible. Even little choices like eating right and exercising regularly can change your outlook on life (and even help reduce the pain). In this chapter, we're your cheerleaders, encouraging you to make some positive changes that can help decrease the hold endometriosis has on your life.

Focusing on Life beyond Endometriosis

What's the first step to improving your life when you have a chronic disease? Change your focus. Stop putting endometriosis in the center stage of your life. Everything doesn't have to be about endometriosis, even if you're in pain, even if you never know how you're going to feel from day to day.

Just by changing your perspective on life, you can make significant changes (and maybe start to feel a bit better). This section shows you how staying positive and adjusting your schedule to allow for good and bad days is a good start.

Keeping a positive attitude

As with any chronic disease process, a positive attitude can't cure endometriosis, but it can make the disease much more tolerable for you and your family and friends. Staying positive may be an easy concept, but when you have to walk the walk (not just talk the talk), the concept isn't that easy. However, you can express a positive attitude simply through an optimistic rather than pessimistic attitude toward life.

We're not the only people in the world to say that a positive attitude can overcome a lot of ills. Consider these studies and their conclusions:

- A Dutch study of more than 900 people found that people who described themselves as being highly optimistic had a 23 percent lower risk of cardiovascular death and had a 55 percent lower risk of all causes of death than people who said they were highly pessimistic.

- A study in the journal *Proceedings of the National Academy of Sciences* links *negative* brain activity with a weakened immune system — and we're discovering that endometriosis may be linked with immune issues.

- A study summarizing more than 30 years of data by the Mayo Clinic reports that people who expect misfortune and who only see the darker side of life don't live as long as people with a more optimistic view.

Dozens of studies similar to these all seem to agree: Optimistic, positive people live longer than negative, pessimistic people.

This news is great if you're already a positive person. But what if you're not? With some work, you can improve your outlook. For example, you can:

- **Quiet your *inner critic*, the little voice that whispers "You can't do it" or "You'll never get all this done."** Teach yourself instead to concentrate on the "I can" messages. You can't do it overnight; it takes time to change your mindset, but you can do it.

✔ **Put everything in perspective.** Ask yourself, "Will this matter in 20 years? Will it even matter next week?" You can easily get discouraged by little events that have no consequence in your overall life, like being cut off by another driver. Put everything in the big picture, and you'll see how unimportant life's little annoyances really are.

✔ **So what about the big stuff?** Everyone has painful traumas in life. Even in the worst of situations, you can make choices. Focus on what you *can* do in difficult situations, not on what you can't change.

✔ **Make positive changes in your life.** Having goals and meeting them give you a sense of control in your life, and when you have a chronic illness like endometriosis, you need to know your life is ultimately still in your own hands. You may always have pain, but you can do things to decrease the pain. You may miss some time at work — but you may miss less this year than last. You may not be able to work at your dream job — but you can work at something you like almost as much. You always have room for improvement, if you're willing to take steps toward it.

This chapter can change your life if you put the principles into practice — just reading them isn't enough! And yes, we know it's not easy. But the results, we promise, are worth the effort.

Scheduling around good and bad days

Keeping a positive outlook isn't always easy because some days with endometriosis are hellish. But some days are also better than others. When you have endometriosis, do some preplanning so endometriosis doesn't ruin every single day.

The good news is that, with endometriosis, you can sometimes project which days are problem days. For example, if you're planning a once-in-a-lifetime visit to Hawaii, don't plan it when you expect your period. Or plan ahead and take medication (birth control pills or progestins) to control your symptoms or hold off your period during your trip. The result? No period cramps and pain and no mess from period bleeding. Two bonuses in one!

Women have scheduled their periods for years for major occasions like weddings, but many women need to think of scheduling their real lives in the same way. Most people have some control over vacation schedules and even the date to have the whole family over to dinner.

Naturally, we don't have this kind of control over attending someone else's wedding or going to school. Birth control pills or progestins (even as long-term injections) can be your best friend in these situations. You can take birth control pills for longer periods of time if you need to get through a special occasion without pain and bleeding. And, of course, birth control pills can help reduce pain and bleeding even when they do occur. (See Chapter 10 for more on how taking birth control pills can benefit endometriosis.)

Coping with Work When You Don't Feel Good

Like it or not, work is a big part of your life (unless you won the lottery and are sitting around eating bonbons all day, which is another issue all in itself). But work brings certain expectations. Bosses expect you to be at work when *they* want you there, and even the most sympathetic bosses need to limit call ins and sick time. Besides, you can't use sick days for predictable monthly aches and pains when you may need those days for another illness or even surgery.

This section helps you analyze what type of job is appropriate for you, discusses whether you need to share your medical history with your prospective boss, and helps you better manage your sick time.

Finding the right job for you

Find a job that has a flexible schedule. However, landing a flexible job is easier said than done. And how many jobs are really flexible? Even traditionally flexible jobs, such as per diem nursing or substitute teaching, aren't totally flexible because you work when *they* need you, not when *you* want to.

Considering different options

A job where you can work when you're well and stay home when you're not is difficult to find. But some jobs may work better for you than others. Obviously, the more flexible a job, the better it is for you. When looking for a job, consider these questions:

- ✔ **Can you switch days with other employees?** Having a co-worker who's willing to trade days can be a big bonus.

- ✔ **Can you work from home?** With computer access, many jobs allow work from home a few days a month. Can you work at home while lying on the couch with a heating pad on days when you're not feeling well?

- ✔ **Can you work per diem, coming in only on days when you feel well?** For example, many hospitals have per diem positions for nurses.

Many jobs come with stress levels through the roof. In fact, some professions promote their long hours and high stress levels as a badge of honor! Women seeking these high-powered careers often work long, hard hours and put off having children, perpetuating the myth that career women are the only ones with endometriosis. Although the myth is hot air (see Chapter 18 for more discussion on this stereotype), stress may be related to endometriosis, and these types of careers can pile it on. (Check out "De-stressing Your Life: More Than Just Breathing in Slowly" later in this chapter for more info.)

Making career sacrifices or not?

If your endometriosis is killing you, your job may be part of the problem. What good is a great career if your life is in shambles? You don't have to give up your stressful job, but you may need to make some concessions.

Look for a way to stay in your chosen field but decrease the stress. This change may mean that you don't make partner or that you don't make the salary you want, so the 80-hour week can be tough to leave (especially if you're a driven person). But your health may depend on it.

Being honest with your potential boss?

Is it better to tell a potential boss that you have a chronic disease, or is it wiser to keep quiet? Several schools of thought exist about disclosing an invisible illness when you're applying for a new job. You certainly won't be the only one having this inner debate; as many as 40 percent of American workers have a chronic illness, and employees justifiably worry about increased health costs and decreased productivity for this 40 percent.

If endometriosis is just an inconvenience in your life (accounting for no more than a few days a year of down time), you probably see no reason to discuss it with a future employer. However, if endometriosis is a major pain for a major part of your life, you may consider bringing it up. You should base part of your decision on how much endometriosis incapacitates you. For example:

- ✔ Do you curl up in a ball on the bed for two or three days every month?
- ✔ Can you keep symptoms under control enough to go to work?
- ✔ Is surgery in your future?
- ✔ Are you thinking of starting a family and do you suspect that you'll need time-consuming, high-tech treatments, such as in vitro fertilization?

Advantages of telling your future boss

The pros for disclosure to your future boss are as follows:

- ✔ Your boss will know why you're out instead of having to guess what your excuses mean.
- ✔ You can tell the truth about your absences.
- ✔ Disclosing a disability or illness to an employer from the beginning may protect your employment under equality legislation.

Knowing your rights under the Employment Equality Act

The Employment Equality Act of 1998, Section 2, outlaws discrimination by employers and employment agencies based on several categories, including chronic illness such as endometriosis. So if you have endometriosis and think that your employer may have fired you because of your disease, you may need to *pull rank* by quoting the Employment Equality Act of 1998, Section 2. We hope you never need to, but it's nice to know your rights. This act defines disability as:

✔ The total or partial absence of a person's bodily functions, including the absence of a part of a person's body

✔ The presence in the body of organisms causing, or likely to cause, chronic illness or illness

✔ The malfunction, malformation, or disfigurement of a part of a person's body

✔ A condition or malfunction that results in a person learning differently from persons without the condition or malfunction

✔ A condition, illness, or disease that results in a disturbance in a person's thought processes, perception of reality, emotions, or judgment

✔ A condition that exists at present, or which previously existed but no longer exists, or which may exist in the future, or which is imputed to a person

Does endometriosis fit these criteria? Yes, under several categories. Is there a catch? Of course. You can be fired for other reasons — a chronic illness doesn't guarantee you a job. However, your place of employment must make an effort to accommodate your disabilities within reason, and, if possible, retrain you if you can't do your current job. Obviously, a mom and pop operation can't provide retraining if it only offers one type of job.

Disadvantages of telling your future boss

The cons for discussing a chronic disease before you're hired are

✔ The employer may not hire you if she suspects you'll miss a lot of work. Although the Equal Opportunity laws say employers can't discriminate because of a disability, the laws don't say you *have* to be hired. Someone else may get the job just because she seems like a *better fit* — and that can mean anything the employer wants it to!

✔ If your superiors think your health may compromise a job, you may face a subtle bias when promotions and assignments come around.

Being aware of your sick time

When you have endometriosis, you may want to call in sick during your down days, right when your period is in full throttle. However, most businesses only allot you X number of sick days a year. How can you manage those eight to ten days so that you don't end up using them all before March?

Although "How much sick time do I get?" can't be the first question out of your mouth during a job interview, you do need to know not only how much time you get, but also how you can use it. For example:

✔ Can you take half a day at a time?

✔ Do you have a waiting period before you can start using sick time?

✔ What happens when you run out of sick time?

✔ Does your time off come out of your vacation time or can you take a day off without pay?

✔ If you're on salary, what is a normal number of sick days and what does the employer consider excessive?

Obviously, the more flexible your sick time, the better off you are. Some workplaces dock vacation time if you take off sick right before or after vacation, even though you're legitimately ill. Find out what the procedure is for sick time. Do you have to call in by a certain time or bring in a doctor's note if you're out more than a day or two? Knowing the rules in advance can help you maximize your sick time.

De-stressing Your Life: More Than Just Breathing in Slowly

If you have a chronic disease, such as endometriosis, de-stressing your life can make a significant difference. Stress can weaken your immune system, and worsen symptoms of endometriosis.

You can rely on yourself to de-stress, or you can seek outside help to avoid internalizing your stress. Studies have shown that people who keep stress inside have more physical and emotional problems than people who vent. This externalization can improve your immune system function and help you psychologically.

Consider the following people when you need to de-stress your life:

✔ **Yourself:** Yes, you can de-stress your life, but you need to teach yourself not to sweat the small stuff (and even some of the big stuff).

Try the following tips to de-stress your life:

- Keep a diary. (See Chapter 2 for more info.)
- Take a long walk while listening to a relaxing CD on headphones.
- Get a massage. (See Chapter 12 for additional treatment options.)

✔ **Friends and family:** You can ask your closest loved ones to help you get through the tough times. Be honest with them about your problem and how you feel at those times. These people can then try to help de-stress your life. If they know when the bad times are and what you go though, they can support you and not add to your stress level. (For more suggestions, see Chapter 17, which is directed to these important folks.)

The same advice is good for your friends and extended family. Again, be upfront with them. You have nothing to hide, you didn't want to have endometriosis, and they can help you avoid stress in you everyday life.

✔ **Co-workers or your boss:** The workplace is another area where you can reduce stress. Don't hide you problem. Let your boss and co-workers know about your bad days — maybe they can help you cope with the stress of work so you don't have to take a day off. (Check out "Coping with Work When You Don't Feel Good" earlier in this chapter for more work-related info.)

✔ **Professional therapist:** If you feel you can't de-stress on your own, professional help is available. Psychologists are trained to help you deal with the stress of endometriosis and make your life more comfortable. Working with a therapist doesn't mean you're crazy, and she can help you avoid driving other people crazy when you're going through a bad time with your disease.

✔ **Spiritual support:** If you have a priest, rabbi, or other spiritual support, seek guidance. He or she may be able to help you deal with the stress of everyday life, marriage, kids, and work, and may help you soothe your stress spiritually.

Changing Your Bad Habits

Everyone has a bad habit or two — behaviors you probably know aren't good for you, like eating the wrong foods, smoking, or overindulging in alcohol. Although the occasional indulgence probably won't hurt you, regular doses of things that aren't good for you can harm your health. When you have a chronic disease like endometriosis, anything that harms your health can worsen your symptoms.

No matter what your bad habit is, this section can help. We provide plenty of information to help you change your eating habits. We also look at your drinking and smoking habits and explain how cutting back can make a difference even if you can't completely stop.

Eating well really can change your life

Everyone has to eat, but, unfortunately, most people don't eat very well. Many people just don't eat the food they should, even though they want to and even try to. And when you have endometriosis, eating well is extra important.

Eating well really does make a difference in how you feel. It can help keep your weight normal, keep your energy levels high, and prevent heart disease and other long-term illness. Many theories on how to eat when you have endometriosis are out there too. Some plans probably work better for some people than others. In general, eating more fresh food rather than processed, and keeping your saturated fats low and your veggie and fruit intake high works for just about everybody.

So are you ready to start eating better (and feeling better)? This section looks more closely at different steps you can take to improve your diet and break the bad habits of eating unhealthy food.

Do certain foods worsen endometriosis?

Many nutritionists and holistic medical practitioners claim to know what foods are best if you have endometriosis, and most of their recommendations are similar. Almost all of these diets stress the following:

- **Eat less dairy.** Dairy products contain saturated fat, which increases the circulation of estrogen and produces *prostaglandin F2-alpha,* a fatty acid that can increase the inflammation and cramping from endometriosis.

- **Eat less meat.** When you do eat meat, eat organic or free-range meat. Meat also contains saturated fat, and many animals were fed hormones to increase their weight.

- **Eat more veggies.** Make sure you wash fruit and vegetables thoroughly and buy organic when you can to avoid pesticides.

- **Drink less alcohol.** Alcohol is hard on your liver, and a stressed liver can't remove toxins and waste products from the body well. (Check out the section "Cutting back on the drinks" later in this chapter for more information on reducing your alcohol intake.)

- **Consume less caffeine.** Caffeine can make you jumpy and irritable; it also dehydrates you and depletes your vitamin B stores.

- **Eat more fiber.** Good sources of fiber include oatmeal, fruits and vegetables, brown rice, beans, and whole grains, excluding wheat.

- **Eat less wheat in any form.** Some doctors who specialize in endometriosis feel that sensitivity to wheat products is increasing, and that removing wheat from the diet can decrease pain for endometriosis.

- **Eat less soy and fewer soy products.** See the "What happened to the joy of soy?" sidebar in this chapter for more information.

What happened to the joy of soy?

Not too many years ago, soy was a near-miracle food. Now, many dieticians and naturopaths suggest you avoid soy. Why the turnaround?

The list of negative effects of soy has now outgrown the list of benefits. Among the reasons to avoid soy products, according to many health aficionados, are

✔ Phytic acid in soy may reduce absorption of calcium, copper, iron, magnesium, and zinc, all essential minerals.

✔ Phyoestrogens in soy may disrupt fertility and increase the risk of breast cancer.

✔ Phyoestrogens in soy disrupt thyroid function.

✔ Soy products contain high levels of aluminum, which is toxic to the kidneys and nervous system.

✔ Soy increases the need for vitamins B12 and D.

Have you been drinking soy and assuming you were health conscious? You may want to reconsider. Check with your doctor for her opinion.

✔ **Eat less refined sugar.** It really has no nutritional benefits, although we don't argue that it tastes good!

✔ **Eat more omega-3 fatty-acid-producing oils.** Good sources of omega-3 include walnut oil, flaxseed oil, evening primrose, and safflower oil.

✔ **Eat less saturated fat, butter, lard, and animal oils.** These fats may increase your chance of developing heart disease.

✔ **Eat foods that boost the immune system.** Healthful, immune-boosting foods include carrots, beans, lentils, onions, ginger, green tea, and rhubarb.

Can you wake up tomorrow and transform yourself into a total health freak? Probably not! In fact, introducing changes slowly, and one at a time, can keep you from feeling deprived and help you to pinpoint changes that really make a difference.

Taking supplemental vitamins and minerals

If you have endometriosis, should you take extra vitamin and mineral supplements? Doing so can't hurt, and they may help — as long as you follow some general guidelines. And as always, discuss it with your physician before you start buying bottles off the health-food shelf. If you take several different supplements, you may be duplicating ingredients. And many vitamins (especially those that are fat soluble) and some minerals are toxic in large amounts. The following list of vitamins and minerals and their benefits may help you get started:

✔ **Vitamin A:** Boosts the immune system; an antioxidant; helps lessen profuse menstrual bleeding

✔ **Vitamin B complex:** Helps break down proteins, carbohydrates, and fats in the body; helps keep estrogen levels naturally low; helps produce good prostaglandins

✔ **Vitamin C:** Helps boost the immune system and fight off disease; antioxidant; helps control excessive bleeding; detoxifies pollutants

✔ **Vitamin D:** Helps retain calcium

✔ **Vitamin E:** Boosts the immune system; helps decrease pain from cramps

✔ **Beta carotene:** Converts to vitamin A in the body

✔ **Calcium:** Deficiency can cause cramping, headaches, and pelvic pain

✔ **Folic acid:** Necessary for making healthy red blood cells

✔ **Iron:** Prevents anemia, weakness, and fatigue due to heavy bleeding

✔ **Magnesium:** Decreases cramping; a muscle relaxant

✔ **Selenium:** Boosts immune system; decreases inflammation when taken with vitamin E

✔ **Zinc:** Boosts immune system

If you're not much of a pill popper, preferring to get your vitamins and minerals from food sources, the following list of foods containing vitamins and minerals can help you:

✔ **Vitamin A:** Apricots, broccoli, cantaloupe, carrots, eggs, milk, pumpkin, spinach, squash

✔ **Vitamin B:** Fortified cereals, beans, red meat, poultry, mollusks, liver

✔ **Vitamin C:** Berries, broccoli, cantaloupe, grapefruit, lemons, oranges, peppers, spinach, strawberries

✔ **Vitamin D:** Butter, cheese, eggs, salmon, tuna

✔ **Vitamin E:** Almonds, avocado, eggs, safflower oil, salmon, sunflower oil

✔ **Beta carotene:** Carrots, spinach, sweet potatoes, tomatoes, cantaloupe

✔ **Calcium:** Almonds, hard cheese, green beans, kelp, milk

✔ **Folic acid:** Asparagus, green leafy vegetables, organ meats

✔ **Iron:** Clams, fortified cereals, liver, oysters, lean red meat, dried beans

✔ **Magnesium:** Bananas, barley, green beans, kelp, sunflower seeds, raspberry leaves

✔ **Selenium:** Cabbage, celery, cucumbers

✔ **Zinc:** Ginger root, oysters, lamb chops, pecans

Prostaglandins: The good, the bad, and the painful

Prostaglandins are fatty acids that the body can manufacture or that you can consume in foods. Prostaglandins have useful functions that you can't live without. But women with endometriosis may produce too many prostaglandins, resulting in inflammation in tissues and painful cramping.

Prostaglandins have an interesting history. A Swedish scientist named Ulf Von Euler discovered them in human semen in the 1930s. He thought prostaglandins came from the prostate, hence their name. But prostaglandins are in just about every type of cell and act as chemical messengers inside the cell. They don't travel around the body.

A number of different prostaglandins, all with differing functions, are in the human body. Some prostaglandins activate immune responses and can cause fever and inflammation. Others help form blood clots in some places and prevent their formation in others. Certain prostaglandins can cause uterine cramping, diarrhea, fever, and pain. Scientists have identified around a dozen different types of prostaglandins.

Good and bad prostaglandins are also in foods. The bad ones are in foods such as dairy and meat. Good prostaglandins are made from fatty acids in some marine plants and fish. These are part of the omega-3 fatty acids. By avoiding the bad prostaglandins and increasing your intake of the good ones, you may help alleviate or lessen your symptoms.

Eating organic

People talk about eating *organic* foods, but what does organic really mean? Some people consider organic foods to be anything they buy from the local fruit and veggie stand. However, in order to be labeled *organic,* foods, including meat, need to meet the following strict criteria of the U.S. Department of Agriculture. The foods must be free from

- Conventional pesticides
- Petroleum-based fertilizers
- Irradiation
- Sewage sludge
- Antibiotics and growth hormones

Whether or not organic foods keep you healthier or decrease endometriosis is a matter of much debate. But if you want to eat as naturally as possible and avoid chemical exposure, organic foods are a good bet. (Check out the nearby sidebar, "Locating organic food" in this chapter.)

Locating organic food

Are you interested in eating more organic food but just don't know where to look? Check out www.localharvest.org on the Internet; by keying in your zip code, you can find places near you that produce organic products. Or you can have organic foods delivered right to your door by going to www.diamondorganics. com. They even have organic takeout!

These are just two of several online sites for organic produce. You can even grow your own organic produce from organic seeds! You pay more for organically produced food, but if you're convinced chemicals are making you sick, your money is well spent.

Cutting back on the drinks

Outside of the obvious risks of overindulging in alcohol, such as liver damage, accidental injury, and making a fool out of yourself at the office holiday party, alcohol may also be harmful if you have endometriosis.

Alcohol may increase estrogen levels, which can worsen endometriosis symptoms and encourage growth of endometrial implants. Will an occasional glass of wine be harmful? Probably not — but monitor your own response. Does drinking alcohol increase your pelvic pain or cause intestinal problems? You may want to avoid alcohol altogether if it aggravates your symptoms.

Snuffing out the smokes

Smoking is a serious and dangerous addiction. Around 48 million Americans smoke, and around 400,000 die each year from causes related to smoking. No direct proof links smoking to causing or worsening endometriosis, although many scientists suspect that it may. Smoking has been associated with changes in the immune system, which is significant because endometriosis is more and more considered to have an autoimmune component. What is known is that smoking decreases fertility, and because many endometriosis patients are also infertility patients, it's certainly in your best interest to quit smoking altogether, or at least cut down.

Exercising for Health and Other Benefits

You probably know you should exercise, but exercise is easy to put off until tomorrow. After all, getting up early to go to the gym or going after work (when all you want to do is collapse on the couch in front of the television) is hard work.

Many people are often too tired to exercise, but the irony is that daily exercise can energize and rejuvenate you. Don't believe it? Many studies show that exercise has benefits beyond the physical. This section looks at how exercise can help you feel better, even when your endometriosis symptoms are acting up.

Understanding the benefits of movement

Do you often find yourself saying, "I'd exercise if I thought it would really accomplish anything."? Or are you just so busy that you don't have even 20 to 30 minutes a day, three times a week to devote to exercising? Well, to prove to you that exercise is good for you, consider the following facts:

- ✔ Women who have exercised more than two hours a week from an early age are less likely to develop endometriosis.

- ✔ Exercise decreases estrogen levels, which may slow the growth of endometriosis. Exercise also increases the body's production of *endorphins,* natural pain-blocking substances.

- ✔ Exercise doesn't have to be strenuous to have benefits. Yoga, swimming, and walking all help release endorphins.

- ✔ Exercise reduces stress and tension and helps you sleep better.

- ✔ Exercise helps keep your bones strong.

You don't need to spend a fortune on equipment and devote hours a day to exercise. Taking even a few small steps toward regular exercise, like a short daily walk, will encourage you to do more as time goes by.

Taking the first step

Jumping head first into an exercise program like some people do isn't a good idea. You know the drill — they decide they should start exercising more, so they rent ten different exercise videos, buy six new color-coordinated exercise outfits and two new pairs of shoes, buy a pedometer and a pulse monitor, pick up a few dumbbells (color-coordinated to match their outfits), buy a treadmill and three new exercise magazines, and then . . . collapse on the couch for a week.

Or a woman may actually start a new exercise program by hitting the gym in the morning, the track at lunch, and the treadmill in the evening for a week. But the next week, she needs to see a chiropractor for her back, a podiatrist for her swollen feet, and an orthopedist for her brand-new stress fracture — not to mention a marriage counselor for driving her spouse crazy by exercising at 5 a.m. each morning and a human resource counselor to find a new job because she's been falling asleep on the job all week.

Exercise is good, but make sure you start slowly. Why? Here are just a few of the reasons:

- ✔ You're less likely to hurt yourself.
- ✔ You're more likely to remain enthusiastic if you don't burn out in the first week.
- ✔ Your muscles need time to get into condition.

However, before you begin any exercise program, talk to your doctor. She can advise you about your exercise plans.

If you're not sure where to start, don't worry. Exercise doesn't have to be complicated; you can start a walking program, exercise to videos, or use a treadmill at home for next to nothing. You don't need to join a gym to get in shape — if you're motivated enough to design and continue your own exercise regimen at home. If you feel you need the extra push (and you know if you do), joining a gym may be your best bet. You may consider one step further: Hire a personal trainer for at least a few sessions. That extra commitment can make exercising a habit and can ensure that you don't jump in over your head just to land on the couch!

Finding Chemically Safe Products

Will cutting down on chemical exposure help control endometriosis? The jury is still way out on whether chemical exposure causes autoimmune diseases like endometriosis. But reducing contact with some chemicals certainly can't hurt. (See Chapter 4 for more on chemical exposure and endometriosis.)

Many of the foods you eat are contaminated with environmental chemicals. Compounds migrate from the items to which they were added and build up in the fat tissue of animals that everyone eats, and eventually end up in people. Although levels of some dangerous environmental chemicals have actually dropped over the last few decades, such as bath and paper products, for example, other chemical levels have risen.

Avoiding chemicals today isn't as hard as 30 years ago, when people didn't know the contents of many products. Every product these days has a label, and — if your eyesight is good enough — you can read it before you decide to buy. These are just a few items you can buy chemical-free:

- ✔ Bath products
- ✔ Bedding
- ✔ Cleaning products
- ✔ Clothing

✔ Paper products

✔ Sanitary products

Although you don't need to buy a gas mask and suit up in chemical gear yet (unless you're a member of Homeland Security), you can take the following steps to reduce your exposure to harmful chemicals in the air, in your food, and on the ground:

✔ Wash fruits and vegetables before eating.

✔ Wash meat, chicken, and fish before eating.

✔ Skin and trim fat from fish because some contaminants congregate there.

✔ Open the windows instead of using artificial air fresheners (unless you live in a polluted area).

✔ Avoid using chemicals on your lawn — are a few dandelions all that bad?

✔ Swat bugs instead of spraying them.

✔ Use natural cleaning products.

✔ Try chemical-free detergent instead of using dryer sheets.

✔ Use nonperfumed toilet paper, paper towels, and other paper products.

✔ Hire a professional instead of trying to remove lead-based paint.

✔ Stain or seal-pressure treated wood, such as decks or walkways, to avoid the chemicals they contain.

✔ Avoid burning trash, even if it's legal in your area.

To buy environmentally friendly, chemical-free household goods and clothing, try the following sources:

✔ www.seventhgeneration.com

✔ www.ecomall.com

Adjusting Your Sex Life

If you have endometriosis, you probably think your sex life needs some adjusting. (Actually, most people feel this way!) Unfortunately, endometriosis can wreak havoc on your sex life by causing pain at a time that should be most pleasurable.

Studies have shown that more than 50 percent of women with endometriosis have pain with intercourse for most of their lives. In addition, women with endometriosis

✔ Have intercourse less often

✔ Have less satisfying orgasms

✔ Feel less relaxed during intercourse

✔ Frequently have to stop in the middle of sex due to pain

However, even if you have *dyspareunia* (pain during sex), you can keep sex in the pleasure, rather than in the pain, category with modifications that are easy to pick up and fun to practice!

We want to give you hope that your sex life can be enjoyable and not so painful. This section gives tips to help you communicate with your partner, looks at how you can enjoy sex more, and offers suggestions for ways to spice things up with new positions. Ooh-la-la! Have fun!

Being upfront with your partner

If you have painful sex as a result of endometriosis, be honest and upfront with your partner. Your partner may think the worst if you don't explain the real reason sex doesn't excite you. Your partner may think that you don't have affectionate feelings toward him or her. Or your partner may believe that you want to be with someone else. And if sex involves pain for you, your partner is likely to feel guilty for causing you pain, thinking he or she is doing something wrong.

Guilt and lack of communication can kill any relationship, so being upfront about endometriosis and its effect on your sex life is paramount. Take your partner with you to the doctor's office if necessary, so you both know what's going on and can get some ideas on how to overcome pain during sex.

Explain to your partner where and when you feel pain. With your partner, find a position or other form of lovemaking that's comfortable for both of you. Maybe all you need is to avoid certain days. When you communicate this to your partner, you lessen misinterpretations about your lack of interest at those certain times.

Getting the most out of sex

Do you have endometriosis and want to improve your sex life? Remember the following:

✔ **Figure out what times of the month are least painful for you.** For some women with endometriosis, ovulation time is least painful. Find what's best for you.

✔ **Take some pain medication before getting started.** But go easy on drugs that make you drowsy!

✔ **Use lots of lubricant.** Water-based or silicone-based lubricants can help decrease dryness and painful entry. Many drugs for endometriosis dry up vaginal secretions.

Trying different positions

When you have endometriosis, just mixing up your sex life and trying different positions can help ease the pain. Deep penetration is most likely to cause pain when you have endometriosis, so try new angles — they may make the difference between pleasure and pain. You may feel much more comfortable if you try:

✔ Being on top

✔ Lying side by side

✔ Any position that makes you happy

✔ Oral sex (giving and receiving)

✔ Hanging from the rafters (okay, maybe not quite so drastic)

These simple changes and any others that make you more comfortable can help, if not save, your sex life. Be sure to discuss these ideas with your partner so he or she understands why you're suddenly kinkier at certain times of the month. Knowing why you're changing the routine can make your partner feel better and just may inspire him or her to find ways to help you feel better too.

Chapter 17

Just for Friends and Family: Help and Support

*H*aving a chronic illness isn't fun. No one can argue that. But it's no fun sometimes to be the significant other of someone who has a chronic disease, such as endometriosis. Living with endometriosis day to day can be stressful, not only for the patient, but also for her family and friends. If you're a significant other, a parent, a friend, or a family member, you may feel even more helpless because you can't take the burden from your loved one or truly understand how she feels.

In this chapter, we discuss the frustrations of living with — and loving — someone who has endometriosis, and discuss ways to make the situation a bit better — for both of you. We cover topics from helping without hindering to improving your sex life. We look at how you can be supportive concerning difficult infertility issues, and we provide information for parents who may have an adult daughter dealing with endometriosis. Finally, we don't forget what support you need. For everyone who cares for someone with endometriosis, this chapter is for you!

Living with Endometriosis — Secondhand

Sometimes watching someone you care about suffer is just as difficult as feeling the pain yourself. If someone you care about has endometriosis, you probably have days where you want to wave a wand and fix all the problems. You can't wave a wand, but you can do the next best thing. You can be supportive when she really needs it, when she questions her own feelings, and when she feels bad about letting you down.

This section tells you how you can be part of the solution without going down with the ship yourself. We help you understand your loved one's pain, provide tips on how you can help without being a nuisance, suggest ways to keep your sex life on fire, and take a close look at financial issues.

Understanding how endometriosis affects her

It's hard to be on the same page with someone whose symptoms are always changing. Picture this: Your partner comes into the kitchen, kicks the cat out of the way, pours herself a cup of coffee, and chugs it in one gulp. You assume that she's having a bad day, so, trying to be empathetic, you say, "Poor baby, are you having cramps again?"

She picks up the nearest newspaper and heaves it at your head. "I don't have cramps at this time of the month," she hisses. "My stomach is killing me!"

Well, how are you supposed to know? You thought endometriosis was mostly about cramps. Don't be embarrassed; many people think that's the only problem. By reading this chapter, you're off to the right start to understand better what your loved one is experiencing. Maybe you're reading it under duress, with your partner glaring at you from across the table. She may even have you chained to a chair. That's okay. We promise you'll be glad you read this chapter (and even the book) in the end.

For starters, you need to know that endometriosis can affect a legion of body functions. For example, endometriosis can cause a number of symptoms. (We start with the most common ones.)

- ✔ Uterine cramps
- ✔ Pelvic pain
- ✔ Pain during sex
- ✔ Pain during orgasm
- ✔ Irregular bleeding
- ✔ Lower back pain
- ✔ Fatigue
- ✔ Infertility
- ✔ Diarrhea and/or constipation
- ✔ Nausea and/or vomiting
- ✔ Painful bowel movements at certain times
- ✔ Intestinal discomfort
- ✔ Bloating
- ✔ Bladder pain or urinary frequency
- ✔ Yeast infections (vaginal and other)
- ✔ Muscle pain (fibromyalgia)
- ✔ Chest pain
- ✔ Asthma
- ✔ Coughing up blood
- ✔ Collapsed lung (rare, but possible)
- ✔ Blood in the lungs (also rare)
- ✔ Allergies and eczema flare-ups
- ✔ Low blood sugar
- ✔ Depression
- ✔ Lack of energy
- ✔ Headache
- ✔ Seizures
- ✔ Leg pain (from endometriosis near the sciatic nerve)

As you can see, endometriosis can definitely be more than "just cramps!" To understand more about how endometriosis can cause pain, check out Chapter 2 for a more in-depth discussion on symptoms.

Helping without being a pain

You don't have endometriosis, but you care about someone who does. You want to help, but some days you feel like you're only irritating your partner. She pushes you away when you offer her a back rub. In fact, she may push you away all together! How do you handle living with a chronic illness that isn't yours?

Being able to empathize with your partner can help. But you may be wondering how to empathize. In truth, the ability to empathize is a rare gift. To empathize is to say, "I don't know what you're going through, but I'm here for you" *without* falling into the "You poor thing" or "I know what you're going through" trap.

When women with endometriosis were asked what they wanted most from family and friends, the answer was *support*. But support is hard to define. The following list includes some suggestions for supporting your loved one:

- **Listen to her (primary to any relationship!).** Listening means more than saying "Uh huh" occasionally; it means really hearing what she's saying — and sometimes reading between the lines to hear what she's afraid to say out loud. Listening takes practice.

- **Believe her when she says she's hurting.** People who live with a lot of pain often become good at hiding it, so don't assume that she's not really in pain because she's not writhing on the floor; she may be writhing on the inside.

- **Be patient with her.** It can be annoying to have plans turned upside down at the last minute by flare-ups, but she doesn't enjoy having life topsy-turvy any more than you do.

- **Learn about the disease yourself.** Understanding what she's feeling is the first step to real empathy.

- **Don't blame her for her symptoms.** No one chooses to have endometriosis, and she feels bad enough about missing events, staying home from work, or missing out on family time as it is.

- **Don't make judgments.** No "If you would only . . . " statements. Even if what you're saying is true, a positive attitude from you will be much more motivating than accusations.

- **Be committed.** No threats to leave when times are bad, which may be one of her biggest fears.

- **Ask what you can do to help — and do it.** Even better, although you've worked a long day, do what needs to be done without asking!

- **Run interference with other family and friends when she doesn't feel up to being with them.** Families can take this as rejection; it may be up to you to clear things up for them.

- **Don't feel like you have to fix everything.** No one can be everything to everyone all the time, and you can wear yourself out trying.

- **Give positive feedback.** Comments such as, "You're handling a hard situation well" work wonders. Praise is a great motivator!

- **Become an expert at giving back rubs or massages.** Good ones can really make a difference!

- **Go to doctor visits with her if she asks.** You may discover helpful information, and understanding what's going on can help you be more empathetic.

Accentuate the positive. Sometimes your partner may not be able to think about the good parts of your lives. But, if you both fall into the same "woe is us" trap, you're going to have a very gloomy household. You don't need to be unrealistic or try and bully your partner into feeling better — which never works anyway. Saying "You *should* . . ." makes her feel like she's getting a lecture, and the natural inclination is to become angry or defensive.

Listen, listen, listen!!! Listening is more than having half an ear tuned in; it's giving all your attention and really trying to hear what she's saying beyond the words themselves. Letting her talk is one of the greatest gifts you can give her.

Coping with the sexual effects of endometriosis

Do you want to talk about sex? Maybe not, but you need to if your partner is suffering from endometriosis. (If the person you love with endometriosis is your friend or daughter, feel free to skip this section!)

Almost 60 percent of women with endometriosis have sexual problems directly related to endometriosis. Of course, sex (or lack of sex or unsatisfying sex) can railroad almost any relationship. So you need to know what you may be up against with sex and endometriosis.

- ✔ **Believe that endometriosis can cause real pain during sex.** Her claims aren't an avoidance tactic.

- ✔ **Ask her what hurts.** The area may vary, depending on the time of the month.

- ✔ **Change positions.** Deep penetration may be very painful for her. Oral sex or sex toys may be a better alternative at times.

- ✔ **Be understanding, even when you're frustrated.** We know this balance is hard to maintain!

- ✔ **Be willing to experiment.** Sometimes figuring out what works for her takes time.

- ✔ **Be committed.** Let her know that sex is just a part of your life together and that you're not going to throw in the towel because of sexual issues.

- ✔ **Don't pressure her.** When you have urgent needs she can't meet at the time, don't storm off threatening to find alternatives. If a cold shower doesn't appeal to you, you can release the tension yourself, so to speak. Okay, it's not as much fun, but masturbation can do the job when necessary.

- ✔ **Sometimes the pain is talking, not the woman who loves you.** Pain makes people say words they don't mean. Add guilt to pain and almost any idea can come out — without really meaning it. Don't take any words from the middle of a painful moment to heart.

Keeping afloat financially

Endometriosis can be a costly disease. Considering the surgeries, medications, doctor's visits, therapy, time off from work, or an inability to keep a job or to work at all — chronic illness can put a big dent in your financial planning. Your partner may feel guilty for not being able to carry her financial share, and you may be frustrated with this situation as well.

Look for ways to work around the financial quagmires. Can your partner work at home? More and more jobs today allow employees to work outside the office, at least part of the time. Ask your loved one to discuss such a possibility with her employer. Many positions, such as medical transcribers, medical billers, phone sales, and so on, are possible to do from home. These jobs may not be ideal, but they can help pay the bills.

When your partner isn't feeling well, she may not be emotionally or physically able to dive into insurance issues and health plans. But a good plan can save you a lot of money, so make sure the plan you choose covers the expenses you're likely to have. Many companies offer more than one option to choose from. The cheapest, not surprisingly, may not be the best for you. Then again, it may be!

Know your insurance coverage so you can fight denials when necessary. Yes, the language is obscure, and calls to insurance companies can eat up hours of time. But saving co-pays or fighting denials can be worth your time and effort, especially if you're on a tight budget.

I have had patients whose insurance companies denied their claims for obscure reasons. In several cases related to endometriosis, I have gone to bat for my patients and helped them get payment. Ask your doctor to help by writing letters, or get a lawyer involved. Sometimes a letter from the doctor or a lawyer can expedite payment.

Keep good financial records and don't throw away any correspondence from your insurance company until you're sure you don't need it. (Keep your records for at least three years, if you're claiming large expenses on your tax returns, three years if you're not claiming a large deduction.) Taking all the legal deductions that you're entitled to on tax returns requires documentation.

Persevering Through Infertility Treatments Together

We've both spent years working with infertile patients and found that this area can really make or break a relationship. Because so many women with endometriosis suffer from some form of infertility, you and your loved one may face this problem as well. Please believe us when we say that your life (and relationship) can be easier if you face the challenges together.

Finding out that you may have trouble conceiving can be devastating. Most people assume that having children is an inalienable right and they're shocked to find out it may not be that easy. Families dealing with infertility go through all the stages of grief: denial, anger, bargaining, and rationalization before acceptance and dealing with the problem face on. (See Chapter 7 for a complete rundown on infertility issues that endometriosis can cause.)

What can you do to help your partner through this difficult time of trying to get pregnant? You can show the same support as you do with the rest of her problems (check out "Helping without being a pain" earlier in this chapter), plus a few more:

- **Avoid the blame game.** Your partner feels bad enough about the infertility. Don't make the matter worse by pointing your finger. Besides, infertility can have many factors, including problems on your part.

- **Keep a positive attitude.** Endometriosis doesn't mean you'll never have children; treatments are available to help you.

- **Expect mood swings if your partner is on hormone medication.** Yes, *more* mood swings! Mood swings are inevitable when you're taking potent hormones.

- **Understand the elements of the process.** You may find parts of the infertility treatment highly unpleasant, such as giving your partner injections and producing semen on demand in the doctor's office. But when you understand why certain steps are necessary, you may accept them more easily.

- **Be aware that infertility treatments can change sex from enjoyment to duty.** Try to keep the romance in sex when you're in the middle of fertility treatments. Your partner may be so focused on the end result (a baby) that she can't see the forest for the trees. Sexual pleasure may be the last thought on her mind when she says, "Tonight's the night!" You may need to make the evening enjoyable and pleasurable, despite the timetable.

Infertility treatments add another layer of pressure to a life that's already stressful. For example, just knowing that you have to give your partner injections can cause your stress level to go through the roof when you're already concerned about the expense, the travel time, lost time from work, the emotional toll, and whether or not the treatment will work.

The middle of infertility treatments isn't the time to remodel the bathroom, plan a cross-country move, or start a new business. Keep outside distractions to a minimum, and both of you will be in much better shape to deal with the stresses of parenthood in a few months! (For more information on fertility issues, check out *Fertility For Dummies* by Jackie Meyers-Thompson and yours truly, Sharon Perkins [Wiley].)

Just for Moms and Dads: Being There for Your Adult Daughter

Parents have a hard time dealing with an adult child's chronic illness. If your child has endometriosis, you may vacillate between an "Oh, poor baby" and a "Just get over it" attitude, with feelings of guilt for good measure. Parents can forget their children are still children and, unknowingly, cause hurt feelings. Believe it or not, even as adults, your children are looking for your approval on some level.

So how do you handle the ongoing issues of endometriosis in your adult child's life? You can

- **Remember that your child is an adult.** This advice means that she has the right to make her own decisions (even if you know they're the wrong ones).

- **Keep your mouth shut when the occasion warrants it.** When is that? Every time you start to say, "I think you should . . ." when your child hasn't asked.

- **Remember that your child still cares about your opinion.** If you think she's making huge mistakes in the way she's dealing with endometriosis, stay quiet unless the result is life threatening or she asks you what you think. When she does ask, be tactful. Talk to her like you talk to a friend, not a toddler.

- **Don't tell a personal story (especially negative ones) every time she starts to tell you about her situation.** Your child may not want to hear about the horrible pain Aunt Jenny had with her periods, or how your friend's insides were all stuck together before she had surgery. Just listen without playing "Can you top this story?"

- **Stay positive, especially if your child is trying to get pregnant.** Don't bemoan the fact that it's taking so long for her to give you a grandchild. *Never ever* offer advice in this area unless specifically asked!

- **Learn about endometriosis.** This book is a good place to start. Researchers have discovered much about this disease in the last 20 years and have made many advances in treatment. The scenarios aren't the same as poor Aunt Jenny's 30 years ago.

- **Try not to feel guilty.** Even if this disease runs in the family, it's not your fault. Many factors influence endometriosis; family history is just one of them. You may be feeling guiltier if you pooh-poohed your daughter's symptoms when she was a teenager. You did the best you could.

Finding Support for Yourself

You may have days where you're feeling left out, wondering why no one cares about *your* feelings and aches and pains. Trust us, someone does. Who? Your mother, for one, and your partner does too, even though she may be in pain. A whole lot of people are in the same boat you are and want to know that their feelings are normal, too. These subjects don't easily come up at work or in the gym, though. People just don't stand around the water cooler, talking about their partner's cramps, irregular bleeding, or infertility issues.

So where can you go to talk about the frustrations and difficulties of dealing with endometriosis secondhand? The easiest way to find people to talk to, even in the wee hours of the morning, is the Internet. You can always access it, and the Internet is popular with insomniacs, so you can almost always find someone who's willing to talk.

The following Web sites are available for information and support just for partners of women with endometriosis:

✔ http://www.geocities.com/HotSprings/Spa/8449/

✔ http://www.endometriosis.org.uk/partners/index.htm

As you can see, there's a need for more Web sites just for support people to talk about endometriosis. Are you an Internet geek? Start a board of your own — or visit the endometriosis sites listed in Appendix B and see if you can start a support-person's site.

In addition, some women's groups welcome family and friends wanting to understand the disease better (although other groups are strictly for the person with endometriosis). Some groups have a moderator, some don't. You can find out a lot just by listening to fellow endometriosis sufferers chatting with each other. They tell each other their thoughts, even ones that they may be embarrassed to tell you!

How else can you help yourself? Try the following:

✔ **Give yourself permission to grieve.** A chronic illness in a loved one means the loss of certain hopes and dreams. The stages of grief — denial, anger, bargaining, rationalization, and acceptance — take time.

✔ **Give yourself permission to be angry at times.** However, keep your anger directed at the disease itself, not at the person who has it.

✔ **Give yourself time off.** Don't allow endometriosis to be the center of your life or your partner's. Plan fun activities to do when she's up to it. Find hobbies that can take you away from the stress of chronic illness.

✔ **Think about the issues one day at a time.** Some of the effects of endometriosis can be devastating, financially and emotionally, for both you and your partner. When you try to think about all the issues at once, the problems can overwhelm you. Long-term plans are fine, but realize that they may need to adapt to unforeseen changes.

✔ **Keep a journal.** Even if you're not the expressive type, getting your feelings down on paper can help. Many men have never kept a journal, but recording your thoughts and emotions can be a great tension reliever. And reading what you wrote a year or two ago can also help you realize that circumstances do change. What upset you a year ago may never enter your mind now. Seeing change and growth in your own life can be positive reinforcement!

Who should you *not* pour out your troubles to? We suggest you not share your feelings with people who may hold your comments against you or your partner, or take sides. This list may include your closest relatives; they have to be very strong people not to fall into the trap of sympathizing with you and holding some type of resentment toward your partner. If you think your own relatives can't listen without becoming judgmental, don't tell all. Yes, tea and sympathy from your nearest and dearest can be wonderful, but not at the expense of their relationship with your partner.

Part V
The Part of Tens

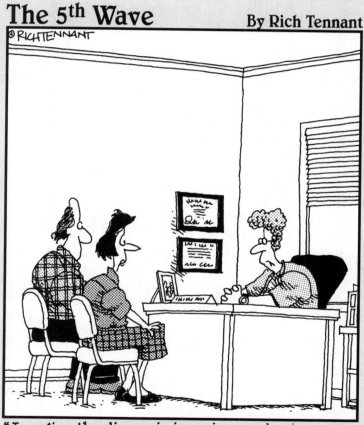

The 5th Wave — By Rich Tennant

"I realize the diagnosis is serious and raises many questions, but let's try to address them in order. We'll look at various treatment options, make a list of the best clinics to consider, and then determine what color ribbon you should be wearing."

In this part . . .

Confused about fact and fiction when it comes to endometriosis? How about a fast look at the future of endometriosis diagnosis and treatment? Want some quick ideas on how to deal with the pain of endometriosis? You can find answers to these questions and more in this Part of Tens section — solid information in a quick-and-easy format.

Chapter 18

Ten Myths about Endometriosis

In This Chapter

▶ Endometriosis is a minor problem

▶ Just certain women get endometriosis

▶ The solutions for endometriosis are simple

▶ You just can't get pregnant if you have endometriosis

Endometriosis is often a misunderstood disease. Ask your friends what they know about endometriosis, and you're likely to hear a list of misconceptions. Even your doctor may not truly understand endometriosis.

This chapter examines ten of the most common misconceptions about endometriosis, so feel free to hand it to anyone who tries to misinform you.

Endometriosis Is All in Your Head

Even doctors used to believe that endometriosis was a psychological disease. The prevailing attitude was that, if you just stopped thinking about yourself all the time, all the pain would disappear. Some doctors actually believed that a woman's positive attitude would make the pain go away. Unfortunately, some professionals still use this rationale today.

Although a positive attitude is certainly good to have throughout your life, you probably know that attitude doesn't decrease your endometriosis one bit. Endometriosis isn't just in your head (although it can be; endometriosis has been found in the brain! See Chapter 6 for more info) — it's in your pelvis, and it hurts.

Endometriosis Is Just Cramps

Although your significant other may think your endometriosis is just a case of really bad cramps, you know the difference. Endometriosis can affect many parts of your body, and symptoms can occur at any time of the month, not just during your period. Endometriosis can cause permanent damage to your ovaries, fallopian tubes, bowels, bladder, and any other body part it attaches to.

Of all the misguided attitudes about endometriosis, this one is the most dangerous because it may lead you to ignore your symptoms until they've done permanent damage. (See Chapter 2 for more on ways to differentiate between endometriosis and other diseases that cause similar symptoms.) As doctors and the public become more educated about the far-reaching consequences of endometriosis, the myth of endometriosis as *just cramps* will be permanently debunked.

If you suffer debilitating cramps, don't wait another minute. Call your gynecologist immediately for an exam to see whether you have endometriosis or some other ailment. The earlier you know, the better.

Only Women Get Endometriosis

Just imagine if men worried about getting endometriosis. Congress probably would pass legislation approving millions of dollars of research for a cure, right? You may be surprised, but men can actually get endometriosis. Of course, these occurrences are rare because endometriosis usually appears in men who take high doses of estrogen hormones for diseases such as prostate cancer, but it can happen.

Teenagers Don't Get Endometriosis

Girls as young as 11 years old have been diagnosed with endometriosis. Because girls now start menstruating at an earlier age than they did in past decades, their endometriosis is occurring at a younger age too. (See Chapter 14 for more info.) And because endometriosis was considered a *career woman*'s disease up until the 1980s, physicians didn't consider looking for it in teenage girls who had the symptoms. In the past, many doctors thought bad cramps were just part of being a woman. Now, however, more and more doctors are testing teenagers who have symptoms, and the diagnosis is frequently endometriosis.

Endometriosis Goes Away at Menopause

Although the symptoms of endometriosis often decrease at menopause because estrogen levels drop, some doctors and researchers have found endometriosis in women in their 70s. In fact, some women are first diagnosed with endometriosis in menopause, usually because endometriosis is found at the time of surgery for chronic pelvic pain or for unrelated reasons.

Endometriosis Is a Career Woman's Disease

The concept of endometriosis being a career woman's disease is an old wives' tale based on the premise that only driven, Type-A personalities got endometriosis. This myth is a twisted version of "it's all in your head," but it adds the dig, "You brought this problem on yourself by being a driven career woman." The attitude probably gained credence when career women started trying to get pregnant at a later age than traditional homemakers. If the older woman had trouble getting pregnant, endometriosis was often the cause.

In fact, no relationship has ever been proven; women from every socioeconomic and racial group can have endometriosis, whether they're working in the office or at home (check out Chapter 1 for more statistics about who gets endometriosis).

Endometriosis Only Exists in Industrialized Countries

This statement is a variation of the career woman myth. In the past, experts believed endometriosis was a disease only in industrialized countries where exposure to toxic chemicals was rampant. But researchers haven't proven this theory. Women in third-world countries have endometriosis, but, without the resources to obtain treatment, they're less likely to be diagnosed. These women also tend to have children at a younger age, which helps keep symptoms at bay longer. (See Chapter 4 for more on how and why pregnancy affects your chances of having endometriosis.)

A Hysterectomy Cures Endometriosis

A *hysterectomy* (the removal of your uterus) doesn't cure endometriosis, unless the endometriosis is only in the uterus. Although a hysterectomy stops menstrual bleeding because the blood comes from the uterine lining, the surgery doesn't change the endometriosis on your ovaries, bowel, bladder, or elsewhere in your pelvic cavity.

However, hysterectomy *with removal of both ovaries* will permanently get rid of endometriosis symptoms in most women, because removing the ovaries removes most of the hormonal stimulation that activates endometrial implants, wherever they're found. Unfortunately, the surgical menopause that results has a multitude of additional symptoms to cope with (refer to Chapter 11 for more info).

Endometriosis Is Easy to See and Remove during Surgery

Although your doctor may be able to see endometriosis during surgery, she may not recognize and thus remove all the implants. Studies have shown that surgeons are able to accurately visualize and diagnose only 60 percent of endometriosis. Unfortunately, endometriosis may look like other conditions, such as scar tissue; furthermore, other conditions, such as tumors, may look like endometriosis and can only be differentiated by biopsy.

You Can't Get Pregnant If You Have Endometriosis

Even if you have endometriosis, you can get pregnant. In fact, 60 to 70 percent of women with endometriosis do conceive, but they may have a harder time than a woman without the disease. Although some women with endometriosis get pregnant easily, others need to see a fertility specialist (see Chapter 7 for more on fertility issues). The bottom line: If you want to have kids and you have endometriosis, see a specialist and, if at all possible, have babies sooner rather than later in life.

Chapter 19

Ten (Or So) Trends in the Future of Endometriosis

· ·

· ·

*W*hat does the future hold for endometriosis? Endometriosis has more research going on now than at any other time in history, and more research means hope for earlier detection, better diagnosis, and more effective ways to treat it without damaging future fertility. Are you ready to jump into the future? Some of this chapter may be too technical for you. However, if you're interested, this chapter shows what the future holds. Hang on; it may be a wild ride!

Determining the Source of Endometriosis

Scientists are now challenging many long-accepted theories about endometriosis. The theory that *retrograde menstruation* (menstrual blood that flows backwards, up, and out of the fallopian tubes; see Chapter 4 for more info) causes endometriosis may be true in some cases, or it may be a contributing factor. But most likely retrograde menstruation isn't the only cause of endometriosis. This one theory can't explain the many variations of endometriosis.

In fact, many experts feel that *endometriosis* may be a generic term to describe two or more diseases. That is, the slow-growing, annoying-but-not-life-altering endometriosis may be a whole different disease than the aggressive, painful, debilitating disease some women have. And why do some women's symptoms recur more quickly and other women's symptoms don't? Is the difference between the women, or is it within the disease? Researchers are working on answering these questions.

Identifying Endometriosis Genes

Endometriosis is likely to involve genetics because a woman has an increased risk of developing endometriosis if a close relative also has it. Studies suggest that the disease involves several different genes, each playing a unique role. But environmental factors may also be necessary to activate the genes that predispose a woman to develop endometriosis (much like some cancers are genetic based and activated by environmental factors). As the ability to find genes and genetic markers evolves, researchers will be able to identify endometriosis genes.

Recent studies have shown that many genes in the endometrium of women with endometriosis act abnormally. Scientists can plot hundreds of genes and their activity during the menstrual cycle. In normal women, certain genes are more active at specific times and then decrease at other times. Research has found that this sequence of gene activation and deactivation is different in women with endometriosis. Our ability to identify and measure these sequences may help diagnose endometriosis in the future.

More recently, researchers have found a chromosome marker in women with endometriosis. This chromosome, specifically 10q26, is probably only one of many that will be found in the future. If researchers can detect this chromosome in the blood, then perhaps diagnosis of endometriosis can be easier, based on a simple blood test.

Other researchers are working on different possible markers in the bloodstream, making them easy to find with a blood test. One of these is elevated in some white blood cells of women with endometriosis. If scientists can establish normal and abnormal levels of these markers and others, they can use them in the future to diagnose the disease earlier and more easily.

Overcoming Infertility in Endometriosis

Researchers have associated endometriosis with infertility for years — a logical connection because 35 to 50 percent of infertile women also have endometriosis. However, new research into the causes of infertility in endometriosis shows that some women with endometriosis lack the molecules that allow embryos to attach to the uterine lining. Obviously, if the embryo can't attach, this problem prevents pregnancy even though fertilization may occur.

This study also indicates that some genes in the uterus of endometriosis patients appear to function abnormally. As a result, infertility in endometriosis patients appears to be much more complicated than originally thought. Infertility isn't just the result of blocked fallopian tubes or other mechanical factors. The uterine lining may also have an inherent defect that prevents pregnancy.

For women with severe infertility problems related to endometriosis, embryo freezing can be a godsend. Eggs can be taken during an egg retrieval cycle and fertilized with the partner's sperm. The embryos produced this way can be stored for many years until the time is right for a pregnancy. This process can help those women who may lose their eggs over time due to endometriosis. Embryo freezing may also allow women to wait for better treatments for endometriosis to be developed in the future. In rare cases, these frozen embryos can be implanted into another woman without the disease, which allows the affected woman to have a child with her own genes even if she has lost her uterus because of endometriosis. *Oocyte* (egg) freezing (cryopreserving just the unfertilized egg; more research is being done in this area) may be a viable alternative for women with endometriosis who don't have a partner, and will have the same benefits as embryo freezing.

Diagnosing Endometriosis Earlier

At one time, scientists thought that teens rarely developed endometriosis and that preteens never did. Researchers have now proven these notions incorrect. The earlier that doctors can diagnose teens and preteens, the earlier treatment can begin and the more damage can be minimized.

Diagnosing and starting treatment early is vital to maintain a teen's future fertility and to decrease symptoms and damage to organs. So, awareness of the disease and its symptoms, along with an accurate family history of the disease, is important. In addition, newer blood tests for chromosomes, antibodies, and other proteins may provide earlier detection.

Refining Medication Treatments

Research into new medications for treatment of endometriosis is exciting. Much research centers on targeting specific causes of endometriosis rather than using medications that may sometimes have harmful systemic effects on body systems outside the reproductive system. In the future, scientists may find additional uses for selective estrogen receptor modulators (SERMs). The SERMs can affect the way estrogen interacts with the cell receptors in endometriosis lesions. Aromatase inhibitors (AI) target *aromatase,* the final enzyme in the estrogen-biosynthesis pathway. These AI medications selectively decrease estrogen production in endometriotic lesions without affecting ovarian function.

Other treatments may block progesterone and other hormones that have an effect on endometriosis. These new classes of medications may have fewer side effects, and patients may tolerate them better than present treatments.

Still newer and different treatments may come. Botox (yes, the wrinkle cure!) has been tried in a small number of patients with some success. We never know what can be next!

Improving Immune Therapy

Immune therapy is still in its infancy in treating endometriosis. (See Chapter 12 for more about immunotherapy.) Although use of immune therapy for cancer treatment is common, doctors don't use it as much as they could to treat autoimmune diseases. This reluctance stems from the potentially serious side effects. After all, who wants to treat a disease and have side effects that are potentially life-threatening and worse than the disease itself? New, less destructive and dangerous drugs may make immune therapy more acceptable for endometriosis.

Gaining Respect for Endometriosis

Endometriosis is a disease that affects more women than any other disease in the United States. But do you see ads for endometriosis awareness on television or telethons to raise money for research? No! Why is that? The answer is simple: In the past, doctors and lay persons alike have treated endometriosis more as an emotional problem than a medical one.

Scientists and medical personnel are just beginning to realize how complicated and debilitating endometriosis can be. In the near future, we hope to see more awareness of the problem and a greater emphasis on its research, understanding, and treatment in both the medical profession and the public.

Starting More Organizations to Help

In Appendix B, we list some organizations that can help people deal with endometriosis. The more awareness women have of the disease, the sooner women can seek help. And the more organizations that develop, the more women can get the help — physically and emotionally — that they need.

No endometriosis associations in your area? Think about starting one! Place ads in local gynecologists' offices or on grocery store bulletin boards and get together with fellow sufferers to talk about endometriosis and compare notes on treatments and medications.

Getting Insurers to Help Cover the Costs

In the past, insurance companies have been leery about covering the costs associated with endometriosis. You may wonder why. Most insurance companies exist to make money. The less they have to pay out in benefits, the more they make. You may have read or seen stories about people fighting with insurance companies to get payment for new or unusual treatments for some disease. These treatments are often expensive and not mainstream, so the insurers try not to pay.

Unfortunately, endometriosis is in this category. So if the public or government doesn't pressure insurers to pay for mental health care or issues that only affect women, not men, these insurers often refuse to cover them. Some states have begun to mandate that insurers cover certain diseases like infertility, and we hope all problems will be insured in the future.

The trick is to convince the insurance companies that they'll still make billions of dollars even if they fully cover endometriosis testing and treatment. This convincing may take governmental prodding, but, as awareness of endometriosis and its impact on women's health grows, we hope the insurers will understand that diagnosing endometriosis early and treating it fully are also in the insurers' best interests.

Transplanting Ovaries and Other Reproductive Organs

Transplantation works for kidneys, hearts, lungs, and corneas. Is the day coming when surgeons can routinely transplant ovaries, uteri, and fallopian tubes as well? Ovarian transplants already exist; in fact, transplanted ovaries have provided eggs for healthy pregnancies. However, in this case the child wasn't genetically related to the woman.

Surgeons have performed at least one uterine transplant, but the uterus worked for only a few months before the patient's body rejected it. One problem with transplanting reproductive organs is that women must take anti-rejection drugs, which have powerful side effects. These drugs also can't be used during a pregnancy because they would harm the fetus. Because having a uterus isn't a necessity unless a woman wants to become pregnant and doesn't want to use a gestational carrier, taking anti-rejection drugs just to keep a uterus transplant isn't practical at the moment. But in the future — anything's possible!

Decreasing Surgical Risks

One risk of surgery to treat endometriosis is that it tends to create more adhesions, or scar tissue. So the treatment itself can cause more problems down the road. The following changes may make surgery less likely to create adhesions in the future:

- ✔ Laparoscopy rather than laparotomy (see Chapter 11 for the differences between the two types of surgeries) for many surgical procedures
- ✔ The development of anti-adhesion barriers like sprays, gels, liquids, and patches to prevent adhesion-formation

Surgical treatment for endometriosis must also take future fertility into account. Surgeons must first understand the disease so they don't do more harm than good. In addition, surgeons need increased training to develop safer surgical skills when dealing with endometriosis.

The riskiest part of any surgery used to be anesthesia. Recent advances in techniques and instrumentation have made laparoscopy possible with lighter and even local anesthesia. Surgeries will become safer and easier in the future as techniques and instruments improve.

Even when a patient needs general anesthesia, newer anesthetics make it very safe and reduce side effects markedly. No longer do anesthesiologists use large doses of narcotics and sodium pentothal (with all the nausea, drowsiness, and other terrible side effects). Now, small doses of quick-acting medications that have minimal side effects have become the standard.

Chapter 20

Ten Strategies to Help with the Pain

. . . .

In This Chapter

▶ Anticipating pain and avoiding the onset

▶ Managing your meds

▶ Pampering yourself to decrease pain

▶ Using your head

. . . .

*P*ain is just that — a pain. It can serve a valuable purpose in life when it lets you know something's wrong, but presumably you're beyond that. What *you* want are some quick ideas for handling pain when you're not in the mood for a long dissertation. This chapter gives you some quick fixes for those days when your pain is nearly unbearable.

Planning to Avoid Pain

You may think avoiding the pain is impossible; after all, if you could avoid pain, you would, right? But are you doing all you can to keep the pain from starting? Are you

✔ **Anticipating when pain may begin?** If you've had pain that starts three days before your period every month for the last 12 months, you can pretty much count on having pain three days before your period this month too. Are you ready?

✔ **Warding the pain off by taking anti-inflammatory drugs, such as ibuprofen, before it begins?** Studies have shown that taking anti-inflammatory drugs before pain starts is more effective in decreasing pain than waiting until it begins. (See Chapter 13 for more on pain relief and endometriosis.)

✔ **Scheduling acupuncture, massage therapy, or whatever works for you before the pain even starts?** See Chapter 12 for more on alternative treatments.

> ✔ **Eating well, exercising moderately, and avoiding stress (as best you can) just before you regularly have pain?** Studies have shown that exercise and stress avoidance can help reduce symptoms.
>
> ✔ **Avoiding your triggers?** By keeping a journal of symptoms, you may discover certain conditions bring on or worsen the pain.

Jumping on Pain the Minute It Begins

All right, so you waited a day too long to ward off the pain, and now it's already started. Don't let it get out of hand. Use your big guns upfront and a little pain may never develop into a bigger one. As soon as you feel a little discomfort, go into de-stress mode:

> ✔ Take a warm bath
>
> ✔ Take an anti-inflammatory medication
>
> ✔ Get a massage
>
> ✔ Forget about that nonessential meeting after work

You may be tempted to ignore a little pain, hoping it'll just go away (even though it never does). Don't ignore it; getting rid of that little pain may be much easier than getting rid of a big one.

Keeping Medications You Need on Hand

Discovering that you're out of your regular pain medication on the Friday evening of a holiday weekend definitely isn't good. In fact, trying to call in a prescription when you're writhing in pain isn't a good idea either. You scream at your doctor's receptionist because you're hurting, so she puts your call on the bottom of the doctor's callback pile. (Not really — most doctors' receptionists are very nice people!)

You're never going to feel like driving to the drugstore when you're in pain, so make sure you always have the pain meds you need.

Soaking in a Hot Tub

Don't jump in the lake — and don't even jump in the tub. Try lowering yourself gently into a warm tub of water up to your chin, and don't forget the pillow for your head, a candle for soft light, and a relaxing CD. Moist heat helps your tense muscles relax.

Don't have a tub? Fill a hot-water bottle, cover it with a towel warmed in the microwave, and lie down. Go one step further and put a warm washcloth across your forehead. Then listen to some relaxing music and use guided imagery to escape to a more pleasant place, where the word *pain* doesn't even exist. Sound corny? Don't knock them till you've tried them; these relaxation tips really may help. (See Chapter 12 for more on techniques to reduce pain without medication.)

Massaging Away the Pain

A gentle massage can help you and your tight muscles relax. Always ask your doctor before you undergo any type of deep massage. Stay away from rough massages, which can send you off the table when you're in pain.

You don't know anyone who can give you a massage? A hand-held massager may not be quite as good as having someone else do the honors, but it can help in a pinch.

Breathing Slow and Easy

Pain may feel like a never-ending cycle. The pain makes you tense, the tension makes you breathe harder, and the hard breathing makes you more tense. To alleviate some of your pain, concentrate on breathing slow and easy.

Have you ever had a child? If so, do you remember the breathing techniques for the pain during childbirth? All right, so they don't work 100 percent, but they can help you relax. Never been to a childbirth class? The technique is simple: Breathe in and out slowly, emptying your lungs completely before taking another breath. And don't worry — no one's going to be grading your technique!

Using Your Imagination

Breathe slowly and pretend you're somewhere else, with no pain or stress. Guided imagery may sound a little hokey, but it really works for many people. Imagine yourself on a quiet, balmy, warm island. If imagining a piña colada in your hand works, feel free. In fact, if you actually *have* a piña colada in your hand, feel free. After all, you're on an island, aren't you?

Talking It Over

Sometimes a listening ear is just what you need. Talking away stress and frustration to your partner, your best friend, your shrink, or a higher power may help you relax. If you want to complain, go ahead. But try not to get all hot and bothered, which can make you tense, which can cause muscle spasms, which can increase the pain — another vicious circle.

Talking online with other people in the same boat or finding a support group that meets monthly can be a godsend when you have that "no one understands what I'm going through" feeling. And that conversation's a lot cheaper than paying someone to listen to you too! (Check out Appendix B for information about online resources.)

Trying a Little Laughter

Studies have shown that laughter really is one of the best medicines; yet one study showed that the average adult laughs only 17 times a day. Children, on the other hand, laugh more than 300 times a day! Laughter can decrease pain by releasing endorphins, relaxing muscle tension, and taking you *out of yourself* for a little while. Some studies show that laughter may even boost your immune system, making you less likely to become ill in the first place! So rent some comedies and save the tear jerkers for another time.

Knowing What Works for You

You're not like everyone else; what works for your Aunt Jane's cramps may do nothing for you. Try different suggestions until you find a plan that works for you, and then stick to it. Don't worry about trying all your relatives' home remedies — you may find out that the medicine bottle Granny Annie sips from all day long is actually straight scotch.

When other people know you're in pain, you end up listening to everyone's suggestions. Giving fresh ideas a try doesn't hurt, as long as you remember that you're the only person who can know what works for you.

Part VI
Appendixes

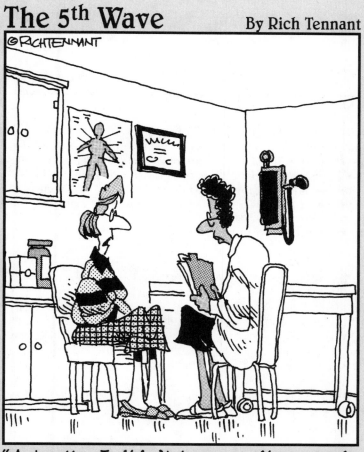

The 5th Wave   By Rich Tennant

"Actually, I didn't become dizzy and nauseous until I started inhaling the scent strips in the waiting room magazines."

In this part . . .

No, not that kind of appendix! This part has the facts you need: definitions of all those long Latin medical terms and a list of resources for more info — just in case you want to know even more about endometriosis.

Appendix A

Glossary

*I*s your Latin a little rusty? Figuring out the meaning of medical terms is a lousy way to spend an afternoon, so we've made it easier to understand this book by including the definitions for some of the terms we use that you don't see every day (Latin and otherwise).

abnormal uterine bleeding (AUB): Also called *dysfunctional uterine bleeding* (DUB); uterine bleeding that's heavier than normal, or occurs at irregular times, or lasts too long.

acupuncture: Oriental system of puncturing the skin with fine needles to treat ailments.

add-back therapy: Hormonal therapy to minimize side effects of medications that suppress *estrogen* (such as leuprolide acetate); add-back therapy usually decreases hot flashes and also helps prevent bone loss.

adenomyosis: A common benign condition of the uterus where the endometrium grows into the uterine wall. Previously this condition was called *endometriosis interna,* although it appears to be unrelated to endometriosis.

adhesions: Bands of fibrous scar tissue.

adrenal gland: Small glands located above each kidney that produce steroid *hormones* that help control bodily functions, such as heart rate and blood pressure.

agonist: Medication that acts like another medication but with different c haracteristics.

allergen: A substance that causes an allergic reaction.

allergy: Symptoms caused by an overreaction of the body's immune system.

androgen: Male sex *hormone.*

angiogenesis: The growth of new blood vessels.

anovulation: A lack of *ovulation;* no *egg* matures or is released.

antagonist: A medication that works against or blocks a substance; *GnRH* antagonists, for example, block the effects of GnRH.

anterior cul-de-sac: A dead end in a woman's body between the pubic bone and the *uterus.*

antibody: Proteins that make the body immune to *antigens.*

antigen: Any substance that the immune system recognizes as foreign.

antiprogestin: A substance that inhibits *progesterone* formation or function.

appendix: A blind-ended, fingerlike projection extending from the cecum (the end of the large intestine where it connects to the small intestine).

aromatase: An *enzyme* that converts other *hormones* into *estrogen.*

ASRM staging system: The system used by the American Society of Reproductive Medicine to describe different degrees of *endometriosis.*

autoantibodies: A body's *antibodies* against its own cells.

autoimmune: Initiating or resulting from the production of *autoantibodies.*

autoimmune disease: A disease in which the body attacks itself.

bilateral: Located on both sides of the body.

bisphosphonate: A medication to improve bone density.

B lymphocyte: A *white blood cell* that matures in bone marrow and produces *antibodies;* also called B cells.

candida albicans: A *yeast fungus* in the *vagina* or *rectum.*

carcinogen: A cancer-causing agent.

cervix: The lower segment of the *uterus* that protrudes into the *vagina;* sometimes called the "mouth" of the uterus or womb.

coagulation: Clotting of the blood.

colostomy: A surgical opening in the abdominal wall for bowel drainage.

contracture: A shortening or distortion of a structure.

cul-de-sac: A dead end in the female pelvis. See *anterior cul-de-sac* and *posterior cul-de-sac*.

cystoscopy: The passing of a lighted tube (cystoscope) into the bladder and *ureters* through the *urethra* to examine for abnormalities.

cytokines: Proteins (produced by *white blood cells*) that act as chemical messengers between cells; can stimulate or inhibit the growth and activity of various immune cells.

deep endometriosis: Endometrial lesions that infiltrate at least 5 mm into vital structures, such as the intestines.

DHEA: A malelike *hormone* (made in the *adrenal gland*) that's not as potent as *testosterone*.

dioxins: Toxic organic compounds that may form as a result of incomplete combustion.

dysfunctional uterine bleeding (DUB): See *abnormal uterine bleeding (AUB)*.

dysmenorrhea: Pain or discomfort before or during a *menstrual* period.

dyspareunia: Pain in the *vagina* or pelvis during intercourse.

ectopic pregnancy: A pregnancy that implants a fertilized *egg* outside the *uterus,* usually in the *fallopian tubes*.

eggs: The *oocyte,* the sex cell produced by females.

embryo: The product of conception from Day 14 after fertilization to Week 8 of pregnancy.

endometrioma: An ovarian cyst containing endometrial *tissue* and blood.

endometriosis: The presence of endometrial *tissue* outside the lining of the *uterus*.

endometrium: The layer of *tissue* that lines the *uterus*.

enzyme: A protein that accelerates the rate of chemical reactions.

estrogen: A sex *hormone* that stimulates the development of female sex characteristics.

fallopian tube: The tube that extends outward from the top of the *uterus* to near the *ovary;* carries an *egg* from the ovary to the uterus.

fibromyalgia: A syndrome (thought to be *autoimmune*) that causes muscle soreness, pain, stiffness, and fatigue.

fimbria: A fingerlike projection at the end of the *fallopian tube,* near the *ovary.* Fimbriae help guide a newly released *egg* into the fallopian tube.

follicle: A small, fluid-filled cyst (in the *ovary*) where an *egg* grows and matures.

follicle-stimulating hormone (FSH): A *hormone* (produced by the *pituitary gland*) that stimulates the growth of *eggs* in the *ovaries.*

follicular phase: The time in a *menstrual cycle* that begins with an *egg's* development and ends with its *ovulation.*

frozen pelvis: A slang term for the presence of *adhesions* that bind together all the *pelvic cavity* organs.

ganglion: A group of *neurons.*

gland: An organ that secretes a substance to be used in the body.

gonadotropin-releasing hormone (GnRH): A hormone made by the *hypothalamus,* GnRH causes the pituitary gland to make *luteinizing hormone* (LH) and *follicle-stimulating hormone* (FSH).

hematosalpinx: A swollen, dilated *fallopian tube* filled with blood; usually caused by an *ectopic pregnancy.*

histologic: The microscopic appearance of a *tissue* structure.

hormone: A chemical produced in a *gland* and transported in the bloodstream to another organ, where it produces specific effects on metabolism.

hydrosalpinx: A swollen, dilated *fallopian tube* filled with fluid; usually caused by blockage (by scar tissue) of the far end of the tube.

hypothalamus: A small *gland* at the base of the brain that regulates many body functions.

hypothalamus-pituitary-ovarian axis: A term describing the combined interactions of these three *endocrine glands,* which normally behave as a single system.

hysterectomy: The surgical removal of the *uterus* through an abdominal incision or the *vagina,* sometimes with the aid of a laparoscope.

hysterosalpingogram: A radiographic diagnostic test to determine whether the *fallopian tubes* are open and whether the *uterus* has any abnormalities.

hysteroscopy: A diagnostic procedure in which a doctor inserts a lighted scope (hysteroscope) through the *cervix* into the *uterus* for viewing the inside of the uterus.

immunoglobulins: A class of *antibodies* released into the bloodstream in response to infections, immunizations, and *autoimmune* diseases.

immunotherapy: Treatment of disease by inducing, enhancing, or suppressing an immune response.

interleukins: *Cytokines* made by *leukocytes.*

irritable bowel syndrome (IBS): A bowel condition that results in irregular and uncoordinated intestinal contractions and often causes diarrhea, constipation, and abdominal pain.

laparoscopic uterosacral nerve ablation (LUNA): A surgical procedure to sever nerves and relax the *ligaments* that attach to the bottom of the *uterus* in an attempt to decrease pain from *endometriosis.*

laparoscopy: The direct visualization of the *ovaries* and exterior of the *fallopian tubes* and *uterus* through a surgical instrument (laparoscope) inserted through a small incision near the navel.

laparotomy: Surgical incision through the abdominal wall; may be up and down *(midline incision)* or across *(bikini incision).*

lesions: Areas of abnormal *tissue* or disease.

leukocytes: *White blood cells.*

ligaments: Strong bands of cordlike *tissue* that connect bone to bone.

luteinized unruptured follicle syndrome (LUF): Failure of the *ovary* to release the *egg* into the abdominal cavity at the time of *ovulation.*

luteinizing hormone (LH): The *hormone* secreted by the *pituitary gland* to stimulate growth and maturation of *eggs* in women.

lymph: An almost colorless fluid that carries *white blood cells* through the *lymphatic system.*

lymphatic system: The circulatory network of vessels carrying *lymph* and the lymphoid organs (such as the lymph nodes, spleen, and thymus) that produce and store infection-fighting cells.

lymphocyte: A type of *white blood cell* that helps the body fight infection.

macrophage: A type of *white blood cell* that surrounds and kills microorganisms, removes dead cells, and stimulates the action of other immune system cells.

menorrhagia: Heavy *menstrual* bleeding.

menstrual cycle: The monthly cycle of hormonal changes in a woman.

mesoderm: The middle layer of cells in an *embryo* that become the musculoskeletal, uretogenital, vascular, and connective *tissue* systems.

metabolism: A biochemical modification in cells and organisms to produce organic compounds and energy.

metaplasia: A change of cells from one type to another, sometimes to a type of cell that doesn't normally occur in the tissue where it is found.

metrorrhagia: Irregular uterine bleeding or uterine bleeding during times other than a normal *menstrual cycle*.

monocyte: A large *white blood cell* that ingests microbes or other cells and foreign particles; develops into a *macrophage* when entering *tissues*.

Mullerian ducts: A system present in both sexes early in fetal development; upon development, this system differentiates into a *uterus, fallopian tubes,* and upper portion of the *vagina*.

myometrium: The muscular outer layer of the *uterus*.

natural killer cells: A type of *white blood cell* containing granules with *enzymes* that kill tumor and microbial cells.

neurons: Cells in the nervous system that receive and conduct electrical impulses.

neutrophil: A *white blood cell* important in ingesting *pathogens*.

nonsteroidal anti-inflammatory drug (NSAID): Medications such as ibuprofen or aspirin.

oligomenorrhea: Scant blood flow during the *menstrual* period.

oocyte: The *egg* produced by a female.

oophorectomy: The surgical removal of the *ovaries*.

ovary: The female reproductive organ that manufactures *estrogen* and *eggs*.

ovulation: The release of an *egg* from the *ovary*.

pathogens: Microorganisms that cause disease.

pelvic cavity: The basin-shaped cavity that holds the reproductive organs.

pelvis: The lower part of the abdomen between the hip bones.

peritoneum: The membrane lining the cavity of the abdomen.

phytoestrogens: Naturally occurring *estrogen*-like compounds.

pituitary: An endocrine *gland* at the base of the brain.

polychlorinated biphenyls (PCBs): Nonflammable chemicals used in industry; known to be long-lasting and to cause cell alterations.

polymenorrhea: Abnormally frequent *menstrual* periods.

posterior cul-de-sac: A dead end in a woman's body behind the *uterus.*

pre-sacral neurectomy: The destruction of the nerves (which run over the sacrum) that carry pain sensations from the pelvis.

progesterone: A steroid *hormone* secreted by the *ovaries.*

prostaglandins: Several types of chemicals (made by cells) that have specific functions, such as controlling body temperature, stimulating smooth muscle, and influencing heat cycles.

rectum: The last few inches of the large intestine, which end at the anus (the outer opening of the intestines).

resection: The cutting out of *tissue* or organs.

retrograde menstruation: The backward flow of *menstrual* blood into the *fallopian tubes;* thought to be a possible cause of *endometriosis.*

sacrum: The curved, triangular bone at the base of the spine; consisting of five fused vertebrae, known as sacral vertebrae.

serosa: The delicate, one-cell-thick outside lining of an organ in the body.

stenosis: The narrowing of any blood vessel or passage.

stratum basilis: The inner layer of the *endometrium.*

stratum functionalis: The outer layer of the *endometrium,* which is sloughed off during a *menstrual* period.

stroma: The connective *tissue* framework of an organ, *gland,* or other structure.

T lymphocytes (T cells): *White blood cells* (produced in the bone marrow) that aid B cells *(B lymphocytes)* in making *antibodies* to fight bacterial infections.

testosterone: The primary male *hormone.*

thyroid: A *gland* (located in the front of the neck) that regulates metabolism.

tissue: A group of similar cells united to perform a specific function.

tumor necrosis factor (TNF): A *cytokine* produced by *T cells* and *macrophages.*

umbilicus: The navel, or belly button.

ureter: One of two 12-inch-long tubes that carry urine from the kidneys to the bladder.

urethra: The canal or duct that transports urine from the bladder to outside the body.

uterosacral ligament: A pair of ligaments that attach the *cervix* to the *sacrum* and are a common place to find *endometriosis.*

uterus: The hollow, muscular, pear-shaped organ in a woman that contains and nourishes a fetus.

vagina: The female organ of sexual intercourse; the birth canal.

vascular system: Vessels and *tissue* that carry and circulate fluids, such as blood and *lymph.*

viscera: The soft internal organs of the body, including the lungs, the heart, and the organs of the digestive, excretory, and reproductive systems.

white blood cells (WBC): A type of blood cell that involves the immune system.

yeast fungus: A microorganism; more evolved than bacteria. *Candida albicans* species is a common yeast fungus in humans.

Appendix B

Resources and Support

*I*f you have endometriosis, suspect you have endometriosis, or even have a loved one who has endometriosis, you probably aren't satisfied with reading one book; you want to know everything you can. Although we provide a lot of information in this book, we realize it isn't comprehensive, especially if you want to know more in-depth information about a particular topic. Just in case you're itching for more stuff, this appendix points out other valuable sources of information, including professional organizations, online resources, books, and so on. In this appendix, we tell you how to uncover next to everything about endometriosis — short of going to medical school and getting a degree in gynecology.

Looking for an Organization

Organizations for people with endometriosis were uncommon just a few decades ago. But endometriosis is now recognized as a real disease. Support continues to build for research and organizations that are devoted to informing and helping those who need it.

The granddaddy of all organizations is the Endometriosis Association founded by Mary Lou Ballweg in 1980. This organization runs support groups, publishes literature, offers tapes and videos, supports research, publishes books, runs chat rooms, and issues a newsletter. You can contact the Endometriosis Association at

Endometriosis Association
International Headquarters
8585 N. Seventy-sixth Place
Milwaukee, WI 53223
Phone 414-355-2200 or
800-992-3636
Fax 414-355-6065
E-mail endo@endometriosisassn.org
Web site www.endometriosisassn.org

Another organization with support groups, Web sites, newsletters, and information is

Endometriosis Research Center
World Headquarters
630 Ibis Drive
Delray Beach, FL 33444
Phone 800-239-7280 or
561-274-7442
Fax 561-274-0931
Web site www.endocenter.org

Going Online

What did we ever do before search engines? A wealth of information on endometriosis is available on the Web, most of it available simply by typing *endometriosis* into your search engine. If you want to go to the latest research and physician studies, go to online medical sites. If you want to chat or join bulletin board groups, plenty of those are available too.

For nonmedical information, check out the following Web sites:

✔ **www.endometriosisassn.org.** This Web site has special chat rooms for teens, many of the latest research articles, and enough information to keep you reading for days. (Check out the information in the previous section about the Endometriosis Association.)

✔ **www.endocenter.org.** This Web site by the Endometriosis Research Center (ERC) organizes support groups, bulletin boards, and educational programs for people with endometriosis. (See additional info in the previous section.)

✔ **www.endometriosis.org.** This is another active Web site with support groups, articles, links to research, and even a schedule of upcoming gynecological conferences around the world.

✔ **www.endo-resolved.com.** If you live outside the United States, you can find help here. This site provides information about support groups in a number of different countries plus lots of other helpful info.

✔ **www.endozone.org.** This site has a multitude of articles and links to new information, as well as chat forums. They'll notify you via e-mail when new information is published.

If you're looking to play doctor or just dazzle yours, check out the following Web sites for professionals:

✔ http://wes.endometriosis.org/index.htm (**world society for gynecologists, endocrinologists, scientists, and biologists**)

✔ http://www.ACOG.org (**a Web site for gynecologists**)

✔ http://www.AAGL.org (**another Web site for gynecologists**)

Flipping through Books

In addition to this helpful book in your two hands, you can find other books on endometriosis, although many of them may have a particular slant. Some emphasize diet and nutrition; some focus on fertility issues. Others emphasize only lung and colon endometriosis or holistic healing and endometriosis. For general endometriosis information, you may want to check out the following:

- *Endometriosis: The Complete Reference for Taking Charge of Your Health* by Mary Lou Ballweg (McGraw-Hill)

- *Coping with Endometriosis: A Practical Guide* by Robert Phillips (Avery)

- *Living Well with Endometriosis: What Your Doctor Doesn't Tell You...That You Need to Know* by Kerry-Ann Morris (Collins)

If you're not satisfied with these books and you're the scholarly type, take a look at these two textbooks on endometriosis. They may satisfy your desire to know everything:

- *Modern Management of Endometriosis* by Christopher Sutton (Taylor and Francis). This 448-page tome for medical professionals can probably answer all your questions — but you may need someone to translate medicalese into English! Most textbooks are quite technical, but if you're determined or have some medical knowledge, you can learn a lot from these books. Although they're not available in your local bookstore, you can order them from most online bookstores. But these textbooks don't come cheap; this one is around $230.

- *Endometriosis in Clinical Practice* by David Olive (Taylor and Francis). Want to know what your doctor reads to learn about endometriosis? Come in with this book under your arm and watch him wince! (Seriously, leave the book at home — a nervous doctor is generally not a helpful doctor. But you can read it surreptitiously before you go into the office and then dazzle him with your knowledge.)

Reading Newsletters

Want to make sure you know the latest news in endometriosis as soon as it becomes available? Newsletters that update you on a regular basis can keep you in the know. In addition to the online groups mentioned earlier in this appendix, the following sites also offer regular newsletters:

- `www.remedyfind.com` is an Internet site providing information on a number of diseases, including endometriosis. If you sign up, they send a free newsletter via e-mail every other month with information on endometriosis.

✔ `www.webmd.com` also offers newsletters on women's health issues as well as articles, bulletin boards, and all the latest information on a number of health issues.

Getting Involved in Clinical Trials

Do you want to become part of cutting-edge technology, help test new drugs, or be involved with research on endometriosis? You don't have to be a scientist — you can participate as a patient in trials all across the country.

Don't know where to look? Start at `www.centerwatch.com/patient/studies/cat60.html` for a list of clinical trials across the United States as well as information on tests and patient requirements. If you've always wanted to do something to further endometriosis treatment and help other women, here's your chance!

Attending Meetings and Support Groups

If you do better with face-to-face contact than chatting online or reading a book, you can search your area for meetings and support groups for endometriosis sufferers. How do you find support groups that meet live and in person? Check your local hospital for monthly meetings, or ask your gynecologist if she knows of any support groups. When all else fails, start your own group!

Asking Relatives and Friends

If you have endometriosis, chances are someone in your family has it too. (See Chapter 4, which discusses the possible hereditary links to endometriosis.) Your mother, aunt, sister, or cousin may be able to give you insight into the disease and how she deals with it. Because you're related, the suggestions may work for you too. Don't be afraid to talk to your relatives about your problems.

Likewise, you may know someone who has endometriosis, and she may be too shy to tell everyone about her disease. If you can bring up your troubles in a subtle way, she may open up to you. By sharing resources, you can help each other deal with endometriosis.

Index

• J •

• K •

• L •

• N •

BUSINESS, CAREERS & PERSONAL FINANCE

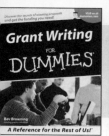

0-7645-5307-0

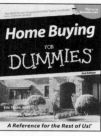

0-7645-5331-3 *†

Also available:

- Accounting For Dummies †
  0-7645-5314-3
- Business Plans Kit For Dummies †
  0-7645-5365-8
- Cover Letters For Dummies
  0-7645-5224-4
- Frugal Living For Dummies
  0-7645-5403-4
- Leadership For Dummies
  0-7645-5176-0
- Managing For Dummies
  0-7645-1771-6

- Marketing For Dummies
  0-7645-5600-2
- Personal Finance For Dummies *
  0-7645-2590-5
- Project Management For Dummies
  0-7645-5283-X
- Resumes For Dummies †
  0-7645-5471-9
- Selling For Dummies
  0-7645-5363-1
- Small Business Kit For Dummies *†
  0-7645-5093-4

HOME & BUSINESS COMPUTER BASICS

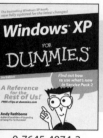

0-7645-4074-2

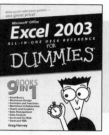

0-7645-3758-X

Also available:

- ACT! 6 For Dummies
  0-7645-2645-6
- iLife '04 All-in-One Desk Reference
  For Dummies
  0-7645-7347-0
- iPAQ For Dummies
  0-7645-6769-1
- Mac OS X Panther Timesaving
  Techniques For Dummies
  0-7645-5812-9
- Macs For Dummies
  0-7645-5656-8

- Microsoft Money 2004 For Dummies
  0-7645-4195-1
- Office 2003 All-in-One Desk Reference
  For Dummies
  0-7645-3883-7
- Outlook 2003 For Dummies
  0-7645-3759-8
- PCs For Dummies
  0-7645-4074-2
- TiVo For Dummies
  0-7645-6923-6
- Upgrading and Fixing PCs For Dummies
  0-7645-1665-5
- Windows XP Timesaving Techniques
  For Dummies
  0-7645-3748-2

FOOD, HOME, GARDEN, HOBBIES, MUSIC & PETS

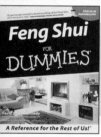

0-7645-5295-3

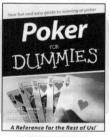

0-7645-5232-5

Also available:

- Bass Guitar For Dummies
  0-7645-2487-9
- Diabetes Cookbook For Dummies
  0-7645-5230-9
- Gardening For Dummies *
  0-7645-5130-2
- Guitar For Dummies
  0-7645-5106-X
- Holiday Decorating For Dummies
  0-7645-2570-0
- Home Improvement All-in-One
  For Dummies
  0-7645-5680-0

- Knitting For Dummies
  0-7645-5395-X
- Piano For Dummies
  0-7645-5105-1
- Puppies For Dummies
  0-7645-5255-4
- Scrapbooking For Dummies
  0-7645-7208-3
- Senior Dogs For Dummies
  0-7645-5818-8
- Singing For Dummies
  0-7645-2475-5
- 30-Minute Meals For Dummies
  0-7645-2589-1

INTERNET & DIGITAL MEDIA

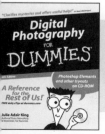

0-7645-1664-7

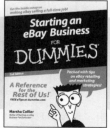

0-7645-6924-4

Also available:

- 2005 Online Shopping Directory
  For Dummies
  0-7645-7495-7
- CD & DVD Recording For Dummies
  0-7645-5956-7
- eBay For Dummies
  0-7645-5654-1
- Fighting Spam For Dummies
  0-7645-5965-6
- Genealogy Online For Dummies
  0-7645-5964-8
- Google For Dummies
  0-7645-4420-9

- Home Recording For Musicians
  For Dummies
  0-7645-1634-5
- The Internet For Dummies
  0-7645-4173-0
- iPod & iTunes For Dummies
  0-7645-7772-7
- Preventing Identity Theft For Dummies
  0-7645-7336-5
- Pro Tools All-in-One Desk Reference
  For Dummies
  0-7645-5714-9
- Roxio Easy Media Creator For Dummies
  0-7645-7131-1

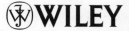

SPORTS, FITNESS, PARENTING, RELIGION & SPIRITUALITY

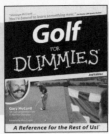

0-7645-5146-9

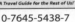

0-7645-5418-2

Also available:

- Adoption For Dummies
  0-7645-5488-3
- Basketball For Dummies
  0-7645-5248-1
- The Bible For Dummies
  0-7645-5296-1
- Buddhism For Dummies
  0-7645-5359-3
- Catholicism For Dummies
  0-7645-5391-7
- Hockey For Dummies
  0-7645-5228-7

- Judaism For Dummies
  0-7645-5299-6
- Martial Arts For Dummies
  0-7645-5358-5
- Pilates For Dummies
  0-7645-5397-6
- Religion For Dummies
  0-7645-5264-3
- Teaching Kids to Read For Dummies
  0-7645-4043-2
- Weight Training For Dummies
  0-7645-5168-X
- Yoga For Dummies
  0-7645-5117-5

TRAVEL

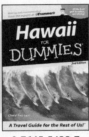

0-7645-5438-7

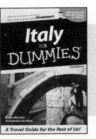

0-7645-5453-0

Also available:

- Alaska For Dummies
  0-7645-1761-9
- Arizona For Dummies
  0-7645-6938-4
- Cancún and the Yucatán For Dummies
  0-7645-2437-2
- Cruise Vacations For Dummies
  0-7645-6941-4
- Europe For Dummies
  0-7645-5456-5
- Ireland For Dummies
  0-7645-5455-7

- Las Vegas For Dummies
  0-7645-5448-4
- London For Dummies
  0-7645-4277-X
- New York City For Dummies
  0-7645-6945-7
- Paris For Dummies
  0-7645-5494-8
- RV Vacations For Dummies
  0-7645-5443-3
- Walt Disney World & Orlando For Dummies
  0-7645-6943-0

GRAPHICS, DESIGN & WEB DEVELOPMENT

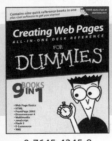

0-7645-4345-8

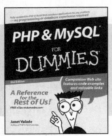

0-7645-5589-8

Also available:

- Adobe Acrobat 6 PDF For Dummies
  0-7645-3760-1
- Building a Web Site For Dummies
  0-7645-7144-3
- Dreamweaver MX 2004 For Dummies
  0-7645-4342-3
- FrontPage 2003 For Dummies
  0-7645-3882-9
- HTML 4 For Dummies
  0-7645-1995-6
- Illustrator cs For Dummies
  0-7645-4084-X

- Macromedia Flash MX 2004 For Dummies
  0-7645-4358-X
- Photoshop 7 All-in-One Desk
  Reference For Dummies
  0-7645-1667-1
- Photoshop cs Timesaving Techniques
  For Dummies
  0-7645-6782-9
- PHP 5 For Dummies
  0-7645-4166-8
- PowerPoint 2003 For Dummies
  0-7645-3908-6
- QuarkXPress 6 For Dummies
  0-7645-2593-X

NETWORKING, SECURITY, PROGRAMMING & DATABASES

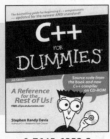

0-7645-6852-3

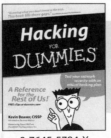

0-7645-5784-X

Also available:

- A+ Certification For Dummies
  0-7645-4187-0
- Access 2003 All-in-One Desk
  Reference For Dummies
  0-7645-3988-4
- Beginning Programming For Dummies
  0-7645-4997-9
- C For Dummies
  0-7645-7068-4
- Firewalls For Dummies
  0-7645-4048-3
- Home Networking For Dummies
  0-7645-42796

- Network Security For Dummies
  0-7645-1679-5
- Networking For Dummies
  0-7645-1677-9
- TCP/IP For Dummies
  0-7645-1760-0
- VBA For Dummies
  0-7645-3989-2
- Wireless All In-One Desk Reference
  For Dummies
  0-7645-7496-5
- Wireless Home Networking For Dummies
  0-7645-3910-8

EALTH & SELF-HELP

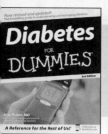

Diabetes FOR **DUMMIES**

0-7645-6820-5 *†

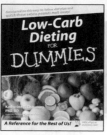

Low-Carb Dieting FOR **DUMMIES**

0-7645-2566-2

Also available:
- Alzheimer's For Dummies
  0-7645-3899-3
- Asthma For Dummies
  0-7645-4233-8
- Controlling Cholesterol For Dummies
  0-7645-5440-9
- Depression For Dummies
  0-7645-3900-0
- Dieting For Dummies
  0-7645-4149-8
- Fertility For Dummies
  0-7645-2549-2

- Fibromyalgia For Dummies
  0-7645-5441-7
- Improving Your Memory For Dummies
  0-7645-5435-2
- Pregnancy For Dummies †
  0-7645-4483-7
- Quitting Smoking For Dummies
  0-7645-2629-4
- Relationships For Dummies
  0-7645-5384-4
- Thyroid For Dummies
  0-7645-5385-2

UCATION, HISTORY, REFERENCE & TEST PREPARATION

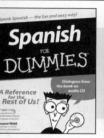

Spanish FOR **DUMMIES**

0-7645-5194-9

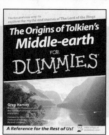

The Origins of Tolkien's Middle-earth FOR **DUMMIES**

0-7645-4186-2

Also available:
- Algebra For Dummies
  0-7645-5325-9
- British History For Dummies
  0-7645-7021-8
- Calculus For Dummies
  0-7645-2498-4
- English Grammar For Dummies
  0-7645-5322-4
- Forensics For Dummies
  0-7645-5580-4
- The GMAT For Dummies
  0-7645-5251-1
- Inglés Para Dummies
  0-7645-5427-1

- Italian For Dummies
  0-7645-5196-5
- Latin For Dummies
  0-7645-5431-X
- Lewis & Clark For Dummies
  0-7645-2545-X
- Research Papers For Dummies
  0-7645-5426-3
- The SAT I For Dummies
  0-7645-7193-1
- Science Fair Projects For Dummies
  0-7645-5460-3
- U.S. History For Dummies
  0-7645-5249-X

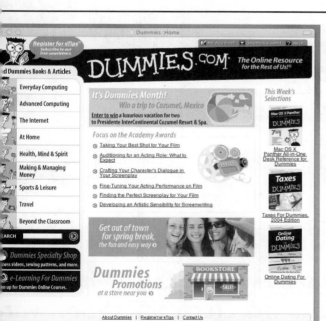

Get smart @ dummies.com®

- **Find a full list of Dummies titles**
- **Look into loads of FREE on-site articles**
- **Sign up for FREE eTips e-mailed to you weekly**
- **See what other products carry the Dummies name**
- **Shop directly from the Dummies bookstore**
- **Enter to win new prizes every month!**

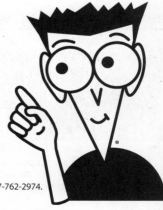

parate Canadian edition also available
parate U.K. edition also available

lable wherever books are sold. For more information or to order direct: U.S. customers visit www.dummies.com or call 1-877-762-2974.
customers visit www.wileyeurope.com or call 0800 243407. Canadian customers visit www.wiley.ca or call 1-800-567-4797.

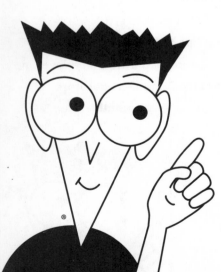
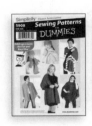
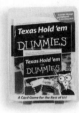
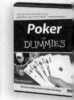
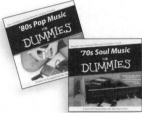
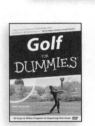
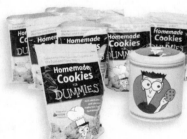
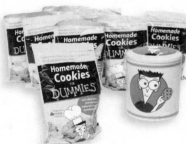
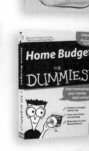